Quality Measures

Deeb N. Salem
Editor

Karen M. Freund • Saul N. Weingart
Associate Editors

Quality Measures

The Revolution in Patient Safety and Outcomes

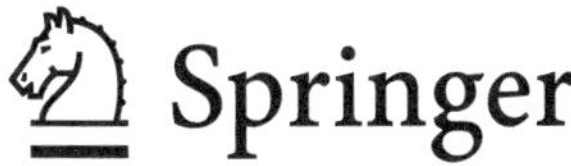 Springer

Editor
Deeb N. Salem, MD
Department of Medicine
Tufts Medical Center
Tufts University School of Medicine
Boston, MA
USA

Associate Editors
Karen M. Freund, MD
Department of Medicine
Tufts Medical Center,
Tufts University School of Medicine
Boston, MA
USA

Saul N. Weingart, MD, MPP, PhD
Department of Medicine
Tufts Medical Center,
Tufts University School of Medicine
Boston, MA
USA

ISBN 978-3-030-37144-9   ISBN 978-3-030-37145-6   (eBook)
https://doi.org/10.1007/978-3-030-37145-6

This Springer imprint is published by the registered company Springer Nature Switzerland AG
The registered company address is: Gewerbestrasse 11, 6330 Cham, Switzerland

We dedicate this book to the hardworking clinicians and administrators that strive daily to create safer care and improved outcomes for all of our patients.

Preface

Over the past two decades, medical quality measures have been implemented nationally in order to establish standards aimed at improving the quality and safety of patient care. This book was conceived to fulfill the need for a comprehensive text that would serve as an authoritative reference for the medical community and general public with an interest in the specifics of quality metrics across a wide range of clinical and administrative settings. It is written to provide scholarly yet practical information to all that are involved in measuring and assessing quality of care. The book recognizes that quality measures themselves may be flawed and must continue to be modified and evolve.

Recognition is due with appreciation to the expert authors who contributed excellent chapters and thereby made this effort possible. The superb organizational skills of Danisha Charles and the helpful assistance of the Springer staff merit grateful acknowledgement.

Boston, MA, USA   Deeb N. Salem, MD

Foreword

One of the most frequently quoted business proverbs declares "what gets measured, gets managed." The quote, often attributed to Peter Drucker, highlights the centrality of metrics in the pursuit of accountability and improvement. In healthcare, there are many facets to manage and improve: clinical outcomes; the experiences of patients, providers, and students; efficiency; and the multiple dimensions of quality. We use measures to drive improvement, to promote accountability, to keep score, and to determine value.

We rely on quantitation to give credibility and gravitas to important assessments – following the mindset of Lord Kelvin that "when you can measure what you are speaking about, and express it in numbers, you know something about it; but when you cannot express it in numbers, your knowledge is of a meagre and unsatisfactory kind." While that may be true, it can be challenging to identify relevant measures that can be created with efficiency and that inform decision-making in ways that promote positive change.

It might be said that the measures we can easily collect aren't necessarily the measures that we want and the measures we want may not be the measures we need to truly understand an issue. We frequently depend on surrogate measures for the things we really want to know about. For example, we measure care processes or control of biomarkers when measurements of relevant clinical outcomes are elusive. We recognize the impact of biological variation on processes or outcomes of interest and yet are challenged to address risk adjustment in a robust manner. We also appreciate that measurement can have perverse consequences, sometimes inducing behavior that achieves better quantitative performance as measured by compromising performance in other important ways. One might consider that all metrics are flawed to some extent but some metrics are useful.

Despite measurements having many limitations, they are a way to articulate what is important and are at the core of determining if a given change is an improvement. Confronting those limitations, articulating the tradeoffs in their specification, and developing measurement systems that balance focus across different perspectives allow us to usefully apply measurement in the interest of improving healthcare. Progress reflects the adoption of incremental changes and innovations that have a positive benefit. If we aim to help people thrive as they strive to stay healthy or as they face injury, illness, and recovery, we have to know how well we are doing and whether the innovative ideas we have for improvement are bearing fruit.

As a compendium of thoughtful analyses on the use of measurement in important domains of healthcare and academic medicine, this book provides a way to understand the evolution, limitations, and applications of metrics that can drive improvement and innovation.

Michael Apkon, MD, PhD, MBA
President and Chief Executive Officer
Tufts Medical Center and Floating Hospital for Children
Boston, MA, USA

Acknowledgment

We are very grateful for the generous support that we have received from the Tupper Research Fund.

Contents

1 The History of Quality Metrics 1
Deeb N. Salem, Sucharita Kher, Danisha Charles,
and Karen M. Freund

2 Pediatric Quality Measures 5
Geoffrey Binney

3 Quality and Safety Improvement in Surgery 23
William C. Mackey

4 Infection Prevention Quality Metrics 47
Susanne Meninger, Hasan Fadlallah, Karen Dowler,
and Shira Doron

5 Evolution of Modern Cardiovascular Quality Metrics 63
Ifeany David Chinedozi and Benjamin Wessler

6 Along the Road to Quality in Cancer Care 85
Joshua Dower, Fei Song, Diane Y. Sun, and Rachel J. Buchsbaum

7 Quality Measures for Palliative Care 99
Tamara Vesel and Jatin Dave

8 Developing a Hospital Quality Metrics System and Dashboard 115
Alexander Pavoll, Catherine Feleppa Camenga,
and Saul N. Weingart

9 Patient Satisfaction Metrics 127
Craig Best

10 Quality Measures in Undergraduate Medical Education 151
David Li, Gordon Wong, and Marcia Boumil

11 Resident Quality Training: More than Metrics 165
Mikhail Romashko and Kari E. Roberts

**12   The Role of the Hospital Board of Trustees in Ensuring
      Quality Care** 181
      Stanley Goldstein and Jeffrey Weinstein

**13   Quality Improvement and Population Management in
      Adult Primary Care** 201
      Julie Tishler, Kristin T. Huang, and Deborah Blazey-Martin

14   Quality of Quality Measures 215
      Yazan Daaboul, Saahil Jumkhawala, and Deeb N. Salem

Index 241

Contributors

Craig Best, MD, MPH Tufts Medical Center Physician Organization, Boston, MA, USA

Geoffrey Binney, Jr MD, MPH Floating Hospital for Children at Tufts Medical Center, Department of Pediatrics, Tufts University School of Medicine, Boston, MA, USA

Deborah Blazey-Martin, MD, MPH Internal Medicine and Adult Primary Care, Tufts Medical Center, Boston, MA, USA

Marcia Boumil, MS, JD, LL.M. Tufts University School of Medicine, Boston, MA, USA

Rachel J. Buchsbaum, MD Department of Medicine, Tufts Cancer Center, Tufts Medical Center, Tufts University School of Medicine, Boston, MA, USA

Catherine Feleppa Camenga, RN, MS Department of Quality and Patient Safety, Tufts Medical Center, Boston, MA, USA

Danisha Charles, BA Tufts Medical Center, Boston, MA, USA

Ifeany David Chinedozi, BA Tufts University School of Medicine, Boston, MA, USA

Yazan Daaboul, MD Department of Medicine, Tufts Medical Center, Tufts University School of Medicine, Boston, MA, USA

Jatin Dave, MD, MPH Division of Palliative Care, Department of Medicine, Tufts Medical Center, Tufts University School of Medicine, New England Quality Care Alliance, Boston, MA, USA

Shira Doron, MD Division of Geographic Medicine and Infectious Diseases, Tufts Medical Center, Boston, MA, USA
Tufts Medical Center, Boston, MA, USA

Joshua Dower, MD Department of Medicine, Tufts Medical Center, Tufts University School of Medicine, Boston, MA, USA

Karen Dowler, RN Department of Infection Prevention, Tufts Medical Center, Boston, MA, USA

Department of Quality and Patient Safety, Tufts Medical Center, Boston, MA, USA

Hasan Fadlallah MD Division of Geographic Medicine and Infectious Diseases, Tufts Medical Center, Boston, MA, USA

Karen M. Freund, MD Department of Medicine, Tufts Medical Center, Tufts University School of Medicine, Boston, MA, USA

Stanley Goldstein, BA Tufts Medical Center, Boston, MA, USA

Kristin T. Huang, MD Internal Medicine and Adult Primary Care, Tufts Medical Center, Boston, MA, USA

Saahil Jumkhawala, BS Department of Medicine, Tufts Medical Center, Tufts University School of Medicine, Boston, MA, USA

Sucharita Kher, MD Department of Medicine, Division of Pulmonary, Critical Care & Sleep Medicine, Tufts Medical Center, Boston, MA, USA

David Li, MD, MBA Department of Dermatology, Brigham and Women's Hospital, Boston, MA, USA

William C. Mackey, MD, FACS Tufts Medical Center, Department of Surgery, Tufts University School of Medicine, Boston, MA, USA

Susanne Meninger, RN Department of Infection Prevention, Tufts Medical Center, Boston, MA, USA

Alexander Pavoll, MPH Department of Quality and Patient Safety, Tufts Medical Center, Boston, MA, USA

Kari E. Roberts, MD Tufts Medical Center, Boston, MA, USA

Mikhail Romashko, MD Tufts Medical Center, Boston, MA, USA

Deeb N. Salem, MD Department of Medicine, Tufts Medical Center, Tufts University School of Medicine, Boston, MA, USA

Fei Song, MD Department of Medicine, Tufts Medical Center, Tufts University School of Medicine, Boston, MA, USA

Diane Y. Sun, MD Department of Medicine, Tufts Medical Center, Tufts University School of Medicine, Boston, MA, USA

Julie Tishler, MD Internal Medicine and Adult Primary Care, Tufts Medical Center, Boston, MA, USA

Tamara Vesel, MD Division of Palliative Care, Department of Medicine, Tufts Medical Center, Tufts University School of Medicine, Boston, MA, USA

Saul N. Weingart, MD, MPP, PhD Department of Medicine, Tufts Medical Center, Tufts University School of Medicine, Boston, MA, USA

Jeffrey Weinstein, LLB Tufts Medical Center, Boston, MA, USA

Benjamin Wessler, MD, FACC Division of Cardiology, Tufts Medical Center, Boston, MA, USA

Predictive Analytic sand Comparative Effectiveness (PACE) Center, Tufts Medical Center, Boston, MA, USA

Gordon Wong, MD, MBA Department of Internal Medicine, UC Davis Medical Center, Davis, CA, USA

Chapter 1
The History of Quality Metrics

Deeb N. Salem, Sucharita Kher, Danisha Charles, and Karen M. Freund

In a humorous, satirical editorial, Dr. Joseph Alpert depicts Socrates conversing with Asculepo, a young medical student, regarding the elements of high-quality medicine [1]. In their discussion, Asculepo states that he is confused about the elements of high-quality medicine that his professors called quality "metrics." Socrates responds that it is "quite strange" that they want to teach you to practice high-quality medicine, but they evidently cannot agree on how to measure this thing called "quality." During the past two decades, quality measures have evolved to play a crucial role in healthcare delivery; but in many ways, we are still not clear about what they should consist of.

Many believe that the modern healthcare movement began in the mid-1960s when Dr. Avedis Donabedian at the University of Michigan School of Public Health published his historic article entitled "Evaluating the Quality of Medical Care" [2, 4]. In this paper, Dr. Donabedian developed the triad of structure, process, and outcome as the metrics of quality of care. This report triggered the widespread development of

D. N. Salem (✉)
Department of Medicine, Tufts Medical Center, Tufts University School of Medicine, Boston, MA, USA
e-mail: dsalem@tuftsmedicalcenter.org

S. Kher
Department of Medicine, Division of Pulmonary, Critical Care & Sleep Medicine, Tufts Medical Center, Boston, MA, USA
e-mail: skher@tuftsmedicalcenter.org

D. Charles
Tufts Medical Center, Boston, MA, USA
e-mail: dcharles@tuftsmedicalcenter.org

K. M. Freund
Department of Medicine, Tufts Medical Center, Tufts University School of Medicine, Boston, MA, USA
e-mail: kfreund@tuftsmedicalcenter.org

© Springer Nature Switzerland AG 2020
D. N. Salem (ed.), *Quality Measures*, https://doi.org/10.1007/978-3-030-37145-6_1

what we now call quality metrics. These tools are meant to aid in quantifying the "what" that surrounds healthcare including its "outcomes, structure, and processes" across the multitude of healthcare organizations.

While a great deal of improvements in process and outcomes has occurred since the onset of the quality metrics era, many feel that there is still a long way to go. Hospitals and clinicians are faced with quality metrics that have been developed by a myriad organizations such as CMS, Leapfrog, AHRQ, The Joint Commission, and Health Grades, just to name a few. Even Consumer Reports has ventured into the healthcare quality metrics field. Their ratings include measurements from readmissions, to proper communication with patients, to the appropriate use of hospital devices and equipment. Consumer Reports promotes its data as "useful information that is accessible and meaningful to consumer" [3]. Recently, the editors of JAMA Internal Medicine have asked for a quality improvement effort for quality improvement studies [7] and the Annals of Internal Medicine have strongly spoken out about the weaknesses of current pay-for-performance models [6]. This example and a number of others attest to the need for hospitals and other medical organizations to weigh the current performance against prospective improvements.

We are approaching two decades since the Institute of Medicine published its landmark report "To Err Is Human"; there is no doubt that the growth of the quality metric movement has played a pivotal role in improving healthcare outcomes. However, we still have a long way to go to ensure the usefulness and accuracy of current measures. Currently, we rely too heavily on claims-based data that was never designed to measure quality and has not been validated for truly measuring quality. Researching, publishing, and implementing faulty, and seemingly bias, claims-based data portray an inaccurate view and connotation of the healthcare organizations and their services. Future measures need to be developed by experts, tested, and subject to peer review to ensure confidence in their reliability by clinicians, institutions, and the public [5]. The acceptance of quality metrics should require peer review processes similar to those that are used in judging the validity of other medical interventions including replicating the studies that they are based on. The methodology used to determine "risk adjustment" must be reported [8], and care must be taken in avoiding a metric to a population that was not included in the studies that a metric was developed from. Assertive, yet progressive, efforts will produce better outcomes for both physicians and patients, alike.

It is our hope and expectation that this book will provide clarity to the debate around quality metrics. We start with discussing the history of quality metrics in medicine. The book then critically focuses on quality metrics that must be considered in various specialties such as pediatrics, surgery, infectious disease, cardiovascular disease, and oncology as well as at the end of life. Metrics focused on patient satisfaction are reviewed. In addition, we tackle the vital issue of training our future generations of medical students and residents in quality metrics. The path to developing a hospital's quality metric system and the role that a hospital governance can play in monitoring the quality measures are reviewed in detail. Finally, who tracks the quality of these quality metrics? The book ends with this important thought on analyzing the quality of the metrics.

In this day and age where there is so much focus on the healthcare processes, outcomes, and structures, this book will serve as the single guide of quality measures for trainees, physicians, nurses, and administrative personnel.

References

1. Alpert JS. Socrates on quality. Am J Med. 2018;131(8):855–6. https://doi.org/10.1016/j.amjmed.2018.03.022.
2. Ayanian JZ, Markel H. Donabedian's lasting framework for health care quality. N Engl J Med. 2016;375(3):205–7. https://doi.org/10.1056/NEJMp1605101.
3. Consumer Reports. How we rate hospitals. 2018 June. Retrieved from http://article.images.consumerreports.org/prod/content/dam/cro/news_articles/health/PDFs/Hospital_Ratings_Technical_Report.pdf.
4. Donabedian A. Evaluating the quality of medical care. Milbank Q. 1966;83(4):691–729. https://doi.org/10.1111/j.1468-0009.2005.00397.x.
5. Esposito ML, Selker HP, Salem DN. Quantity over quality: how the rise in quality measures is not producing quality results. J Gen Intern Med. 2015;30(8):1204–7. https://doi.org/10.1007/s11606-015-3278-6.
6. Frakt AB, Jha AK. Face the facts: we need to change the way we do pay for performance changing how we do pay for performance. Ann Intern Med. 2018;168(4):291–2. https://doi.org/10.7326/M17-3005.
7. Grady D, Redberg RF, O'Malley PG. Quality improvement for quality improvement studies quality improvement for quality improvement studies editorial. JAMA Intern Med. 2018;178(2):187. https://doi.org/10.1001/jamainternmed.2017.6875.
8. Hwang SW, Salem D, Thaler D, Heilman CB. A review of stroke DRG mortality rate as a quality of care measure. AAANS Bulletin. 2007;16(2):28–31.

Chapter 2
Pediatric Quality Measures

Geoffrey Binney

Introduction

As in other areas of medicine, the number and variety of pediatric quality measures have exploded over the past several decades. The source of these measures and metrics is highly variable, and many measures have been extrapolated from adult measures. For numerous reasons related to factors unique to the pediatric population, the development of quality measures of children's health and health care has lagged behind the development of adult measures. Examining the source of quality measures and their classification in pediatrics will help illustrate some of the important aspects of quality measures in pediatrics and their use and impact on children's health and care.

Source of Pediatric Quality Measures

Like measures formulated for the adult population, quality measures for pediatrics have been developed and promulgated by a large and diverse set of organizations and sources. Many of the national measures have originated at the federal government level. The Agency for Healthcare Research and Quality (AHRQ) has a mission to "produce evidence to make health care safer, higher quality, more accessible, equitable, and affordable and to work within the U.S. Department of Health and Human Services and with other partners to make sure that the evidence is understood and used." [1] Many of its programs are involved with developing and

G. Binney (✉)
Floating Hospital for Children at Tufts Medical Center, Department of Pediatrics,
Tufts University School of Medicine, Boston, MA, USA
e-mail: gbinney@tuftsmedicalcenter.org

© Springer Nature Switzerland AG 2020

D. N. Salem (ed.), *Quality Measures*, https://doi.org/10.1007/978-3-030-37145-6_2

implementing measures that assess aspects of both health and also the health care delivery system. One such program, AHRQ Quality Indicators™, which uses hospital inpatient administrative data to measure and track clinical performance and outcomes, includes a set of measures focused on pediatric health care. The Pediatric Quality Indicators (PDI) include measures that assess hospital level performance as well as area level health status (Fig. 2.1).

Since the Centers for Medicare and Medicaid Services (CMS) have a responsibility to ensure that the services and health care supported by the federal government is high quality, CMS conducts a number of activities where quality measures are needed, such as continuous quality improvement, pay-for-performance, and public reporting activities.

In order to ensure that the measures appropriately assess the quality of health care for children, the government has developed pediatric-specific agencies and systems. The Children's Health Insurance Program Reauthorization Act of 2009 (CHIPRA) helped create more opportunities to develop and promote standardized pediatric quality metrics. CHIPRA contained several provisions related to quality. The law required that a core set of children's quality measures be developed for

---

Pediatric Quality Indicators

Hospital-Level Indicators

- NQI 01 - Iatrogenic pneumothorax in neonates
- NQI 02 - Neonatal mortality
- NQI 03 - Bloodstream infections in neonates
- PDI 01 - Accidental puncture or laceration
- PDI 02 - Pressure ulcer
- PDI 03 - Retained surgical item or unretrieved device fragment
- PDI 05 - Iatrogenic pneumothorax
- PDI 06 - Pediatric heart surgery mortality
- PDI 07 - Pediatric heart surgery volume
- PDI 08 - Postoperative hemorrhage or hematoma
- PDI 09 - Postoperative respiratory failure
- PDI 10 - Postoperative sepsis

- PDI 11- Postoperative wound dehiscence
- PDI 12 - Central venous catheter-related bloodstream infections
- PDI 13 - Transfusion reactions
- PDI 19 - Pediatric Safety for Selected Indicators

Area-Level Indicators (e.g., county, State)

- PDI 14 - Asthma admissions
- PDI 15 - Diabetes short-term complications
- PDI 16 - Gastroenteritis admissions
- PDI 17 - Perforated appendix admissions
- PDI 18 - Urinary tract infection admissions
- PDI 90 - Pediatric Quality Overall Composite
- PDI 91 - Pediatric Quality Acute Composite
- PDI 92 - Pediatric Quality Chronic Composite

QI Web Site: qualityindicators.ahrq.gov

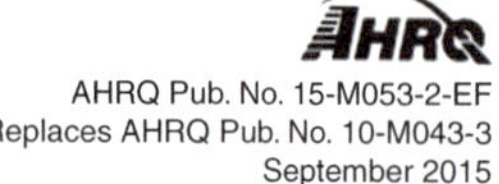

AHRQ Pub. No. 15-M053-2-EF
Replaces AHRQ Pub. No. 10-M043-3
September 2015

Fig. 2.1 AHRQ Pediatric Quality Indicators. Pediatric Quality Indicators are obtained from hospital inpatient administrative data and include measures that assess both hospital performance and area health status. (Image obtained from a September 2015 AHRQ pamphlet, "AHRQ Quality Indicators™: Pediatric Quality Indicators" [2])

states to use on a voluntary basis to report on the quality of care provided to Medicaid and Children's Health Insurance Program (CHIP) beneficiaries. The Secretary of Health and Human Services first published the initial Child Core Set in December 2009. This first set included 24 measures, which encompassed elements addressing the physical and mental health of children. These measures were used by Medicaid and CHIP programs on a voluntary basis [3]. Since its establishment, the Child Core Set has been refined and updated annually as required by CHIPRA. The most recent update, the 2019 Child Core Set, was published in November 2018 in a Center for Medicaid and CHIP Services (CMCS) Informational Bulletin [4]. The current Child Core Set includes 26 measures that address a variety of topics (Fig. 2.2).

Acknowledging that existing measures were insufficient for the pediatric population, CHIPRA also established the Pediatric Quality Measurement Program (PQMP). The PQMP was charged with improving and strengthening existing quality metrics and also with increasing the portfolio of pediatric quality measures. One mechanism established to help in this effort was the creation and funding of 7 PQMP Centers of Excellence in 2011. The centers have been working to develop and refine child health measures in high priority areas.

Other national quality metrics have originated from certifying or accrediting organizations such as The Joint Commission (TJC) or the National Committee for Quality Assurance (NCQA). As with the governmental metrics, the number pediatric measures developed from these sources is lower than the number developed for adults. In 1987 The Joint Commission set forth its *Agenda for Change*, which aimed to modernize its accreditation process, and introduced the idea of including standardized core performance measures as part of the accreditation process. This quality improvement initiative, eventually named ORYX®, became operational in 1999 and initially allowed a fair amount of flexibility in what measures could be reported. Over time, ORYX® has developed into a standardized set of performance measures, the majority of which are endorsed by the National Quality Forum (NQF) [6]. Although many of these measures can be applied to pediatrics, the first performance measurement set designed specifically for the pediatric population by The Joint Commission was the Children's Asthma Care (CAC) set. Introduced in 2007, the 3 CAC measures reported on the use of relievers (CAC1) and systemic corticosteroids (CAC2) for inpatient asthma, and the provision of a home management plan of care to the patient or caregiver (CAC3) prior to discharge.

While asthma is clearly a major pediatric issue and measuring the quality of care provided to children with asthma is desirable, choosing appropriate measures to judge quality is crucial. The two CAC measures looking at medication usage reported on practices that were already almost universally in use at the time. In 2008, reliever and corticosteroid use in inpatient asthma was already used more than 99% of the time in hospitals reporting this performance measure. There is such uniformity in the use of these medications that measuring usage does not help identify where improvement is needed. On the other hand, the third measure – reporting that the patient or caregiver received a home management plan of care (CAC3) – was only used 40.6% of the time by reporting hospitals in 2008 [7]. The data indicated that this process had room for improvement, and by 2014 hospitals had

2019 Core Set of Children's Health Care Quality Measures for Medicaid and CHIP (Child Core Set)

NQF#	Measure steward	Measure Name
Primary Care Access and Preventive Care		
0024	NCQA	Weight Assessment and Counseling for Nutrition and Physical Activity for Children/Adolescents – Body Mass Index Assessment for Children/Adolescents (WCC-CH)
0033	NCQA	Chlamydia Screening in Women Ages 16-20 (CHL-CH)
0038	NCQA	Childhood Immunization Status (CIS-CH)
0418/0418e	CMS	Screening for Depression and Follow-Up Plan: Ages 12-17 (CDF-CH)
1392	NCQA	Well-Child Visits in the First 15 Months of Life (W15-CH)
1407	NCQA	Immunizations for Adolescents (IMA-CH)
1448*	OHSU	Developmental Screening in the First Three Years of Life (DEV-CH)
1516	NCQA	Well-Child Visits in the Third, Fourth, Fifth and Sixth Years of Life (W34-CH)
NA	NCQA	Adolescent Well-Care Visits (AWC-CH)
NA	NCQA	Children and Adolescents' Access to Primary Care Practitioners (CAP-CH)
Maternal and Perinatal Health		
0139	CDC	Pediatric Central Line-Associated Bloodstream Infections (CLABSI-CH)
0471	TJC	PC-02: Cesarean Birth (PC02-CH)
1360	CDC	Audiological Diagnosis No Later Than 3 Months of Age (AUD-CH)
1382	CDC	Live Births Weighing Less Than 2,500 Grams (LBW-CH)
1517*	NCQA	Prenatal and Postpartum Care: Timeliness of Prenatal Care (PPC-CH)
2902	OPA	Contraceptive Care – Postpartum Women Ages 15-20 (CCP-CH)
2903/2904	OPA	Contraceptive Care – All Women Ages 15-20 (CCW-CH)
Care of Acute and Chronic Conditions		
1800	NCQA	Asthma Medication Ratio: Ages 5-18 (AMR-CH)
NA	NCQA	Ambulatory Care: Emergency Department (ED) Visits (AMB-CH)
Behavioral Health Care		
0108	NCQA	Follow-Up Care for Children Prescribed Attention-Deficit/Hyperactivity Disorder (ADHD) Medication (ADD-CH)
0576	NCQA	Follow-Up After Hospitalization for Mental Illness: Ages 6-17 (FUH-CH)
2801	NCQA	Use of First-Line Psychosocial Care for Children and Adolescents on Antipsychotics (APP-CH)
NA	NCQA	Use of Multiple Concurrent Antipsychotics in Children and Adolescents (APC-CH)
Dental and Oral Health Services		
2508*	DQA (ADA)	Dental Sealants for 6-9 Year-Old Children at Elevated Caries Risk (SEAL-CH)
NA	CMS	Percentage of Eligibles Who Received Preventive Dental Services (PDENT-CH)
Experience of Care		
NA	NCQA	Consumer Assessment of Healthcare Providers and Systems (CAHPS®) Health Plan Survey 5.0H – Child Version Including Medicaid and Children with Chronic Conditions Supplemental Items (CPC-CH)

More information on 2019 Updates to the Child and Adult Core Health Care Quality Measurement Sets is available at https://www.medicaid.gov/federal-policy-guidance/downloads/cib112018.pdf.
*This measure is no longer endorsed by NQF.
CDC = Centers for Disease Control and Prevention; CHIP = Children's Health Insurance Program; CMS = Centers for Medicare & Medicaid Services; DQA (ADA) = Dental Quality Alliance (American Dental Association); NA = Measure is not NQF endorsed; NCQA = National Committee for Quality Assurance; NQF = National Quality Forum; OHSU = Oregon Health and Science University; OPA = U.S. Office of Population Affairs; TJC = The Joint Commission.

Fig. 2.2 2019 Child Core Set. The 2019 Child Core Set includes measures in several different content areas. Most measures have been endorsed by the National Quality Forum (NQF). The organizations who have developed the measures and are the stewards for each measure are also listed. (Core set obtained from Medicaid.gov website [5])

improved their documentation of having provided a home management plan of care markedly to 91% [8]. Unfortunately, evidence linking the provision of a home management plan of care to an improvement in outcomes for children with asthma is lacking. The use of the emergency department following discharge or readmissions for asthma did not change in hospitals even as they showed improvement in CAC3 [9]. At the end of 2015, all three CAC measures were retired as the burden of continuing data collection on these measures was no longer felt worth the potential benefit of measuring these processes.

Another national accrediting organization, The National Committee for Quality Assurance (NCQA), is a non-profit, independent organization that was founded in 1990 initially to measure the quality of health plans. Its Healthcare Effectiveness Data and Information Set (HEDIS) now includes 90 measures in 6 domains (Effectiveness of Care, Access/Availability of Care, Experience of Care, Utilization and Risk-Adjusted Utilization, Health Plan Descriptive Information, and Measures Collected Using Electronic Clinical Data Systems) [10]. Of those measures only 25 are relevant to pediatric providers [11]. One of the pediatric-focused measures in HEDIS is its "Weight Assessment and Counseling for Nutrition and Physical Activity for Children/Adolescents (WCC)" measure set. This measure reports on how frequently children/adolescents who receive primary care have their BMI documented and receive counseling for nutrition and physical activity. This measure is highly aligned with the AAP's *Bright Futures: Guidelines for Health Supervision of Infants, Children, and Adolescents* recommendations promoting healthy weight and physical activity [12]. As was noted for asthma and the CAC measures, evidence linking the WCC measures and improvement in children's health is sparse. Obesity rates in children continue to rise despite evidence that shows that both BMI documentation and counseling are being done more frequently [13, 14]. Although there has not been any demonstrable change in obesity rates, there is still widespread belief that checking and discussing BMI as part of routine well child care and providing counseling regarding nutrition and physical activity are beneficial, so measurement of these processes continues (Fig. 2.3).

Other sources of quality metrics in pediatrics tend to be more specialty specific and have been developed by subspecialty organizations. Benchmarking databases and disease registries have been the source of many quality measures and quality improvement activities in pediatrics. In neonatal-perinatal medicine, the Vermont Oxford Network (VON) was established in 1989 to collect data from its member centers and benchmark outcomes in order to promote improvement. There are now more than 1200 centers participating in the network and reporting data related to demographics, treatment, and outcomes of newborns in neonatal intensive care units (NICUs) around the world. Initially NICUs simply used the network to examine trends in their own performance, benchmark their performance against other centers, and use that information to help identify areas for improvement. Now VON leads quality improvement collaboratives and educational activities to drive change

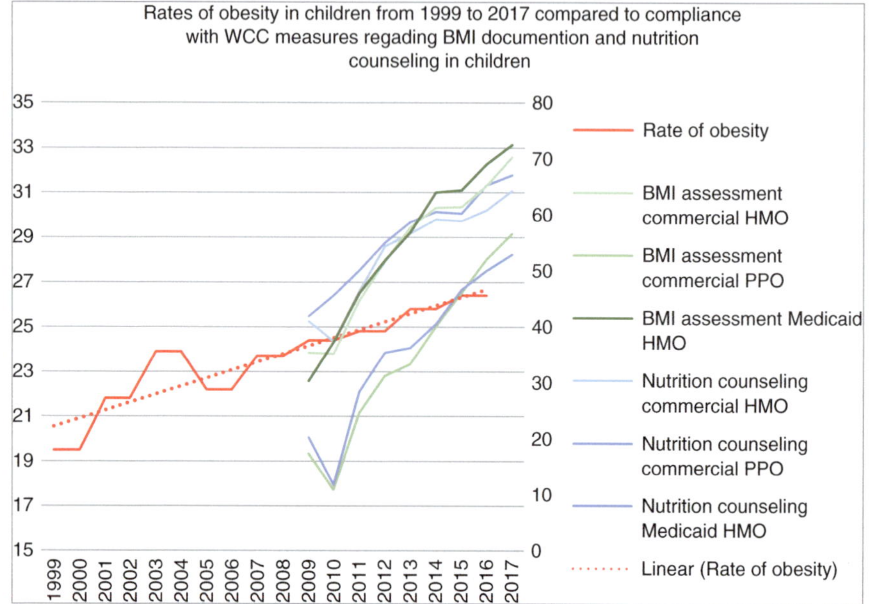

Fig. 2.3 Data comparing the rate of obesity in children aged 2–19 obtained from NHANES 1999–2016 as reported by Skinner et al. to rates of reporting BMI percentile assessment and counseling for nutrition in children aged 3–17 as reported in HEDIS [13, 14]. Despite sharp improvements in compliance with these process measures, there has been little change in the desired outcome of reducing rates of obesity in children at this point in time

with resulting measurable improvement in outcomes. VON is currently the steward of 2 NQF endorsed quality measures (Risk-adjusted Late Sepsis or Meningitis in Very Low Birth Weight Neonates NQF #0304, and Proportion of Infants 22 to 29 Weeks Gestation Screened for Retinopathy of Prematurity NQF #0483) and 2 measures used by the Leapfrog group (Risk-adjusted Death or Morbidity, and Proportion of Infants Who Receive Antenatal Steroids) [15].

Similar to VON, VPS (Virtual Pediatric Systems) provides comparative benchmarking data for more than 135 hospital pediatric intensive care units and is actively positioning itself as an advocate for the improvement of the quality of critical care for children [16]. Databases like VPS address some of the issues that make assessing quality in pediatrics difficult. Compared to adults, the number of children that require critical care is low and the variety of cases treated in any one pediatric intensive care unit (PICU) is relatively large, so obtaining meaningful data about any one particular disease or outcome is difficult [17]. Since all institutions in VPS report a dataset of required elements, pooled data is available that allows comparative measurement between centers.

Both VON and VPS were developed by pediatric subspecialists specifically for their respective populations, but other databases have been derived from previously developed adult databases. The Society of Thoracic Surgeons (STS) National

Database was established in 1989 as a quality improvement initiative among cardio-thoracic surgeons. Then, in 2007, a task force was created to develop quality measures for pediatric and congenital cardiac surgery. The STS Congenital Heart Surgery Database (CHSD) was subsequently developed, and by 2018 more than 475,000 congenital heart surgery records had been collected [18]. STS has developed a number of quality performance measures that have been endorsed by the NQF including 5 measures related to congenital and pediatric heart surgery.

Another pediatric surgical quality program, ACS NSQIP Pediatric was developed after its precursor, the American College of Surgeons National Surgical Quality Improvement Program (ACS NSQIP®), was developed and had demonstrated its value in improving the quality of adult surgical care [19]. NSQIP initially grew out of the Veterans Administration efforts in the 1990s to improve surgical care in its VA hospitals. After NSQIP showed the value of measuring outcomes and focusing on improvement in the VA, hospitals began enrolling in ACS NSQIP® in 2004. The program then expanded to children in 2008 when a pilot program was started. After the pilot, ACS NSQIP Pediatric was formed, and by 2019 more than 130 hospitals were enrolled in the program [20].

The development of ACS NSQIP Pediatric illustrates many of the difficulties in simply extrapolating adult measures to pediatrics. It is more complex than just adjusting for differences in surgical operations, volume, and outcome. Perioperative mortality for most pediatric surgical cases, excluding cardiac procedures, is very low in pediatrics. Developmental changes that occur in children also complicate the measurement and interpretation of aggregated data, since it is expected that outcomes may differ depending on age, size, and physiologic maturity. The surgical procedures and techniques as well are likely to be more varied due to the marked differences in size and development seen in pediatrics. The cognitive limitations expected in neonates, infants, and toddlers also make it more difficult to determine pre-morbid limitations and comorbidities than in older children or adults. Also postoperative complications and quality of life assessments in this population are harder to obtain since they rely on parental or caregiver report and interpretation instead of direct report from the patient. Finally statistical analysis is more challenging due to the low volume, high level of variability of procedures and low mortality rates more commonly seen in children [21].

In addition to subspecialty programs, some benchmarking registries and quality improvement efforts have arisen centered around pediatric-specific diseases or condition (Table 2.1). Like VON and VPS, these types of networks rely on registry data to form the basis of quality improvement work. The data in these registries is usually obtained from a combination of standard health record data and registry-specific data abstracted manually at each participating center. The measures of interest vary based upon the registry and focus of the network. Some of the better-known pediatric disease-focused networks are more research based in mission, such as the Children's Oncology Group. Others, like the Cystic Fibrosis (CF) Foundation, are involved in accrediting treatment centers and initially worked to create standardized treatment regimens. The CF Foundation Patient Registry, created in 1966, has been able to track improvements in the health of patients receiving care within the Care

Table 2.1 Sample of pediatric specialty- or condition-focused networks, care registries, or patient databases

Network, database, or registry		Subspecialty area or disease focus
ACS NSQIP Pediatric	American College of Surgeons National Surgical Quality Improvement Program – Pediatric	Pediatric surgery
ACS TQIP	American College of Surgeons Trauma Quality Improvement Program – Pediatric	Pediatric trauma surgery
CF Foundation Patient Registry	Cystic Fibrosis Foundation's Patient Registry	Cystic fibrosis
CPQCC	California Perinatal Quality Care Collaborative	Neonatal-perinatal care
ELSO	Extracorporeal Life Support Organization Registry	Extracorporeal membrane oxygenation (ECMO)
HRIF	High Risk Infant Follow-Up Program	Neonatal-perinatal care
ICN	Improve Care Now	Pediatric gastroenterology (inflammatory bowel disease)
NPC-QIC	National Pediatric Cardiology Quality Improvement Collaborative	Hypoplastic left heart syndrome
STS-CHSD	Society of Thoracic Surgeons – Congenital Heart Surgery Database	Pediatric cardiothoracic surgery
VON	Vermont Oxford Network	Neonatal critical care
VPS	Virtual Pediatric Solutions	Pediatric critical care

This is a small sample of some of the larger and more commonly used databases used for quality improvement and benchmarking activities in pediatrics. Some have arisen from particular subspecialties, and some are related to specific disease processes

Center Network and has been able to correlate the impact of setting care standards with improvements in the health of this population. As quality improvement science expanded its reach into other areas of medicine in the early 2000s, the CF Foundation launched an initiative to accelerate improvement in CF care using a comprehensive quality improvement framework and leveraging the Care Center network to spread QI methods, disseminate best practices, promote greater involvement of patients with CF and their families, and provide greater familiarity and the use of the data available at the patient and center level. All centers accredited by the CF Foundation must incorporate QI efforts into their clinical practice, and the outcomes reported by the Patient Registry are now evaluated routinely as part of accreditation [22].

Improve Care Now (ICN), a pediatric QI network formed in 2007 "to transform the health, care and costs for all children and adolescents with Crohn's disease and ulcerative colitis (Inflammatory Bowel Disease or IBD) by building a sustainable collaborative chronic care network," exemplifies another pediatric condition-focused QI network that combines a quality improvement focus with a disease-specific data registry [23]. By collecting standardized data during each patient encounter, the network allows reporting on center level process and outcome measures and comparison with aggregate network data. Concurrently the network is trying to establish care guidelines that are evidence based when possible or based upon expert consensus if evidence is lacking. By examining how outcome measures correlate with process measures, networks like ICN are hoping to optimize care practices and adjust those practices as new treatment or diagnostic options arise and are incorporated into clinical care [24, 25].

As the demand for useful information about health care quality increases, the number and variety of quality measures needing to be reported have correspondingly increased. Providers of health care must report multiple measures to numerous entities, and there is not always full alignment among the measures or reporting requirements. Acknowledging the complexity, administrative burden, and difficulty of obtaining and analyzing data that is not uniformly collected, a group of health care stakeholders (including CMS, commercial payers, providers, consumers, and other care service groups) have come together in the Core Quality Measures Collaborative (CQMC) to identify core sets of quality measures that governmental and private payers will commit to use for reporting purposes. The Collaborative split into workgroups to develop consensus regarding measures in 8 key areas: Accountable Care Organizations (ACOs), Patient Centered Medical Homes (PCMH), and Primary Care; Cardiology; Gastroenterology; HIV and Hepatitis C; Medical Oncology; Obstetrics and Gynecology; Orthopedics; Pediatrics. The Pediatric CQMC group developed a set of 9 measures, 7 of which are also in the Medicaid and CHIP Child Core Set; therefore, there is hope that reporting at the national and state level will be more aligned going forward [26, 27].

Classification of Quality Measures

Quality measures in pediatrics can be classified in a number of different ways. In 1966 Donabedian first proposed classifying quality measures into 3 categories: structure, process, and outcome [28]. This framework continues to be useful today. House et al. applied this framework to categorize national pediatric measures in use in 2015 [11]. Examining 15 national quality measure collections, they found that 24% of the 1613 measures in use were relevant to pediatric providers and that the majority of these pediatric measures (59%) were process measures. Only 9% of the measures reported on structure, while the remaining 32% pertained to outcome. The National Quality Forum found a similar distribution of measures when they examined the 123 measures in their portfolio of endorsed measures: 60% were process measures, 3% were structure measures, and 36% were outcome measures [29].

Process Measures

Process measures can be further divided by type: do they measure underuse, overuse, or misuse? [30] The bulk of national pediatric quality measures in 2015 measured underuse (77% of process measures) even though overuse or overtreatment is one of the major contributors to waste in health care [31]. As part of the *Choosing Wisely* initiative – an initiative of the ABIM (American Board of Internal Medicine) Foundation that seeks to advance a national dialogue on avoiding unnecessary medical tests, treatments and procedures – the American Academy of Pediatrics (AAP) created a list, in 2012, of 5 treatments or tests that should not be used or may not be necessary [32]. Since then the list has expanded to 10 items for Pediatrics, and the AAP has created lists for 5 additional subspecialties: Infectious Diseases, Nephrology, Orthopedics, Endocrinology, and Neonatal Perinatal Medicine [33]. In 2015, only one of these overuse issues – antibiotics should not be used for viral respiratory illnesses – was addressed in the national pediatric process measures examined by House.

It is not surprising that most quality measures are process measures. In general, process measures offer more information about potential targets for intervention, and data regarding processes is usually easier to obtain. It is relatively easy to determine if a patient received a specific treatment or test. Did a child receive their immunizations at the recommended time? Was tobacco use status documented? For some processes, the correlation between the process and improved health is well established. Immunizations have been shown to decrease the incidence of numerous life-threatening illnesses, and the process of giving the immunization correlates directly with the mechanism conferring immunity. On the other hand, there is no direct evidence supporting the assumption that documenting tobacco use status leads to improved health. There is an assumption that if tobacco use status needs to be documented, then this requirement will lead to a productive exchange of information between clinician and patient, which in turn will lead to a change in behavior and prompt smoking cessation if tobacco use is discovered, but there is no evidence confirming this assumption.

The CF Foundation has been able to document major improvement in many process measures and remarkable improvements in many outcome measures. Process measures looking at items such as follow-up visits, influenza vaccination, dietician evaluation for children with body mass index (BMI) <50th percentile, and usage of chronic therapies have all improved over time. At the same time, outcome measures such as survival rates, height and weight percentiles for age, and pulmonary function testing results have also dramatically and significantly improved. These general results are encouraging, but do not establish causality between the process measures studied and the particular desired outcomes [34].

When the linkage of process measures to outcomes relies on too many assumptions and poor evidence, the value of collecting the measures becomes suspect. For clinicians or centers looking at disease specific measures and choosing to participate in collaboratives or networks electively, the decision to collect the data about particular process measure may be worthwhile and acceptable, but when the process measure is chosen by external bodies for accountability reasons, such as pay for performance or public reporting, the collection of process measures may be much less acceptable. For this reason, Chassin et al. proposed that 4 criteria should be met for process measures to be used by national accountability programs: (1) there is strong evidence that the process leads to improved outcomes, (2) the measure accurately captures that the process has been done, (3) there are few intervening care steps between the process and the desired outcome, and (4) implementation of the measure has little or no chance of inducing unintended adverse outcomes [35].

Outcome Measures

Outcome measures report on the impact of the care delivered. Outcome measures can assess how health is improved or worsened after interaction with the health care system, or they may be more subjective and assess how the interaction was perceived by the patient or consumer. These types of patient experience metrics are becoming increasingly important in health care. Commonly reported outcome measures include hospital-acquired conditions such as catheter-associated urinary tract infections, central line–associated blood stream infections, pressure injuries, surgical site infections, adverse drug events, and venous thromboembolism. Admission rates for certain diseases such as asthma, UTI, or heart failure and readmission rates for specific conditions or all causes are also commonly reported outcome measures. In 2009, CMS made the readmission rate for certain conditions (pneumonia, acute myocardial infarction, or heart failure) an accountability quality measure for adults by first including it in public reporting and then by using those measures to impact reimbursement. While much data exists regarding readmission rates in adults, there is less evidence linking readmission rates to quality of care in children, and the value of readmission rate measures is still being assessed [36, 37].

It is much easier for the health care system to report on short-term outcomes, so most outcome measures assess the impact of health care on particular, time-limited events. For example, short-term survival after a surgical intervention is a commonly used outcome measure. This measure is easy to collect and offers good evidence about the immediate impact of the service under review. It is therefore not surprising that when STS proposed 21 quality performance measures for congenital and pediatric surgery in 2011, just under half (48%) were outcome measures [38].

For overall health, however, longer-term outcomes are ultimately more important. Did the surgery lead to an improved quality of life and greater longevity? In pediatrics, this discrepancy between short-term outcome and long-term outcome is particularly important but often much more difficult to assess. In neonatology, for example, extrauterine growth failure is a commonly measured outcome. Reducing the number of infants with poor short-term growth has been the goal of many quality initiatives. One way to increase short-term growth is to increase caloric intake, so for many years there was a shift toward increasing overall caloric intake to avoid short-term growth failure. The quality measure chosen to assess short-term growth failure was often extrauterine weight gain without fully understanding the risks and benefits of the long-term impact of this growth. After achieving success in reducing short-term growth failure, neonatology is now hearing from their pediatric and adult colleagues that former premature infants with excessive early weight gain may be more prone to metabolic syndrome later in childhood and as adults [39, 40].

Structure Measures

In the Donabedian framework of measures, structure measures represent the next category of metrics. These measures report on the aspects of the health care system and usually report on static attributes of the setting in which care is delivered. These measures can describe physical items, such as facilities or materials, or they can assess organizational items, such as manpower or access to care. Are the appropriate systems in place to collect health-related data? Are systems in place to ensure safety? Increasingly, structure measures are reporting on whether items are in place to promote quality improvement. In pediatrics, for example, some measures report on participation in national databases for general pediatric or cardiac surgery. Other measures report on electronic health record (EHR) capabilities. Is there ability to receive data electronically into the EHR or laboratory? Is the appropriate skill mix of clinicians in place? How many hours of nursing care are in place? Are interpreter services available? Although structure measures are often the easiest to assess, they are usually used much less than process or outcome measures.

Other Classification Methods

Another way to classify quality measures is to categorize them by topic or content addressed by the measure. Does the measure report on primary care, mental health services, and diagnostic or therapeutic services? Does the measure address care provided in the hospital, outpatient setting, home setting, or elsewhere? Does it address medical or surgical care or outcome? Is the measure focused on health status or care provision? In the most recently released Child Core Set, the measures are broken into 6 topic areas (Table 2.2).

Another way to categorize quality measures would be to classify them according to the aims or priorities set forth in the National Quality Strategy. In March 2011, the Agency for Healthcare Research and Quality (AHRQ) published the National Strategy for Quality Improvement in Healthcare [42]. The National Quality Strategy (NQS), as it is now known, was developed with input from a range of stakeholders representing

Table 2.2 Topics addressed in 2019 Child Core Set measures

Topic	Number of measures
Primary care access and preventative care	10
Maternal and perinatal health	7
Care of acute and chronic conditions	2
Behavioral health care	4
Dental and oral health services	2
Experience of care	1

List of topics and number of measures addressing each topic in the *2019 Core Set of Children's Health Care Quality Measures for Medicaid and CHIP (Child Core Set)* [41]

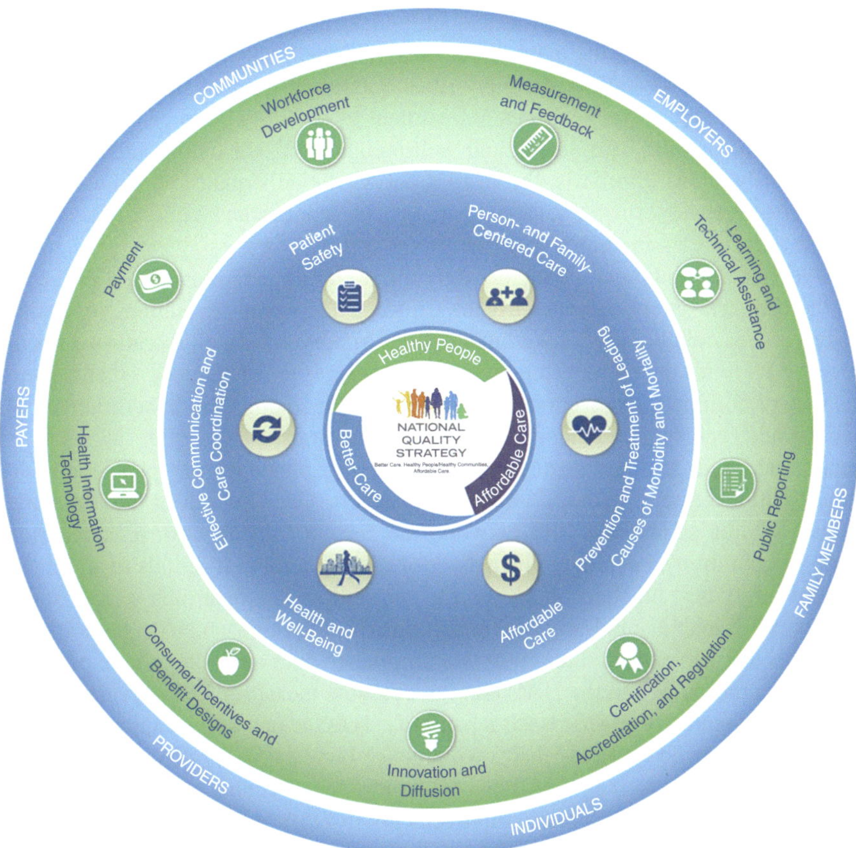

Fig. 2.4 National Quality Strategy. This image presents the 3 aims of the National Quality Strategy surrounded by 6 priorities that can be influenced by 9 levers, which can be used by various stakeholders interested in child health. (The image is taken from a slide set overview of the NQS [44])

the health care industry and general public. The strategy established a set of three overarching aims supported by six priorities to address the most common health concerns faced by Americans (Fig. 2.4). The NQS also identified nine levers that can be used to drive improvement. The three broad aims of the NQS were built upon the Institute for Healthcare Improvement Triple Aim: improve population health, improve experience of care, and reduce per capita cost of care. The NQS restates those aims:

1. "Improve overall quality of health care, by making it more patient-centered, reliable, accessible, and safe."
2. "Improve the health of the U.S. population by supporting proven interventions to address behavioral, social, and environmental determinants of health in addition to delivering higher-quality care."
3. "Reduce the cost of quality health care for individuals, families, employers, and government."

Thus one could examine pediatric quality measure and classify them based upon which of the three aims the metric addresses (better care, healthy people, or affordable care) or upon which of the 6 priorities it assesses (patient safety, person- and family-centered care, prevention and treatment of leading causes of morbidity and mortality, affordable care, health and well-being, or effective communication and care coordination). Similarly, the Institute of Medicine's quality domains (timeliness, effectiveness, efficiency, safety, patient centeredness, and equity) offer another framework for classification [43].

Patient safety has become increasingly important in pediatrics, and at the center of the pediatric safety movement is the Children's Hospitals' Solutions for Patient Safety (SPS) collaborative. Like other quality improvement collaboratives in pediatrics, SPS relies on the reporting of quality measures to drive improvement toward its goal of eliminating preventable harm in hospitalized children. In addition to collecting and reporting on outcome and process measures, SPS uses an "all teach, all learn" paradigm to disseminate high reliability organization principles along with quality improvement methods among its members. Growing out of the 8-member Ohio Children's Hospitals SPS network, the current SPS network includes more than 135 children's hospitals. The network expects member hospitals to adopt culture of safety best practices in addition to submitting data regarding serious safety events (SSE) and hospital-acquired conditions (HAC). For each HAC, participating hospitals are also expected to report on compliance with a bundle of care practices (a process measure) and the HAC rate (an outcome measure). When evidence supporting the bundle of practices for a particular HAC is not well established, hospitals are encouraged to devise their own practice bundles. As evidence accumulates for each HAC, the elements of the HAC bundle then become set by the network. Overall, SPS has seen dramatic improvements in most HACs and claims that the network saved more than 11,000 children from serious harm between 2012 and the end of 2018 [45]. SPS has also demonstrated that bundle compliance is positively correlated with outcome (Fig. 2.5) [46, 47].

Purpose of Quality Measures

Quality measurement may be used to advance the quality of pediatric care and promote better health for children, but it is important that the measures in use are appropriate and meaningful to the pediatric population. Throughout health care, measures are used for a variety of reasons: to drive quality improvement, to benchmark and establish standards of care, to assess health status, to help with accreditation and regulation, to engage consumers through public reporting, and to influence health expenditures with pay-for-performance activities. Although some people have argued that the rapid rise of quality measures is creating undue burden, the number of measures continues to grow [49]. Although more resources and focus have been expended on creating adult measures, pediatric measures have also increased and will continue to increase as long as their value can be demonstrated.

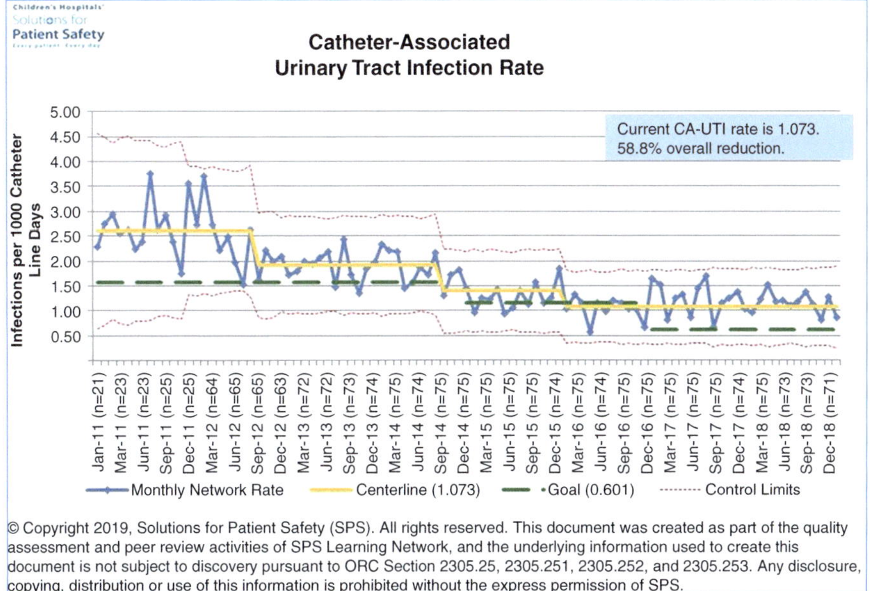

Fig. 2.5 Results from Solutions for Patient Safety's efforts to reduce the Catheter-Associated Urinary Tract Infection Rate 2011–2018. Collecting process measure data (compliance with a bundle of practices) and outcome measure data (catheter-associated urinary tract infection (CAUTI) rate), SPS has shown great improvements in several hospital acquired conditions. This graph shows improvement of the network's CAUTI rate over a 7-year period [48]

It is therefore important to understand how the pediatric population differs from the adult population and to ensure that measures developed and implemented for pediatrics take those differences into account. When comparing adult and pediatric health care, it is important to consider the 5 Ds: developmental change, dependency, differential epidemiology, demographic patterns, and dollars [50]. The needs, physiology, and abilities of children change drastically from infancy to young adulthood, and measures must recognize how each stage of development may impact the health or care being assessed. Furthermore there is increasing evidence that many adult conditions may begin during childhood and that lifelong health may be impacted by changes that begin in childhood. Families and caregivers are integral parts of the health care team since most pediatric patients are dependent upon others for all care and support unlike most adults. Not only are the medical conditions faced by children different than those faced by adults, but the overall state of health differs. Children are generally healthier than adults and maximizing health rather than treating illness or preventing morbidity is a major goal of pediatric care. While some chronic diseases do begin in childhood, such as diabetes, obesity, and asthma, compared to adults, the number of children with chronic conditions is much less. Unfortunately those children with complex medical needs are growing in need and number. The pediatric population in America is the most diverse age group in regard to race and ethnicity, and there is also more poverty among children than adults, so measures assessing social determinants of health may be more meaningful for children. Finally, health care financing and costs for children differ in several crucial ways. The overall costs are lower, but many would argue that the lifetime return on investment of care is greater. The source of funding for health care also differs. While both populations have private insurance payers, state Medicaid and CHIP play significant roles in financing pediatric care but Medicare does not. Because Medicaid programs vary by state and not all require reporting on the Child Core Set measures, this difference between Medicaid and Medicare financing has important implications regarding the national reporting of pediatric quality indicators.

Quality measures may be used for regulation and accreditation, reporting and surveillance, and payment. In these spheres, it is more likely that the quality measures were not developed specifically for children or pediatric practice. With wide variation in measures and the call for reporting quality measures coming from many directions, it is important that more work is done to align measures and reduce the potential burden that collection may impose on the health care system for children [51].

Quality measures to promote improvement in pediatric care and children's health have been able to demonstrate major impact in some areas, especially when selection and implementation are specific to the pediatric population. Synergistic efforts by bodies like the Accreditation Council on Graduate Medical Education (ACGME), which require quality improvement to be a core competency of pediatric trainees, and the American Board of Pediatrics (ABP), which includes quality improvement in its part 4 Maintenance of Certification activities, have expanded the reach of quality measures across the field. These measures are developed most effectively when the needs of pediatric clinicians, trainees, patients, and their families are paramount.

References

1. Internet citation. https://www.ahrq.gov/cpi/about/mission/index.html.
2. Agency for Healthcare Quality and Research. AHRQ Quality Indicators™: Pediatric Quality Indicators. 2015 Sept. Downloaded from https://www.qualityindicators.ahrq.gov/Downloads/Modules/PDI/V50/Pediatric_Ind.pdf
3. Internet citation. https://www.medicaid.gov/medicaid/quality-of-care/performance-measurement/child-core-set/index.html.
4. Mayhew M. CMCS Informational Bulletin. SUBJECT: 2019 Updates to the child and adult core health care quality measurement sets. Department of Health & Human Services Centers for Medicare & Medicaid Services, Baltimore, MD. 2018 Nov 20. Available at: https://www.medicaid.gov/federal-policy-guidance/downloads/cib112018.pdf.
5. Downloaded March 23, 2019 from https://www.medicaid.gov/medicaid/quality-of-care/downloads/performance-measurement/2019-child-core-set.pdf.
6. The Joint Commission. Specifications manual for joint commission national quality measures (v2018B1). 2018 Nov 1. Available at: https://manual.jointcommission.org/releases/TJC2018B1/ Last Accessed on 23 Mar 2109.
7. The Joint Commission. Improving America's hospitals – The Joint Commission's annual report on quality and safety 2012. 2012 Sept 18. Available at https://www.jointcommission.org/improving_americas_hospitals_joint_commission_annual_report_quality_safety_2012/.

8. The Joint Commission. America's hospitals: improving quality and safety: The Joint Commission's annual report 2015. 2015 Nov 16. Available at https://www.jointcommission.org/tjc_annual_report_2015/.
9. Morse RB, Hall M, Fieldston ES, et al. Hospital-level compliance with asthma care quality measures at children's hospitals and subsequent asthma-related outcomes. JAMA. 2011;306(13):1454–60. https://doi.org/10.1001/jama.2011.1385.
10. Internet citation. https://www.ncqa.org/hedis/. Last accessed 23 Mar 2019.
11. House SA, Coon ER, Schroeder AR, Ralston SL. Categorization of national pediatric quality measures. Pediatrics. 2017;139(4):e20163269.
12. Hagan JF, Shaw JS, Duncan PM, American Academy of Pediatrics, Issuing Body. Bright futures: guidelines for health supervision of infants, children, and adolescents. 4th ed. Elk Grove Village: American Academy of Pediatrics; 2017. Web.
13. Skinner AC, Ravanbakht SN, Skelton JA, et al. Prevalence of obesity and severe obesity in US children, 1999–2016. Pediatrics. 2018;141(3):e20173459.
14. Internet citation. https://www.ncqa.org/hedis/measures/weight-assessment-and-counseling-for-nutrition-and-physical-activity-for-children-adolescents/.
15. Internet citation. https://public.vtoxford.org/.
16. Internet citation. https://www.myvps.org/.
17. Bennett TD, Spaeder MC, Matos RI, Watson RS, Typpo KV, Khemani RG, Ecrow S, Benneyworth BD, Thiagarajan RR, Dean JM, Markovitz BP. Existing data analysis in pediatric critical care research. Front Pediatr. 2014;2:79.
18. Internet citation. https://www.sts.org/registries-research-center/sts-national-database/sts-congenital-heart-surgery-database.
19. Hall BL, Hamilton BH, Richards KY, Bilimoria KE, Cohen M, Ko C. Does surgical quality improve in the American College of Surgeons National Surgical Quality Improvement Program: an evaluation of all participating hospitals. Ann Surg. 2009;250(3):363–76.
20. Internet citation. https://www.facs.org/quality-programs/childrens-surgery/pediatric.
21. Dillon P, Hammermeister K, Morrato E, Kempe A, Oldham K, Moss L, Marchildon M, Ziegler M, Steeger J, Rowell K, Shiloach M, Henderson W. Developing a NSQIP module to measure outcomes in children's surgical care: opportunity and challenge. Semin Pediatr Surg. 2008;17(2):131–40.
22. Mogayzel PJ, Dunitz J, Marrow LC, et al. Improving chronic care delivery and outcomes: the impact of the cystic fibrosis Care Center Network. BMJ Qual Saf. 2014;23:i3–8.
23. Internet citation. https://www.improvecarenow.org/purpose-success.
24. Crandall W, Kappelman MD, Colletti RB, Leibowitz I, Grunow JE, Ali S, Baron HI, Berman JH, Boyle B, Cohen S, del Rosario F, Denson LA, Duffy L, Integlia MJ, Kim SC, Milov D, Patel AS, Schoen BT, Walkiewicz D, Margolis P. ImproveCareNow: the development of a pediatric inflammatory bowel disease improvement network. Inflamm Bowel Dis. 2011;17(1):450–7.
25. Egberg MD, Kappelman MD, Gulati AS. Improving Care in Pediatric Inflammatory Bowel Disease. Gastroenterol Clin N Am. 2018;47(4):909–19.
26. Internet citation. https://www.cms.gov/Medicare/Quality-Initiatives-Patient-Assessment-Instruments/QualityMeasures/Core-Measures.html.
27. CQMC. Consensus core set: pediatric measures, version 1.0. Updated 3/24/2017. Available at https://www.cms.gov/Medicare/Quality-Initiatives-Patient-Assessment-Instruments/QualityMeasures/Downloads/Pediatric-Measures.pdf.
28. Donabedian A. Evaluating the quality of medical care. Milbank Mem Fund Q. 1966;44(3):166–206.
29. National Quality Forum. Pediatric measures: final report. 2016 June 15. Available at: http://www.qualityforum.org/Publications/2016/06/Pediatric_Measures_Final_Report.aspx. Accessed 15 Mar 2019.
30. Newton EH, Zazzera EA, Van Moorsel G, Sirovich BE. Undermeasuring overuse - an examination of national clinical performance measures. JAMA Intern Med. 2015;175(10):1709–11.
31. Berwick DM, Hackbarth AD. Eliminating waste in US health care. JAMA. 2012;307(14):1513–6. https://doi.org/10.1001/jama.2012.362.

32. American Academy of Pediatrics. Ten things physicians and patients should question. Choosing wisely, an initiative of ABIM Foundation. Released February 21, 2013 (1–5) and March 17, 2014 (6–10); #1, 3, 9 updated July 13, 2016; #1, 2, 4, 5 and 10 updated June 12, 2018. Downloaded from internet: https://www.choosingwisely.org/wp-content/uploads/2015/02/AAP-Choosing-Wisely-List.pdf.
33. Internet citation. https://www.aap.org/en-us/about-the-aap/aap-press-room/campaigns/choosing-wisely/Pages/default.aspx.
34. Marshall BC, Nelson EC. Accelerating implementation of biomedical research advances: critical elements of a successful 10 year Cystic Fibrosis Foundation healthcare delivery improvement initiative. BMJ Qual Saf. 2014;23:i95–i103.
35. Chassin MR, et al. Accountability measures – using measurement to promote quality improvement. NEJM. 2010;363(7):683–8.
36. Axon RN, Williams MV. Hospital readmission as an accountability measure. JAMA. 2011;305(5):504–5.
37. Berry JG, Toomey SL, Zaslavsky AM, et al. Pediatric readmission prevalence and variability across hospitals. JAMA. 2013;309(4):372–80.
38. Jacobs JP, Jacobs ML, Austin EH. Quality measures for congenital and pediatric cardiac surgery. World J Pediatr Congenit Heart Surg. 2012;3(1):32–47.
39. Gluckman PD, Hanson MA, Cooper C, Thornburg KL. Effect of in utero and early-life conditions on adult health and disease. N Engl J Med. 2008;359:61–73.
40. Belfort MB, Gillman MW, Buka SL, Casey PH, McCormick MC. Preterm infant linear growth and adiposity gain: trade-offs for later weight status and intelligence quotient. J Pediatr. 2013;163(6):1564–9.
41. Internet citation. https://www.medicaid.gov/medicaid/quality-of-care/downloads/performance-measurement/2019-child-core-set.pdf.
42. Internet citation. https://www.ahrq.gov/workingforquality/index.html.
43. Alessandrini E, Varadarajan K, Alpern E, Gorelick M, Shaw K, Ruddy R, Chamberlain J. Emergency department quality: an analysis of existing pediatric measures. Acad Emerg Med. 2011;18(5):519–26.
44. Image taken from Slide 30 of slide set: National Quality Strategy Overview. Content last reviewed January 2017. Agency for Healthcare Research and Quality, Rockville, MD. Downloaded from http://www.ahrq.gov/workingforquality/nqs-tools/briefing-slides.html.
45. Children's Hospitals Solutions for Patient Safety. SPS Network. 2018 Year in review. Downloaded from: https://www.solutionsforpatientsafety.org/wp-content/uploads/2018-Year-in-Review.pdf.
46. Lyren A, Brilli RJ, Zieker K, Marino M, Muething S, Sharek PJ. Children's hospitals' solutions for patient safety collaborative impact on hospital-acquired harm. Pediatrics. 2017;140(3)
47. Martin BS, Arbore M. Measurement, standards, and peer benchmarking: one hospital's journey. Pediatr Clin N Am. 2016;63(2):239–49.
48. Image downloaded on March 22, 2019 from https://www.solutionsforpatientsafety.org/our-results/.
49. Berwick DM. Era 3 for medicine and health care. JAMA. 2016;315(13):1329–30.
50. Stille C, Turchi RM, Antonelli R, Cabana MD, Cheng TL, Laraque D, Perrin J, The Academic Pediatric Association Task Force on Family-Centered Medical Home. APA Policy Statement: The family-centered medical home: specific considerations for child health research and policy. Acad Pediatr. 2010;10(4):211–7.
51. Adirim T, Meade K, Mistry K, AAP Council on Quality Improvement and Patient Safety. A new era in quality measurement: the development and application of quality measures. Pediatrics. 2017;139(1):e20163442.

Chapter 3
Quality and Safety Improvement in Surgery

William C. Mackey

Introduction

Prior to the twenty-first century, surgical quality and safety were measured, reported, and managed locally by individual surgery departments through traditional morbidity and mortality conferences. Peer review protections promoted open discussion at such conferences but hindered institutional oversight and inter-institutional data sharing. In its most robust manifestations, the traditional M + M provided detailed case review, established the causes of complications and deaths, and formulated opportunities for improvement. While the M + M conference remains a critically important tool for surgery quality and safety monitoring and for education, its shortcomings are all too apparent. The case-based format of M + M conferences leads to focus on single cases and not on the identification of trends or benchmarking of outcomes. Without trend analysis and benchmarking, systematic quality and safety improvement programs are impossible.

Acknowledgement of the prevalence of medical errors and complications through such reports as "To Err is Human" led to societal pressure to improve surgical safety and quality and provided the impetus for surgical specialty groups to design large-scale databases to track outcomes [1]. General dissatisfaction with coding-based outcome measures, which lacked granularity and did not permit risk adjustments, added additional motivation for surgeons to take the lead in designing their own reporting tools. Presently, the most sophisticated of these data sets is the American College of Surgeons' National Surgical Quality Improvement Project (NSQIP). Such large-scale specialty society-initiated data sets allow individual surgical departments or divisions and even individual surgeons to track and benchmark their

W. C. Mackey (✉)
Tufts Medical Center, Department of Surgery, Tufts University School of Medicine, Boston, MA, USA
e-mail: wmackey@tuftsmedicalcenter.org

© Springer Nature Switzerland AG 2020
D. N. Salem (ed.), *Quality Measures*, https://doi.org/10.1007/978-3-030-37145-6_3

outcomes over time to allow identification of areas for improvement. While there are many other similar datasets that permit benchmarking and trend analysis, Society for Thoracic Surgery Database, Vascular Quality Initiative, Trauma Quality Improvement Project, to name a few, I will focus on NSQIP since it is the largest, most sophisticated, most accessible, and most user friendly.

Accurate granular risk-adjusted data, benchmarking, and trend analysis are essential but not sufficient elements for robust quality improvement programs. Surgery departments must be organized in a manner that facilitates data acquisition, analysis, and dissemination. In addition, departmental leadership must consistently focus on quality and safety and drive quality improvement initiatives. Departmental structures and functions promoting quality and safety will be discussed in detail.

Several tools are required to maintain and improve quality and safety in surgery. Stringent credentialing and privileging processes are critical. Checklists, dashboards, preoperative briefings, postoperative debriefings, along with standardized hand-offs, and escalation triggers are essential tools discussed in detail.

Even with abundant data, a supportive department structure, and robust tools for quality and safety maintenance, optimal results will remain elusive unless the department's culture is optimized. Blaming and shaming result in under-reporting and defensiveness, which stifle quality and safety improvement efforts. While individual accountability undergirds the surgical ethos, dispassionate analysis of failures need not be a personal attack. Application of psychological safety and just culture principles leads to open and objective QI processes. Departmental cultures conducive to optimal quality and safety initiatives are discussed.

Optimal data, departmental structure, and culture provide the environment in which meaningful quality and safety improvement can thrive. Without well-organized QI improvement processes, however, these critical factors are insufficient. This chapter will conclude with a case study of a QI project.

Data Sources

Intra-institutional

Without question, the most detailed case analyses occur in properly managed morbidity and mortality conferences and root cause analyses. These analyses allow highly granular analysis of individual cases, assessment of the nature and severity of the complication, and identification of the causes of complications and of opportunities for improvement. Such conferences are most effective when a standard format is used, consensus conclusions are required, and detailed minutes are kept. A standard record form from our M + M conference is shown in Fig. 3.1. Following detailed case discussion, the nature of the complication is clearly identified and its severity assessed using the Clavien-Dindo classification, an international standard classification system that has been repeatedly validated (Fig. 3.2) [2]. More controversial often will be the assignment of the cause of the complication. For example,

MR#

Diagnosis:

Date of Surgery:

Attending Surgeon: Resident Surgeon:

Procedure:

Complication:

Severity of Complication:

Cause: Error in Diagnosis   Systems Failure

       Error in Technique   Communications Failure

       Error in Judgment   Patient Disease

       Error in Management   Other: _______________________

Discussion:

Opportunities for Improvement:

Fig. 3.1 Morbidity and mortality conference minutes

Grade I: Any deviation from a standard course that does not require non-routine pharmacologic, radiologic, endoscopic, or surgical intervention.

Grade II: Any deviation from expected course requiring non-routine pharmacologic intervention (including unexpected blood transfusions or need for total parenteral nutrition)

Grade III: Any deviation from expected course requring radiologic, endoscopic, or surgical re-intervention.

     IIIA) Not requiring general anesthesia
     IIIB) Requiring general anesthesia

Grade IV: Life threatening complications (including CNS complications) requiring escalation of care to intensive care unit.

     IVA) Single organ system dysfunction
     IVB) Multi-system organ dysfunction.

Grade V: Death of Patient

(Subheading "d" for disability will be appended to complcation of any grade resulting in need for non-routine follow-up care specifically for the complication.)

Fig. 3.2 Clavien-Dindo classification of surgical complications [1]

by convention, anastomotic leaks, postoperative bleeding, and wound infections are generally classified as errors in technique; however, in re-operative surgeries and in severely compromised patients undergoing salvage surgeries for immediately life-threatening conditions, such complications may occur despite optimal technique. In addition, in areas where there are no evidence-based "best practices," there may be legitimate debate over putative errors in management or judgment. Still, in order to identify all potential areas for improvement, it is important to attribute the complication to one or more potentially correctable causes and to minimize the use of "patient disease" as the sole cause.

For the analysis of particularly impactful complications, a root cause analysis is most appropriate. Such analyses are best conducted by a multidisciplinary team including hospital risk managers, quality and safety officers, as well as surgical, anesthesiology, and nursing personnel. The format for root cause analyses has been well described and allows for a deep dive into all factors contributing to an adverse outcome [3]. Usually an independent referee, not involved in the patient's care, is assigned to perform a detailed analysis of the facts of the case including a timeline of all relevant events. Once the facts of the case are reviewed and the nature of the complication identified, all potential contributing factors are presented and their relative importance discussed. In order to allow for open discussion and avoidance of defensiveness, care is taken to avoid overt blaming, though in a well-conducted root cause analysis, system, team, and individual accountability are clearly established.

Other potential intra-institutional data sources include incident reports and "word on the street". Many hospitals now employ electronic incident reporting systems. Desirable attributes of such systems include:

1. Ease of access for entry of incident for all personnel throughout hospital
2. Ease of use
3. Optional anonymity
4. Drop-down lists for incident categorization (hospital department, nature, and severity)
5. Requirement for brief narrative description of incident
6. Robust data security
7. Ease of distribution to those responsible for investigating event
8. Easy but secure communication among those investigating events
9. Standardized conclusion format including event severity, primary cause, contributing causes, likelihood of event recurrence, actions necessary to prevent recurrence, assignment of responsibility for carrying out these actions and for tracking their completion
10. Final event closure format when steps in #9 completed
11. User-friendly index of events to track trends by provider, service, type of event, etc.

The hospital's and surgery department's culture as well as the quality of the reporting system will, to some extent, determine the usefulness of the incident reporting system. Most importantly, the system will only be useful, and in fact, only be used if its use results in readily apparent changes in care delivery.

Over-use and inappropriate use are often an issue with incident reporting systems. Rather than using the system to report incidents that affected or could have affected patient safety, frustrated staff will often use the system to vent. It is important to encourage all staff to report actual or potential patient safety issues, and it is equally important to give the staff a means for reporting systems or personnel issues that were frustrating but not actually or potentially dangerous. In our operating rooms, we encourage all staff to use the patient safety incident reporting system for all events with actual or potential patient harm. We also have an electronic "learning board" through which staff, using an application on their mobile devices can enter a report regarding delays, equipment issues, facilities issues, and other conditions that did not jeopardize patient safety but should be corrected. These reports are posted publically in the OR and management's response and actions taken are posted as well. When used properly, our learning board prevents the over-use of our patient safety reporting system. Staff are encouraged, when in doubt, to use the patient safety reporting system.

"Word on the street" is a prevalent, variably reliable, and always subjective tool in surgical quality and safety improvement. With readily available incident reporting systems, word on the street is rarely essential for significant single events but may be useful in uncovering chronic issues that may undermine safety and quality. Surgical leaders must stay attuned to what is said about their staff members by anesthesiologists, OR, ICU, and ward nurses, as well as other ancillary personnel. Single off-hand remarks should be remembered. A few similar off-hand comments should prompt questioning of staff. The identification of patterns of performance and behavior that may undermine safety and quality should prompt a discussion with the subject of these comments and could lead to remedial actions. Word on the street is most often useful in uncovering behaviors detrimental to team functions and therefore to patient safety but may also uncover technical performance issues related to medical problems, substance abuse, or other psycho-social stressors.

Extra-institutional Data Sources

AHRQ Data

The Agency for Healthcare Research and Quality (AHRQ) is a federal agency charged with improving the safety and quality of America's health care system. Their mission is "to produce evidence to make healthcare safer, higher quality, more accessible, equitable, and affordable and to work within the U.S. Department of Health and Human Services and with other partners to make sure that the evidence is understood and used." [[4] (AHRQ website, U.S. Department of Health and Human Services. 2018)]. Major functions of AHRQ related to surgery include the AHRQuality Indicators™. Most relevant among these indicators are the Inpatient Quality Indicators and the Patient Safety Indicators. Both data sets rely on data obtained from hospital coding and therefore are considered to be administrative data sets. Inpatient Quality Indicators track mortality rates and volume for selected higher risk procedures such as open AAA repair, esophagectomy, pancreatectomy, and carotid endartertectomy. AHRQ patient safety indicators include specific complications such as iatrogenic pneumothorax, retained surgical item, perioperative hemorrhage or hematoma, accidental puncture or laceration requiring re-operation, perioperative deep venous thrombosis, and mortality rate for low-risk Diagnosis Related Groups (DRGs). Since these data are derived from hospital coding data meant to be used for billing purposes, they are completely dependent on thorough and accurate medical record documentation.

Press Ganey® designs and administers surveys of patients and providers designed to "help health care organizations reduce patient suffering and enhance provider resilience to improve the safety, quality, and experience of care." Rather than dealing with hard outcomes such as mortality and complication rates, their surveys emphasize patient and care provider experiences. Patient experience domains queried include physician communication quality, office staff quality, access, and care coordination along with summary ratings (overall provider and would recommend this provider). Narrative comments are also collected. While these data are helpful in identifying areas for improvement in physician and office staff behavior, access, inter-provider communication, and care coordination, response rates are variable and may not be representative. Those patients having an especially negative or positive experience appear most likely to respond.

Provider surveys collect information on physician engagement and alignment. Areas queried include collegiality, ancillary service functions, OR functions, physical plant and other infrastructure, and electronic medical record. Recently added are questions designed to measure burnout. Given current data linking patient satisfaction and outcomes to provider engagement, these data are becoming increasingly important.

National Surgery Quality Improvement Program (NSQIP)

Derived from the Veterans' Administration Surgical Risk Study (NVASRS) initiated in 1991 and starting with data from 44 VA medical centers, the National Surgical Quality Improvement Program (NSQIP) has grown to include more than 600 U.S. hospitals, 62 Canadian hospitals, and approximately 25 hospitals in other countries. NSQIP is managed by the American College of Surgeons' Quality Programs Division. As NSQIP participants, each hospital submits detailed data on an approximately 20% sample of selected cases. The data are extracted from medical records by trained surgical clinical reviewers (SCRs) who use standardized definitions for each complication and who obtain 30-day follow-up for every case. The data include detailed demographic and comorbidity data to allow robust risk adjustment. Comparison of NSQIP data with data derived from administrative (claims) methods revealed that NSQIP methods detected 61% more complications and 97% more surgical site infections than claims data.

NSQIP methods allow robust risk adjustment and statistical analysis reported back to each participating hospital twice annually. A typical report graph from a NSQIP semi-annual report (SAR) is shown below (Fig. 3.3).

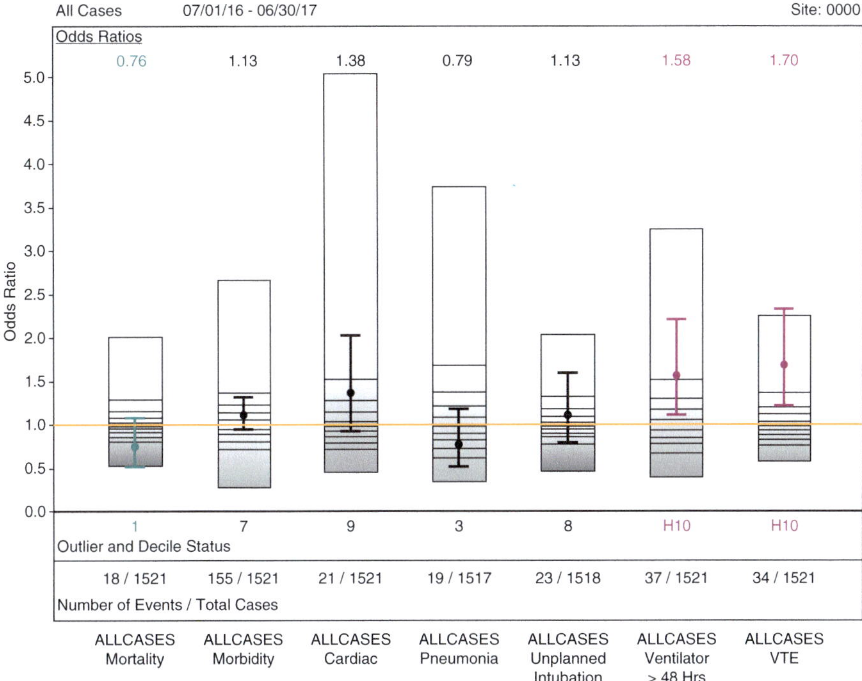

Fig. 3.3 Sample data display from NSQIP semiannual report. (Reproduced with permission from the American College of Surgeons)

This sample report covers cases for 7/1/16–6/30/17. Observed/expected odds ratios (O/E) for each complication are listed at the top of the slide. The boxes represent the range of results across all participating hospitals. Thus, for mortality, the range of O/E outcomes is approximately 0.5–2.0. The horizontal lines within the boxes represent deciles of O/E performance. The reporting center's O/E performance is shown with standard error isobars. Thus, in this illustrative example there are 24% fewer mortalities than would be expected placing the hospital in the top 10% of participants, though, because the isobar crosses the O/E = 1 line, the hospital's results are not statistically significantly different from expected. On the other hand, for unplanned intubations and VTE events, this hospital's O/E ratios of 1.58 and 1.7 are in the 10th decile (worse than 90% of participating hospitals) and since the isobar does not cross the O/E = 1 line, the results are statistically significantly worse than expected. Robust risk adjustment along with reliable data extraction using uniform definitions makes these data highly reliable and useful.

In addition, data can be accessed in real time and compared with national norms, though without the same robust risk adjustment incorporated into the 6 month reports. The sample report below shows the hospital's performance trend with

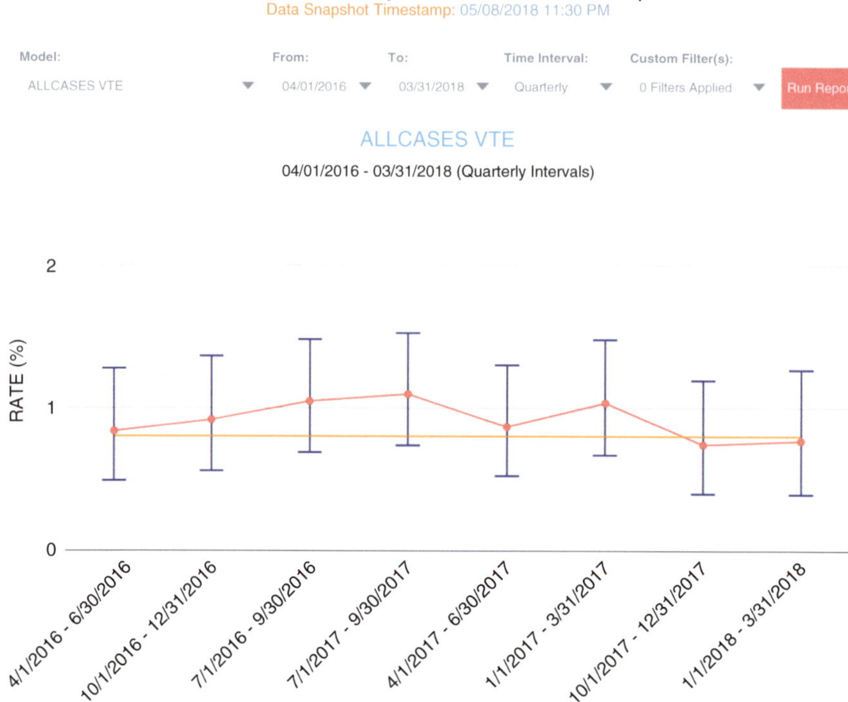

Fig. 3.4 Sample real-time data display comparing individual hospital performance with that of all NSQIP participating hospitals over time. (Reproduced with permission of the American College of Surgeons)

respect to venous thromboembolic (VTE) complications by quarter over a 2 year period in comparison to the 2 year rate of all participating hospitals (Fig. 3.4, reproduced with permission of ACS). While these real-time reports lack the risk adjustment of the semi-annual report shown above, they are useful in determining trends to assess the outcomes of ongoing quality improvement projects.

NSQIP includes most surgical sub-specialties and specialties (gynecology, neurosurgery, orthopedics, otolaryngology, urology) but excludes transplantation, cardiac surgery, and trauma for which there is a parallel program (TQIP). Similar representative specialty-specific surgical quality improvement data sets include:

Cardiac Surgery: Society for Thoracic Surgeons (STS) Database
Surgical Oncology: National Cancer Database
Transplantation Surgery: Scientific Registry of Transplant Recipients (SRTR)
Vascular Surgery: Vascular Quality Initiative (VQI).

Because it is axiomatic that you cannot improve outcomes without accurately measuring them, NSQIP and the other multi-institutional specialty-specific outcomes data sets are essential quality improvement data sources.

Departmental and Institutional Structure

Accurate data are essential but alone are insufficient for optimal surgical quality improvement. Focused and effective leadership as well as active and engaged committees within the surgery department, hospital administration, and even hospital governance are essential to insure the optimal use of safety and quality data.

Each department must appoint a Surgical Quality Officer (SQO). In smaller departments, the Chief of Surgery may fill this role, but in larger departments it is unlikely that the Chair will have the necessary bandwidth. The SQO responsibilities may reside with the Vice-Chair for Clinical Affairs. The SQO should chair the Surgical Quality and Safety Committee. The responsibilities of the SQO are best described in the America College of Surgeons Optimal Resources for Surgical Quality and Safety [7]:

- Provide leadership in surgical quality and safety
- Establish a structure for leading surgical safety and quality efforts that are integrated within the existing governance structure
- Develop mechanisms to improve surgical quality and safety through performance improvement, project management, and QI principles
- Cooperate with other institutional leaders to establish quality and safety goals
- Seek out best practices and QI techniques to share with colleagues
- Demonstrate to external stakeholders such as accrediting bodies, regulatory agencies, payors, and patient advocates that the department and institution are committed to quality and safety by leading collaborative efforts with these bodies
- Understand and address along with other hospital quality and safety officials the regulatory metrics applied to surgical patients

Ideally, the SQO should be an experienced, well-respected active clinician, who demonstrates personal accountability, reliability, outstanding communication skills, charisma, and effective leadership skills. The SQO must be able to communicate effectively her or his compelling vision for the creation of an optimally safe and high quality surgical environment. In addition, the SQO should have formal training in QI processes and a familiarity with the quality- and safety-related data sets such as NSQIP.

In addition to chairing the Surgical Quality and Safety Committee, the SQO should have the oversight of all surgery-related institutional and extra-institutional data sources (M + M conferences, root cause analyses, AHRQ data, NSQIP data, etc.). The SQO will interface with the Medical Staff Office to insure adequate quality and safety data are available for credentialing and re-credentialing decisions. The SQO will also interface with the Surgical Education Office to insure robust quality and safety education for all staff.

The Surgical Quality and Safety Committee

The purpose of the Surgical Quality and Safety Committee (SQSC) is to provide leadership in the measurement of surgical safety and quality and in the implementation of quality and safety improvement efforts. Chaired by the SQO, the committee should be truly multidisciplinary: Our committee includes:

- Surgeon-in-Chief (SQO at our institution): Chair
- Anesthesiologist in Chief
- Representatives from Adult and Pediatric Surgical Services
- Infection Control Representative
- Perioperative Nursing Leader
- OR Administrator
- Director of Office of Quality and Safety
- Chief Medical Officer
- Nursing Director of Center for Pre-operative Assessment
- Head Nurses from Surgical Floors
- Pharmacy Representative
- Risk Manager
- Surgical Chief Resident
- Director of OR Nursing Professional Development

Other participants (blood bank, environmental services, medical engineering, pathology, etc.) are invited as needed to address specific issues.

Our key committee metrics include:

1. Surgical Outcomes as defined by NSQIP, AHRQ measures, National Healthcare Safety Network (NHSN) infection data and others as deemed appropriate by the committee
2. Results of Annual Culture of Safety Survey conducted by hospital
3. Results of internal audits, incident reports, root cause analyses, and other internal data
4. Patient experience data
5. Staff engagement data

Committee success criteria include demonstrable and sustained improvements in quality and safety determined by the above metrics, absence of "never events," decrease in medicolegal claims, improvements in staff engagement and satisfaction, and improvements in patient satisfaction.

The monthly agenda includes a review of all key metrics, especially if any new reports are available since the prior meeting, review of internal audit data, discussion of the progress of any ongoing QI projects, and a case report of an adverse event or near miss that occurred since the prior meeting. The meeting concludes with an invitation for any committee member to bring forth any concerns for discussion and potential action.

Examples of QI projects launched recently by our committee include our Perioperative Pneumonia Prevention Project, which will be discussed as the case study at the conclusion of this chapter, and most recently a revision of our venous thromboembolism risk assessment tool and order sets.

Culture

While individual accountability has always been a major component of the surgical ethos, blaming and shaming discourage disclosure and are likely counterproductive. On the other hand, individual errors of omission and commission still harm or threaten to harm patients, so surgery departments cannot adopt a blame-free culture. Creating the correct balance between individual and corporate accountability is the goal of a just culture [9].

In a just culture, errors causing adverse outcomes and near misses are thoroughly investigated and characterized according to one of many hierarchical schemes. For example in Leonard and Frankel's system errors are characterized as [10]:

Type of error	Response
Unintentional	Caregiver to participate in investigation and subsequent remediation and education
Resulting from risky actions	Caregiver coached and participates in ongoing staff education regarding event
Resulting from reckless actions	Caregiver may be disciplined and subject to re-training Caregiver to help educate staff
Resulting from malicious actions	Disciplinary and potential legal action. Immediate suspension
Resulting from impaired judgment	Performance evaluation, offer, or mandate help events Discipline may be warranted for egregious or repeated events

In addition, Leonard and Frankel recommend subjecting errors in the first three categories to a test to evaluate for potential systemic causes for the error. If three other caregivers with similar expertise would have done the same thing in similar circumstances, then the system supports errors, supports risky actions, or supports reckless actions and requires fixing. In these cases, the system leaders share the accountability.

A just culture will thrive only in circumstances where all team members are empowered to speak up about errors made by themselves or others whether or not the errors resulted in harm to a patient. A prerequisite for such an open and empowering environment is psychological safety. A psychologically safe environment is one in which individuals feel safe to take interpersonal risks by sharing information, questioning prevailing methods, recommending improvements, and taking initiative to implement these improvements [11]. Abundant data support strong roles for psychological safety in promoting upward communication in an organization and in enhancing learning in an environment requiring collaboration. In the operating room, both effective upward communication and collaborative learning are essential for safe and high-quality outcomes. Creating a psychologically safe environment in the operating room is the surgeon's responsibility. Hostile or passive aggressive interactions among members of the team preclude psychological safety, inhibit communication and learning, and will lead to suboptimal outcomes.

Safety and Quality Improvement Tools

Credentialing and Privileging

Credentialing is the process through which a hospital or other health care facility determines whether a practitioner's education, training, and background meet the facility's standards for staff membership. Privileging is the process through which staff members are granted permission to use specific techniques or to treat specific conditions at the facility. Criteria for physician/surgeon credentialing are usually established at the institutional level and apply across all specialties, while privileging is specialty specific and usually determined at the department level. Usual criteria for credentialing usually include a valid medical degree (MD, DO, or equivalent), a valid state medical license, specialty board certification (or board eligibility for entry level physicians), absence of adverse licensure actions, passage of a criminal background check, possession of valid state and federal licenses for the prescription of controlled substances, possession of intact medical liability coverage, and completion of a questionnaire regarding drug and alcohol use and general physical and mental health. Most facilities require re-credentialing at 2-year intervals.

Privileging is much more complex, especially in the procedural specialties, because of the rapid evolution of technology. For broad-based skill sets and the management of common conditions, privileging is often rolled up into the credentialing process. For example, a surgeon, board certified in general surgery, when credentialed, will often be given "Core General Surgery Privileges," which cover the commonly seen surgical conditions and commonly performed procedures. Surgery department leadership will decide what is included in these core privileges. Certain high-risk procedures may be excluded and privileging in these areas reserved for those with advanced training or a proven track record. For example, core general surgery privileges may include colectomy for colon cancer or diverticulitis, but may reserve low anterior resections and pouch reconstructions for inflammatory bowel disease for surgeons with advanced training in colorectal surgery.

Emerging technologies pose real challenges in privileging. Currently robotic and endovascular technologies are progressing so rapidly surgeons are forced to learn on the fly. While some new technologies and procedures are so similar to previously mastered earlier versions that learning on the fly is safe and simple, others require new knowledge and skill sets. The American College of Surgeons Committee on Emerging Technologies and Education (ACS-CESTE) has promulgated the following requirements for privileging in procedures requiring new technology didactic educational training [8]:

1. Skills training (inanimate simulation)
2. Skills training (supervised/proctored)
3. Incorporation into practice
4. Measurement of results

The details applied to these requirements such as the required number of proctored cases vary based on the complexity and risk of the procedure. Proctors must be unbiased in offering privileging recommendations based on their observations.

Initial privileges for procedures requiring new technology should be conditional and based on acceptable performance and outcomes in a specified number of cases. In order to maintain privileges without additional proctoring, surgeons should be required to perform a specified number of the new cases annually and provide detailed results reporting including follow-up data. It is likely that in the future patient-reported outcomes data will be incorporated into decisions regarding continuation of privileges.

Renewal of privileges should be based on acceptable performance in a specified number of cases over a specified period (usually 2 years). Renewal of privileges usually coincides with re-credentialing and requires submission of case volume and case outcomes. Our process requires submission of a case log (generated by the OR billing system), a summary of all cases reported at morbidity and mortality conference, and AHRQ patient safety indicators, along with a statement from the department chair attesting to the surgeon's performance. This constitutes the Ongoing Professional Practice Evaluation (OPPE) required by the Joint Commission. At any time, evidence for substandard performance can trigger an off-cycle review of credentials and privileges or Focused Professional Practice Evaluation (FPPE).

Checklists, Briefings, Debriefings

In *The Checklist Manifesto*, Atul Gawande points out that "the volume and complexity of what we know has exceeded our individual ability to deliver its benefits correctly, safely, or reliably." [12] Nowhere is this more evident than in the operating room. In the planning and conduct of a modern surgical procedure, there are so many details that require attention it is inconceivable that any one person or even any one team can keep them all at top of mind. Even before a patient enters the OR, myriad details require attention. At our institution, entry into the OR requires a completed "Ticket to Safety" (Fig. 3.5):

The preoperative holding area nurse, surgeon, anesthesiologist, and circulating nurse must each complete their sections on pages 1 and 2 before the patient can be moved into the OR. In addition, the attending surgeon must personally sign the ticket to confirm that she/he is on site and available. Page 3 is the template for documentation of the pre-induction team briefing, the pre-incision time-out, and the post-procedure debriefing.

While it is surprisingly difficult to get precise statistics on wrong site, wrong patient, wrong procedure surgical events in the U.S, the NHS in the UK reported 172 such events between April 1, 2017 and January 31, 2018 [13]. That such events keep happening, despite the current ubiquity of surgical safety checklists, suggests that this tool, while necessary, is insufficient. Just having a checklist is not enough.

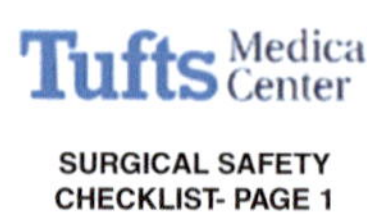

SURGICAL SAFETY CHECKLIST		Alternative Site Marking
Pre-op Nurse	**Initials**	(per policy # 4029)
Verify patient identification with name and date of birth using active communication • Documentation, labels, ID band		
Confirm the procedure, side, and site • With the patient • With the consent (dated within 90 days) • With the H&P		
H&P completed within 30 days		
Pre-op Nursing Assessment Complete		
Report Given to:		

Pre-Op Nurse's Printed Name: _______________________________________

Pre-Op Nurse's Signature: ______________________ Date: _______ Time: _______

Surgeon	**Initials**
Verify patient identification with name and date of birth using active communication • Documentation Hospital generated labels, ID band	
Confirm the procedure, side, and site • With the patient • With the consent (dated within 90 days) • With the H&P	
H&P completed within 30 days I have re-examined the patient and there are no changes noted ☐ Changes Noted; see progress note ☐	
Updated Medication Reconciliation present	
Relevant laboratory and radiologic imaging stucflti available and reviewed Yes ☐ N/A ☐	
Required implants, devices and/or special equipment is available Yes ☐ N/A ☐	
Required Blood Products Ordered Yes ☐ N/A ☐	
Antibiotic Prophylaxis Ordered Yes, Pre-induction ☐ Yes, Post-Op per MD orders ☐ Not Required ☐	
DVT Pharmacologic Prophylaxis Ordered Yes, Pre-induction ☐ Yes, Post-Op per MD orders ☐ Not Required ☐	
Surgical Site Marked Yes ☐ Additional Marking Required Pre-induction ☐	
CONFIRMATION: The Attending Surgeon is on site and available for the planned procedure time.	

Surgeon or Designee's Printed Name: ______________________ Pager #: _________

Surgeon or Designee's Signature: ______________________ Date: _______ Time: _______

Fig. 3.5 Surgical safety checklist

Circulating Nurse	**Initials**
Verify patient identification with name and date of birth using active communication • Documentation Hospital generated labels, ID band	

Confirm the procedure, side, and site
   •   With the patient
   •   With the consent (dated within 90 days)
   • With the H&P	

H&P completed within 30 days	

Required blood products, implants, devices and/or special equipment are available
             Yes ☐
             N/A ☐	

Pre-Op Nursing assessment reviewed	

Surgical Site marked by Performing Physician
             Yes ☐
             N/A ☐	

Circulating Nurse's Printed Name: _______________________________________

Circulating Nurse's Signature: _________________________ Date: _________ Time: _________

Anesthesia Provider	**Initials**
Verify patient identification with name and date of birth using active communication • Documentation Hospital generated labels, ID band	

Confirm the procedure, side, and site
   •   With the patient
   •   With the consent (dated within 90 days)
   • With the H&P	

Pre-anesthetic assessment completed including review of relevant laboratory tests	

DVT Prophylaxis Plan Confirmed
            Yes ☐
            N/A ☐	

Blood sample to Blood Bank
            Yes ☐
             To be drawn in OR ☐
            N/A ☐	

Blood products available if applicable
            Yes ☐
            N/A ☐	

Antibiotic Administration Plan Confirmed
            Yes ☐
            N/A ☐	

Anesthesiologist's Printed Name: ____

Anesthesiologist's Signature: _________________________________ Date: _________ Time: _________

Attending Surgeon Presence:

I confirm that I will remain on the Hospital Campus and am available for the planned procedure.

STOP   Attending Surgeon: _________________ Signature: _________________ Date: _________ Time: _______

DO NOT PROCEED TO THE OPERATING ROOM UNTIL ALL SECTIONS ARE COMPLETE

Attestation: I have reviewed the Surgical Safety Checklist and I confirm that all sections are complete.

Signed: ____ Date: _________ Time: _______

Fig. 3.5 (continued)

PRE-INDUCTION BRIEFING
BEFORE INDUCTION OF ANESTHESIA IN THE OPERATING ROOM

Pre-Induction Briefing Checklist	Sign-off
Patient is Identified with Name and Date of Birth	**BRIEFING WAS PERFORMED** ☐
Procedure Site and Side Confirmed	
Procedure is Verified with the Consent, Specific Details are Discussed and Concerns Addressed	Circulating RN:
Allergies Noted if Applicable	
Airway Concerns	______________________
EBL and Required Blood Products	
Required Equioment and/or Implants	
Patient Positioning	Date: ______________
Medications: glycemic control, beta blockers, special considerations	
Antibiotic Status	Time: ______________
DVT Prophylaxis	
Other Procedure or Patient Specific Concerns	

TIME OUT
BEFORE INCISION
The Clinician performing the procedure is responsible for initiating the Time-Out

Time Out Checklist	Sign-off
STOP and call the **TIME OUT**, Eliminate noise/distractions	**TIME OUT WAS PERFORMED** ☐
Patient Identified with name and date of birth	
Procedure, Site and Side are verified with the Consent	Circulating RN:
All present in the OR are introduced by Name and Role	
Surgical Site marking is visible after prepping and draping	______________________
Patient positioning is confirmed	
IF NO DISCREPANCIES are noted, PROCEED with planned procedure	Date: ______________
THE TIME OUT SHOULD BE REPEATED WHENEVER 1. The patient's position changes 2. A new clinician takes over the case 3. Another surgical procedure is performed	Time: ______________

POST-OP DEBRIEFING
PRIOR TO THE ATTENDING SURGEON LEAVING THE OPERATING ROOM

Verification of Procedure Performed	**DEBRIEFING WAS PERFORMED** ☐
Sharp, Sponge and Instrument Counts complete and reconciled	
Specimens Reconciled	Circulating RN:
All procedure specific documentation Reconciled (Wound Classification, ASA, etc.)	
Unexpected Issues Discussed	______________________
Recovery and Post-op management addressed	
Identification of Equipment and/or Case Specific Issues	Date: ______________
Patient Transferred to:	
Report Given to:	Time: ______________

Fig. 3.5 (continued)

If the checklist is treated as just another obstacle to getting a case started, it will be filled out carelessly. The optimal use of checklists, such as our Ticket to Safety, requires complete buy-in by all team members. To achieve sustainable buy-in surgeons, as team leaders, must set an example. Errors in completing the checklist, either failure to complete properly or entry of erroneous data, must be taken seriously and characterized as unintentional, risky, reckless, or (rarely) malicious, and addressed accordingly. Audits of checklist completion should be routine and results reported regularly to all staff. Performance evaluations should include checklist compliance and accuracy. Those with perfect records should be rewarded and those with repeated deficiencies disciplined. An adverse event should not be the only trigger for action.

Checklist fatigue is a real phenomenon characterized by an increasingly lackadaisical attitude toward checklist completion. Those with checklist fatigue treat this critically important process as just another barrier preventing them from getting their cases done. In order to prevent checklist fatigue and insure active engagement by all team members, pre-induction briefings are critically important. Led by the surgeon, these briefings start with the introduction of all team members and are then scripted to include confirmation of patient identity, procedure, site, and side, site marking, patient positioning, anticipated airway and other anesthesia related concerns, allergies, availability and visibility of necessary imaging studies, presence of essential implants or other equipment, anticipated need for blood products and their availability, anticipated high risk portions of the procedure, and the fire risk assessment score. The script for the pre-induction briefing at our institution is shown in the figure below (Fig. 3.6). A poster size copy of this image is posted in each OR at our institution. It is essential that after the scripted portion of the briefing all team members are encouraged to voice any concerns and to ask for clarification of any ambiguities. At briefing completion, all team members should be asked to confirm their understanding and agreement.

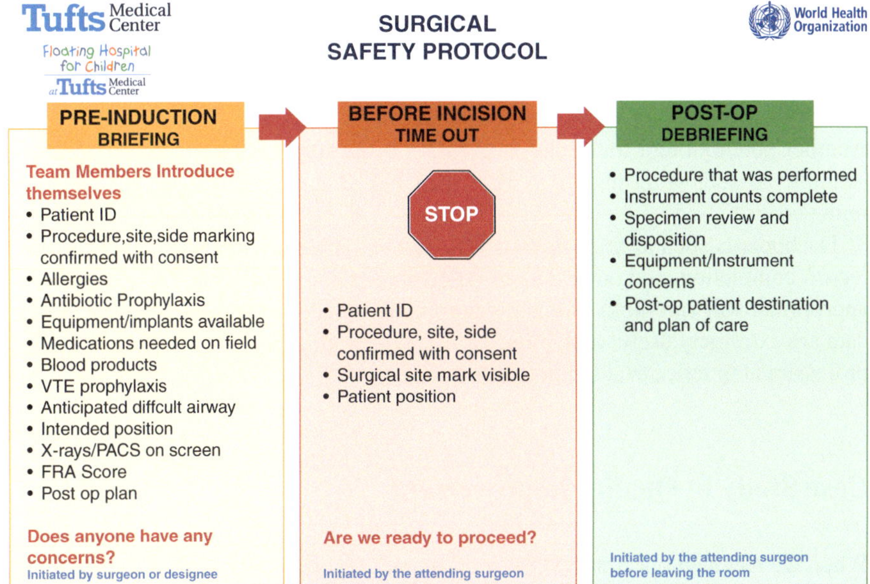

Fig. 3.6 Script for briefing, time-out, and debriefing

After a properly done pre-induction briefing, the pre-incision "time-out" becomes a very brief pause as a final check on patient identity, procedure, site, and side (Fig. 3.6). After the surgeon conducts the "time-out," the anesthesia and OR nursing teams should voice their agreement or any concerns prior to initiation of the case. The surgeon should be handed the scalpel only after all have expressed agreement.

The postoperative debriefing is also an essential element in OR communication. The script for the debriefing is also shown in Fig. 3.6. Prior to leaving the room, the attending surgeon should initiate the debriefing to confirm procedure, accuracy of counts, specimens and their appropriate handling (including appropriate completion of pathology requisition), and postoperative plan for the patient including a detailed discussion of potential areas of concern with detailed instructions as to what to be on the look-out for. In addition, any problems with the case related to equipment or unanticipated events should be discussed. The debriefing is also an opportunity for the surgeon to thank his/her team, to compliment those whose performance was excellent, and to discuss areas in which improvement is expected during the next similar case.

From the scripts shown in Fig. 3.6, it might seem that the briefing and debriefing will take so much time and effort as to be disruptive of efficiency. With appropriate case planning and preoperative evaluation and in the absence of any major discrepancies discovered during the briefing, it should take less than 2 minutes. Of course, if issues are uncovered during the briefing, it may delay the case, but such delays are warranted and in the long run will improve both efficiency and safety. Likewise, in the vast majority of cases, a thorough debriefing will take less than 2 minutes. This is time very well spent!

Performance Dashboard

Another potential tool for quality and safety is the surgeon-specific dashboard. An example of such a dashboard is shown in Fig. 3.7, with the surgeon identifiers removed.

Dashboards such as this allow quality, safety, patient experience, length of stay, record completion, and other data to be displayed in one location. Development of appropriate software links can allow automatic updates at regular intervals. These data are extremely useful at the time of re-credentialing or if the need for a focused professional practice evaluation (FPPE) arises.

Case Study in Quality Improvement

When we received our first NSQIP semi-annual report (SAR), we were shocked to see that our rate of perioperative pneumonia placed us in the 9th decile among participating hospitals. Truthfully, perioperative pneumonias had not even been a con-

MDName		Outpatients	Inpatients	Avg LOS	Avg Exp LOS	LOS Index	Div LOS Index	Mortalities	Mort Rate	Exp Mort	MD Mort Index	Div Mort Index
		1579	156	6.25	6.47	0.97	1.07	1	0.64 %	1.41 %	0.46	0.66

Notes Completion				Readmissions								
MDName	On Time Percent	On Time Notes	Total Notes	MDName	Live D/C's	Related#	MD Relaled	Div Related	All Cause #	MD All Cause	Div AU Cause
	98 %	206	210		155	4	2.6 %	4.4 %	21	13.5 %	12.0 %

Top 5 MSDRG Codes (Inpatient)		
ISDRG	Cases	LOS Index
30-Major small & large bowel procedures w CC	57	0.97
31-Major small & large bowel procedures w/o CC/MCC	31	0.85
29-Major small & large bowel procedures w MCC	14	1.00
49-Anal & stomal procedures w/o CC/MCC	5	1.19
48-Anal & stomal procedures w CC	4	1.46
53-Infectious & parasitic diseases w O.R procedure w MCC	4	1.25

Top 5 CPT Codes (Outpatient, since June 2016)	
CPT	Cases
46606-ANOSCOPY W/BX SINGLEIMUL TIPLE	25
46505-CHEMODENERVATION INTERNAL ANAL SPHINCTER	18
46260-HEMORRHOIDECTOMY INT & XTRNL 2/> COLUMN/GRO	14
46922-DSTRJ LESION ANUS SIMPLE SURG EXCISION	12
46270-SURG TX ANAL FISTULA SUBQ	11

Patient Experience: Outpatient (CGCAHPS) & Inpatient (HCAHPS)			
HORT NAME	Patients	MD Rate	Specialty Rate
CG-MD Easy Instructions	54	79.6 %	83.3 %
CG-MD Explained	60	78.3 %	81.6 %
CG-MD Know PMx	59	67.8 %	73.5 %
CG-MD Listened	60	80.0 %	83.5 %
CG-MD Respectful	58	79.3 %	85.1 %
CG-MD Spent Time	59	78.0 %	83.5 %
CG-Overall Rating	60	78.3 %	81.7 %
MD Explains	24	75.0 %	76.5 %
MD Listens	24	87.5 %	82.4 %
MD Respectful	24	83.3 %	85.3 %
Overall Hospital Rating	24	58.3 %	61.8 %
Recommend Hospital	24	66.7 %	67.6 %

AHRQ Patient Safety Indicator	Numerator	At Risk	MD Rate per 1000	Div Rate per 1000
03-Pressure Ulcer	0	79	0.0	0.0
04-Death among Surgical Inpatients w/Treatable …	1	4	250.0	222.2
06-Iatrogenic Pneumothorax	0	158	0.0	0.0
07-CVC Bloodstream Infections	0	83	0.0	0.0
08-Postoperative Hip Fracture	0	139	0.0	0.0
09-Periop Hemorrhage or Hematoma	1	142	7.0	14.2
10-Postop Physio Metabol Derangement	0	109	0.0	0.0
11-Postop Respiratory Failure	0	107	0.0	6.8
12-Periop PE or DVT	0	155	0.0	0.0
13-Postop Sepsis	0	34	0.0	0.0
14-Postop Wound Dehiscence	0	121	0.0	0.0
15-Accidental Puncture/Laceration	1	160	6.3	7.8

Fig. 3.7 Surgeon performance dashboard

cern. Initially we questioned the validity of the findings and then pulled each pneumonia patient's record for thorough review. While trying to explain why our rate was so high relative to most other hospitals (O/E = 1.34), we got our next SAR, which was no better. Working with pulmonology, anesthesiology, OR nursing, our center for preoperative assessment nurses, and pulmonary physiotherapists, we got to work to develop what became the Tufts Perioperative Pneumonia Prevention Program or T4P.

All surgical patients evaluated in our Center for Preoperative assessment underwent a pneumonia risk assessment using an evidence-based pulmonary risk assessment tool shown below (Fig. 3.8).

This risk stratification program linked directly to preoperative, intraoperative, and postoperative order sets and management guidelines shown below (Fig. 3.9).

The Breathe Protocol referenced in the above figure consisted of:

B Brush teeth in AM and PM and use antiseptic mouthwash.
R Really deep breaths repeatedly.
E Exercise lungs by using incentive spirometer 10 times per hour.
A Active coughing clears lungs.
T Take a walk at least three times per day.
H Head of bed elevated to at least 30° at all times.
E Education regarding the importance of above measures.

T4P
Pulmonary Risk Stratification

Risk Factor	Points
Age	
>65	1
>80	2
ASA>3	2
ADLs	
Independent	0
Partial dependency	1
Dependent	2
Type of Surgery (upper abd, chest, Neuro, airway)	2
COPD, Pulm Hypertension, OSA Severe Asthma	2
Smoking	1
Impaired Sensorium, Neuro-muscular Disease, Swallowing Difficulty	1
Unintentional weight loss >10%	1
BM1<22	1
General Anethesia	2
Surgery > 2 hours	1

Risk Stratification
Green <7 Points
Yellow 7-12 Points
Red >12 Points

Tufts Medical Center

Fig. 3.8 Pneumonia risk stratification scoring system

T4P

Interventions

	Green	Yellow	Red
CPA/Pre-op	Stop smoking Learn **BREATHE PROTOCOL**	Stop smoking Learn **BREATHE PROTOCOL** Incentive spirometer Oral hygiene	Stop smoking Learn **BREATHE PROTOCOL** Incentive spirometer Oral hygiene PFTs/ ? Pulm Consult
Intra-op		Goal directed fluid therapy Lung protective ventilation Selective use NG/OG tubes Special ET Tubes if prolonged intubation anticipated	Goal directed fluid therapy Lung protective ventilation Selective use NG/OG tubes Special ET tubes
Post-op Not Intubated		Mandatory Incentive Spirometry Early removal NG/OG Consult pain management **BREATHE Protocol**	Daily respiratory therapy visits (IS and Acapella) Early removal NG/OG Consult pain management **BREATHE Protocol**
Post-op Intubated	VAP bundle Early mobilization Avoid Circuit Disconnection Earl removal NG/OG	VAP bundle Early mobilization Avoid circuit disconnection Earl removal NG/OG Special ET Tubes	VAP bundle Early mobilization Avoid circuit disconnection Earl removal NG/OG Special ET Tubes

Tufts Medical Center

Fig. 3.9 Pneumonia prevention measures based on risk score

Nurses, respiratory therapists, and patients teamed up to make sure that all components of the protocol were followed carefully.

Initial success with the T4P protocol was remarkable with the O/E ratio for all cases at our institution falling to 0.99 (5th decile) within 12 months of its implementation. However, over the ensuing year, we noted that the O/E crept back up to 1.2 (8th decile) and remained high. In accordance with Plan, Do, Check, Act methodology, we reviewed all 21 pneumonia cases from the most recent report year and found that 17 of them occurred in urgent or emergent cases that did not go through the standard preoperative assessment process. Based on this information, we taught our surgery residents to perform the assessment and initiate the appropriate order set for all patients, even though these urgent and emergent cases would not benefit from the preoperative pulmonary measures offered to those undergoing elective surgery. Review of our most recent data revealed significant improvement with our O/E ratio for pneumonia again approaching 1.

From this experience we learned three lessons. First, without accurate data with benchmarking, we would not have even known that we had a problem with postoperative pneumonias. Second, a multidisciplinary team can develop an effective program to drive improvement and lower complication rates. Third, continued vigilance is essential so that quality improvement programs can be modified in order to sustain progress. We are now using these lessons to develop a similar program to improve our outcomes with respect to postoperative VTE rates and have seen dramatic progress.

Summary and Conclusions

An effective surgery quality and safety improvement program requires accurate data with benchmarks, a supportive departmental organization, a just and open culture that preserves individual accountability, and tools (checklists, dashboards, as well as appropriate credentialing and privileging functions). While the traditional morbidity and mortality conference is still quite important as an educational tool for residents and faculty, it is much less effective as a tool for quality assessment and improvement. Individual cases reported at M + M conference or at root cause analyses are anecdotes, which, though instructive, only occasionally provide a basis for sustainable systematic improvement. Reliable data with robust risk adjustment allow benchmarking and tracking of progress over time. Department organization must reflect the critical importance of quality and safety improvement by including a Surgical Quality and Safety Officer, who chairs a robust Quality and Safety Committee, charged with data analysis as well as the planning, implementation, monitoring, and, when necessary, modification of safety and quality improvement programs. Safety and quality programs will not thrive in an environment that is threatening and unforgiving. While individual accountability remains critically important in surgery, unintentional errors should be treated as opportunities for learning and improvement and not for blaming and shaming. A just culture with well-defined, transparent, and fair policies and procedures for dealing with error and behaviors leading to errors is essential. A variety of evidence-based effective tools are available to promote safety and quality in surgery. Stringent credentialing and privileging processes to insure that surgical staff are appropriately trained and sufficiently experienced are essential. Checklists, briefings, time-outs, and debriefings are critical in the operating room. Longitudinal assessment of performance is facilitated by the use of division-specific and surgeon-specific dashboards. With robust data, appropriate departmental organization, a just culture, and well-designed tools, measureable and sustainable continuous improvement is achievable.

References

1. Institute of Medicine. To Err is human: building a safer health system. Washington, DC: The National Academies Press; 2000. https://doi.org/10.17226/9728.
2. Dindo D, Demartines N, Clavien P-A. Classification of surgical complications: a new proposal with evaluation in a cohort of 6336 patients and results of a survey. Ann Surg. 2004;240(2):205–13.
3. Chung KC, Kotsis SV. Complications in surgery: root cause analysis and preventive measures. Plast Reconstr Surg. 2012;129(6):1421–7.
4. AHRQ Website. U.S. Department of Health and Human Services. 2018. https://www.ahrq.gov.
5. NSQIP Website. https://www.facs.org/quality-programs/acs-nsqip.
6. Steinberg S, Popa M, et al. Comparison of risk adjustment methodologies in surgical quality improvement. Surgery. 2008;144(4):662–7.

7. Ashley SW, Ellison C, Moffatt-Bruce SD. Surgical quality officer. In: Hoyt DB, Ko CY, editors. Optimal resources for surgical quality and safety. Chicago: American College of Surgeons; 2017. p. 37–50.
8. Bass BL, Stain SC. Surgical credentialing and privileging: ensuring that surgeons are capable of providing optimal care. In: Hoyt DB, Ko CY, editors. Optimal resources for surgical quality and safety. Chicago: American College of Surgeons; 2017. p. 69–84.
9. Boysen PG. Just culture: a foundation for balanced accountability and patient safety. Ochsner J. 2013;13:400–6.
10. Leonard MW, Frankel A. A path to safe and reliable healthcare. Pateint Educ Couns. 2010;80:288–92.
11. Edmundson AC, Lei Z. Psychological safety: the history, renaissance, and future of an interpersonal constriuct. Annu Rev Organ Psych Organ Behav. 2014:23–43.
12. Gawande A. The checklist manifesto: how to get things right. New York: Henry Holt and Company; 2009.
13. National Health Service improvement newsletter. 2018 Feb. https://improvement.nhs.uk/documents/2479/Never_Events_1_April_2017_-_31_January_2018_FINAL_v2.pdf.

Chapter 4
Infection Prevention Quality Metrics

Susanne Meninger, Hasan Fadlallah, Karen Dowler, and Shira Doron

It is estimated that healthcare-associated infections occur in 1 out of every 31 hospital patients [1]. Healthcare-associated infections may cause patients to suffer emotionally, physically, and financially. Often, patients with healthcare-associated infections feel "dirty" or shunned, are afraid to infect family members, and are restricted from group supports and access to common areas of the very healthcare institutions in which their healthcare-associated infections were acquired [2]. It is, therefore, imperative that we use our resources wisely to ensure that we are reducing the number of humans affected by these infections. Infection prevention quality metrics are designed to achieve this goal.

S. Meninger
Department of Infection Prevention, Tufts Medical Center, Boston, MA, USA

H. Fadlallah (✉)
Division of Geographic Medicine and Infectious Diseases, Tufts Medical Center, Boston, MA, USA
e-mail: hfadlallah@tuftsmedicalcenter.org

K. Dowler
Department of Infection Prevention, Tufts Medical Center, Boston, MA, USA

Department of Quality and Patient Safety, Tufts Medical Center, Boston, MA, USA

S. Doron
Division of Geographic Medicine and Infectious Diseases, Tufts Medical Center, Boston, MA, USA

Tufts Medical Center, Boston, MA, USA

© Springer Nature Switzerland AG 2020
D. N. Salem (ed.), *Quality Measures*, https://doi.org/10.1007/978-3-030-37145-6_4

History of Infection Prevention Quality Metrics

In 1847, Ignaz Semmelweis presented evidence that "childbed fever" was spread from person to person on the unclean hands of healthcare workers [3, 4]. His findings led the way to the appreciation of hand hygiene as vital to infection prevention. Surgeons gradually adopted aseptic techniques that helped reduce patient susceptibility to postoperative infections. During the 1950s, epidemic penicillin-resistant *Staphylococcus aureus* infections led to public awareness of healthcare-associated infections [5].

By the mid-twentieth century, infection prevention initiatives were being carried out sporadically in hospitals [6, 7], mainly led by physicians in large academic medical centers. Their focus was on prevention of infections in individual patients. Unlike the present day, healthcare-associated infections were not viewed as a public health issue, and public health resources were not allocated to these prevention efforts.

By the 1960s, viewpoints began to change, as hospitals began to be seen as communities requiring interventions utilizing public health principles, strategies, and resources to control healthcare-associated infections. A model for prevention was built that consisted of: (1) systematic surveillance to identify healthcare-associated infections; (2) ongoing analysis of surveillance data to recognize potential problems; (3) application of epidemic investigation techniques to healthcare-associated infections; and (4) implementation of hospital-wide interventions to protect patients, staff, and visitors deemed to be at particular risk [4]. Although closer to the modern-day approach, there was a striking lack of collaboration between hospitals and public health authorities, with the public health departments being seen strictly as regulators rather than colleagues with a common cause, a dynamic that has shifted and improved over time.

The Centers for Disease Control and Prevention (CDC) began to conduct public health research and development activities related to healthcare-associated infections in hospitals in the mid-1960s. One such activity was the launch of the National Nosocomial Infection Surveillance program in 1970. A national network of hospitals voluntarily conducted healthcare-associated infections surveillance using CDC methodology and reported infection rates to the CDC each month [4]. The National Healthcare Safety Network (NHSN) replaced this program in 2005 and continues to provide information to the public about the changing patterns of healthcare-associated infections [4].

By the early 1970s, despite the increase in public and professional concern over healthcare-associated infections, there was no clear mandate that hospitals should have infection prevention programs and no clear uniform criteria for an appropriate structure. Some hospitals had no program at all. Research was needed to provide evidence that infection prevention programs were effective in preventing healthcare-associated infections. The Study on the Effectiveness of Nosocomial Infection Control (SENIC), conducted in the early 1970s, was a rigorous investigation that compared outcomes in hospitals with and without infection prevention programs utilizing CDC standards [8]. The 338 participating hospitals were randomly selected and stratified by criteria such as geography, inpatient bed capacity, and teaching status. The study successfully demonstrated that hospitals with infection prevention programs (almost half of the study hospitals) had significantly lower rates of healthcare-associated infections than hospitals without programs [9]. In light of the study results, in 1976, The Joint Commission made it an accreditation requirement that hospitals have infection prevention programs that follow a set of CDC standards [10]. With this increased regulatory burden came the birth of two new career paths. The Infection Preventionist carries out the day-to-day tasks related to healthcare-associated infection prevention and is supervised by the Hospital Epidemiologist. A typical day for an Infection Preventionist includes time spent entering data reports; rounding on patient care units to assess for proper practice related to devices and appropriate precautions related to specific pathogens; inspection of environments; writing and revising evidence-based policies, protocols and guidelines; conducting training sessions with staff; performing root cause analyses; gathering and presenting data to committees and task forces; creating action plans; assessing and monitoring construction plans and activities; and professional development [21].

Around the turn of the twenty-first century, two crucial pieces of journalism, the Institute of Medicine (IOM) report "To Err is Human" in 1999 and a *Chicago Tribune* article series on hospital infections in 2002 [11], served to shape infection prevention and healthcare epidemiology into their modern-day form. The IOM report stated that medical errors in hospitals, with healthcare-associated infections being at the top of the list in terms of frequency, were leading to thousands of preventable deaths and injuries among hospitalized US patients each year [12]. Soon after, a series of investigative articles in the *Chicago Tribune* criticized hospitals for failing to prevent these infections and started an active debate about a more transparent healthcare-associated infections prevention strategy [11]. As policy makers and consumers realized that a big portion of infections can be prevented by evidence-based infection prevention programs, laws were made at the state level to enact public reporting of healthcare-associated infections.

In recognition of this growing interest in public reporting, experts at the CDC began working with the Healthcare Infection Control Practices Advisory Committee to develop recommendations to help guide future legislation [13]. Later, federal lawmakers also became involved in the issue of healthcare-associated infections. In 2008, as part of the larger deficit reduction act, Congress mandated that the Centers for Medicare and Medicaid Services (CMS) stop giving hospitals increased payments to cover the additional cost of care for patients who develop healthcare-associated infections [4]. In order to implement this strategy, CMS worked closely with CDC to identify healthcare-associated infections that were "reasonably preventable" [4]. In 2010, Congress incorporated healthcare-associated infections prevention into the value-based purchasing program of the Affordable Care Act [4]. CMS also began to require reporting of healthcare-associated infections to the National Healthcare Safety Network, beginning with central line–associated bloodstream infections (CLABSIs) in 2011, with data being publically available [4]. These requirements have led to a dramatic expansion in National Healthcare Safety Network enrollment, from roughly 300 hospitals in 2006 to approximately 3500 in 2010 [4].

Current State: The National Action Plan

The Department of Health and Human Services has several operating divisions united in the National Action Plan to reduce healthcare associated infections (HAIs), [14] including the CDC, the Agency for Healthcare Research and Quality (AHRQ), the National Institutes of Health (NIH), and CMS. At its core, the National Action Plan seeks to improve patient safety and reduce healthcare costs by reducing rates of HAIs [15]. It sets goals for the reduction of central line–associated bloodstream infections (CLABSI), catheter-associated urinary tract infections (CAUTI), specific surgical site infections (SSIs), methicillin-resistant *Staphylococcus aureus* (MRSA) bacteremia, and infections caused by *Clostridioides difficile* (*C. difficile*) [15]. The infection reduction goals were first set in 2009 and were revised in 2015 [15]. Progress was made on the 2013 targets in reducing CLABSI by 50% and SSI by 30% but not in reducing CAUTI, *C. difficile*, or MRSA bacteremia [17]. Some felt the goals were too difficult to achieve given the complexity of patients cared for [16], while some patient advocacy groups felt the reduction goals were not aggressive enough [16]. As a result, data reports, infection definitions, and goals are annually evaluated in an effort to optimize reliability, comparability, and utility [16].

Healthcare-associated infections are incorporated into the annual National Patient safety goals of the Joint Commission, the accrediting organization for all hospitals in the US. CMS uses healthcare-associated infections in their value-based purchasing program [18] as do many commercial payers. CMS requires public reporting of healthcare-associated infections at the federal level. All 50 states (as well as the District of Columbia and Puerto Rico) have their own healthcare-associated infections reduction action plans, which vary in goals and targets; however, most include six basic elements: CLABSI, CAUTI, SSI, MRSA bacteremia, *C. difficile* infection, and healthcare worker influenza vaccination [15]. These plans also qualify states to receive Preventive Health and Health Services Block Grants [15].

Reporting of Healthcare-Associated Infections

In 2005 the CDC released a report recommending that states require healthcare institutions to publicly release healthcare-associated infections rates [13]. The report also advised that one or more of the following should be reported: (1) central line insertion practices; (2) compliance with surgical antimicrobial prophylaxis standards; (3) influenza vaccination rates among patients and healthcare personnel; (4) CLABSI rates; and (5) SSI rates following select operations [13]. As of 2016, there were more than 6000 US hospitals reporting through NHSN [20].

Although the intention of the NHSN guidelines is to provide standardization and consistency in reporting, there is nevertheless widespread variation in surveillance and reporting methodology. New York public health officials reviewed SSI data from coronary artery bypass cases and found that the categorization of the infections as superficial versus deep was only 86% accurate [23]. When they conducted a similar validation of CLABSI data, correcting errors increased the state's CLABSI rate by 5.6% [24]. An analysis performed by Bagchi reviewed CLABSI validation data from 23 states and found an overall reporting error rate of 4.4% [25]. Reporting errors usually involve under-reporting as was seen in a Connecticut state validation of colon surgery infections where 34% of the 102 infections found in the validation had not been reported [26]. This potential variability in surveillance and reporting [22–26] reduces the validity of a metric for use in a program such as value-based purchasing.

Diagnostic Stewardship

Diagnostic stewardship is defined as coordinated systems or user-based interventions designed to promote evidence-based utilization of diagnostic tests, with the primary goals of improving value and care quality and safely reducing cost [28]. Diagnostic tests are ordered routinely in healthcare settings, but the process of ordering and interpreting tests is complex and can result in diagnostic errors. The thought process around ordering tests should take into account the clinical scenario and pretest probability of the condition for which the test is obtained. False positives can occur, especially when clinicians order tests for patients without symptoms or risk factors specific for the disease process. Microbiologic tests including cultures and *C. difficile* tests that are performed on patients without clinical evidence of infection are often positive, reflecting colonization by bacteria or fungi, a condition that does not require treatment. Despite the absence of true infection, prescription of antimicrobials to patients with positive tests is common. Antimicrobial therapy, whether necessary or unnecessary, results in disturbance of the microbiome, can lead to development of antimicrobial resistance and/or *C. difficile*, and incurs cost. When these false-positive microbiologic tests are in the context of evaluation for infection in a hospitalized patient, they may meet criteria for a reportable infection, regardless of whether or not the clinician caring for the patient decides to initiate therapy. Urine cultures obtained from patients without urinary symptoms are the most common example of inappropriate testing for infection, as these positive tests do not represent true infection requiring treatment [27, 29]. Proper use of diagnostics is therefore an essential element in both successful infection prevention and antimicrobial stewardship programs. When diagnostic stewardship is applied to the evaluation of infection, it can be a valuable tool in the effort to lower reportable healthcare-associated infection rates [27, 28].

Examples of diagnostic stewardship interventions used to decrease reportable HAIs include education on test ordering and result analysis, protocols for proper specimen collection, laboratory policies, and computerized decision support designed to limit tests. Diagnostic stewardship has been described by Morgan et al. [28, 30] to occur in three stages: pre-analytic (test-related decision making and specimen collection), analytic (relating to laboratory practices including protocolized or reflex test algorithms), and post-analytic (selective reporting, such as the reporting of susceptibility to only a limited number of antimicrobials to encourage the use of narrower spectrum agents). Diagnostic stewardship has been shown to effectively reduce a variety of unnecessary general inpatient medicine tests, from excessive or redundant daily inpatient labs to diagnostic imaging [28, 31, 32]. Diagnostic stewardship strategies are varied and include user-based approaches (e.g., auditing, price display, and provider feedback) and systems-based approaches (e.g., modifications to the computerized physician order entry system requiring selection of an indication for testing and inappropriate specimen rejection) [28].

There is discordance between surveillance-based definitions of infection and clinically relevant criteria for the diagnosis and treatment of infection. For example, current National Healthcare Safety Network surveillance definitions for hospital onset *C. difficile* infection require only a positive test for *C. difficile* from an unformed stool specimen on or after hospital day 4, irrespective of patient symptoms or possible alternative diagnoses, whereas clinical practice guidelines are much more restrictive as they acknowledge the large proportion of patients who have asymptomatic carriage of *C. difficile* [28, 33, 34]. Furthermore, the highly sensitive nature of new diagnostics, such as polymerase chain reaction–based testing for *C. difficile*, may be even more likely to identify colonized rather than clinically infected patients than traditional tests [28]. That can cause an artificial increase in healthcare-associated infection rates as laboratories update their technology. On the other hand, efforts to reduce unnecessary testing can lead to inadvertent harm to patients if infections are missed. Thus, a major objective for diagnostic stewardship for healthcare-associated infections is to identify the "sweet spot" of test utilization that minimizes over diagnosis and false positive results while maximizing appropriately indicated testing and true positive results [28]. This spot likely will be infection and population (e.g., disease prevalence) specific [28]. Another potential harm of diagnostic stewardship relates to clinician frustration with perceived restrictions to their autonomy in choosing diagnostic tests. This can be overcome by transparent education and open dialogue. Importantly, diagnostic stewardship should be flexible allowing for exceptions and offer solutions rather than obstacles in situations where it is appropriate. For example, a hospital laboratory may require a positive urinalysis before processing a urine culture, with the ability to order urine cultures without urinalysis in pregnant women or patients undergoing invasive urologic surgery, because treatment of asymptomatic bacteriuria is appropriate in these situations [28].

As with any quality improvement effort, in developing a diagnostic stewardship program, measurement of process measures is vital to ensure that stewardship interventions are having their intended effects. This would include an assessment of testing rates, including tests that are rejected from processing [28].

Healthcare-Associated Infection Metrics

Comparative databases for healthcare-associated infections use a variety of metrics to report infections. An incidence rate is calculated using a numerator representing the number of infections, and a denominator, which differs depending on the infection type. Denominators can be device days, patient days, or the number of surgeries of a specific type, often multiplied by 100 or 1000. While incidence rates are useful when compared between time periods in the same unit, they are less useful for comparisons between different units with different patient populations and virtually irrelevant for comparing different hospitals, where patient populations can differ widely. On the other hand, the standardized infection ratio (SIR) is a newer metric that is used to provide risk-adjusted comparisons between facilities. The SIR represents the observed number of infections divided by the expected number of infections as determined by the NHSN based on a set of adjustment variables [35]. Each healthcare-associated infection metric has a different set of variables that are used to calculate the expected number of infections. Device-related infections are risk adjusted at the hospital and unit level (see Table 4.1 for a summary of healthcare-associated infection metrics that are included in the CMS Hospital Compare publicly reported data). An SIR value of 1.0 represents the expected rate of infection [35]. Values higher than 1.0 are considered to be indicative of worse than expected performance, and values below 1.0 indicate better than expected performance with respect to reduction of infection. SIRs are reported along with a statistical significance indicator. When an SIR is not statistically significant, it is interpreted as not different than expected [35]. There are several important limitations to the use of SIRs. First, they are not available when a metric's number of expected infections is less than one [35], so this measurement becomes less relevant as healthcare environments reduce infection or when denominators are small. Second, the SIR is based on the number of expected infections as calculated from a baseline time period that is typically several years in the past. The 2018 SIRs are derived from infections reported in 2015 [35]. These will be used until 2020, at which point the baselines will be re-evaluated and most hospitals' SIRs will reset to close to 1.00. As we approach the 2020 goal date, the SIR becomes less meaningful and more difficult to interpret, being based on a 5-year-old comparison. For example, the goal for CLABSI is for all US hospitals to achieve an SIR of 0.5 by 2020. When a new baseline is set in 2021, a hospital that reached the DHHS 2020 goal will suddenly have an SIR of 1.0 or even higher.

The CDC provides tools to assist with prevention efforts. One such tool is known as the Targeted Assessment for Prevention strategy report [36]. This allows a hospital to rank its units from worst to best performing with the idea that concentrating deployment of resources to the worst performing units (targeting efforts) will be most effective in reducing healthcare-associated infections overall [36]. The report also compares units to like units nationwide. Data are presented in terms of the cumulative attributable difference (CAD), which is the number of infections that must be prevented to achieve the DHHS goal [36]. The cumulative attributable difference metric may be easier for providers and administrators to understand than rates or SIRs. While the report is a helpful tool, it can take only one or two infections in a short period of time for the best performer to become the worst. Even the best performers need to be monitored for practice drift. No indicator is ideal for every situation or patient population, but standard surveillance criteria and definitions that have evolved and are corroborated with other professional metrics are making comparison among institutions more reliable. This has allowed DHHS to set national infection reduction targets for performance improvement and to monitor progress.

Performance Improvement

A variety of strategies have been demonstrated in well-conducted studies to effectively decrease healthcare-associated infection rates. Some examples of evidence-based interventions are listed in Table 4.1. These include the use of central line insertion checklists to reduce CLABSI, the use of early catheter removal protocols to reduce CAUTI, adherence to pre-operative antibiotic timing standards for SSI, and enhanced disinfection of surfaces for *C. difficile* infection. Often the interventions being used by a facility to achieve a specific quality of care outcome are grouped together into a bundle. Bundles can be an effective way to roll out a set of interventions using streamlined resources (a single audit tool can be used to assess adherence, for example). Measurement of compliance with bundles (such as the ventilator-associated pneumonia process measures) is mandated by some states, yet studies have not been done that definitively show which elements of the bundle are actually responsible for preventing infection, or whether any of these elements can be dropped with the same outcome [37]. For example, some hospitals have adopted the use of ultraviolet (UV) light-emitting disinfecting robots for the prevention of *C. difficile* transmission with subsequent decreases in *C. difficile* infection rates. If those same hospitals then convert to hospital-wide sporicidal chemical disinfection and achieve a further decrease in *C. difficile* infection rates, can those hospitals discontinue UV disinfection without seeing a rise in infections, or are both interventions contributing to the improved outcomes? Given the impact of other factors on infection rates (e.g., time of year, staffing ratios, and patient acuity), randomized controlled clinical trials are the only way to assess whether bundles and/or their specific elements are effective. These studies are becoming increasingly challenging to carry out as regulators mandate bundle compliance, and as outcomes (i.e., infections) become less prevalent.

Performance improvement tools are frequently employed as a means to reduce healthcare-associated infections. Though interventions often involve checklists, reminders, education, and policy revisions, in the hierarchy of intervention effectiveness (Fig. 4.1), those methods are considered people dependent and therefore

Table 4.1 Summary of healthcare-associated infection metrics

	Central Line–Associated Bloodstream Infection (CLABSI)	Catheter-Associated Urinary Tract Infection (CAUTI)
Denominator	1000 line days Each nursing unit counts the number of patients with at least one central line each day (patients with more than one line are counted as one)	1000 catheter days Each nursing unit counts the number of patients with an indwelling urinary catheter each day
Case finding	Blood cultures. Central line has to be in place two calendar days	Urine cultures. Indwelling urinary catheter has to be in place two calendar days
Risk adjustment	Negative binomial regression model based on variables including: medical school affiliation, unit type, hospital type, hospital size, birth-weight category (for neonates)	Negative binomial regression model based on variables such as: medical school affiliation, unit type, hospital type, hospital size, average length of stay
Defining infection	Certain organisms and certain line types are excluded. A patient who injects into their own line is excluded. Infection can be attributed to infection at another site and thus excluded if it meets criteria for that infection as set forth in the NHSN manual. Oncology patients with graft vs host disease or neutropenia can be classified as "mucosal barrier injury"–type infection and thus excluded	Certain organisms are excluded (yeast). Urine cultures with more than 2 organisms are excluded. Symptoms are required and fever alone meets the definition. Cannot attribute to an infection at another site
Recent changes	Each year the organism list expands. Line types evolve. New patient care setting exclusions are added, such as patients on extracorporeal membrane oxygenation therapy	Yeast excluded as pathogen. Fever as a symptom can be age dependent
DHHS 2020 goal (set in 2015)	50% reduction	25% reduction
2016 progress (1 year)	11% reduction	7% reduction
Evidence-based interventions	Central line insertion checklists with close attention to sterile technique Antimicrobial coated central lines Antimicrobial impregnated central line dressings Daily assessment of line necessity and prompt removal Diagnostic stewardship (limit blood draws through lines as they may be colonized)	Close attention to sterile technique during the placement of catheters Maintenance of the urine collection bag below the level of the bladder Use of alternative urine collection devices Diagnostic stewardship (avoidance of the "pan culture" approach to fever work-up)

(continued)

Table 4.1 (continued)

	Surgical site infections (SSI)	Laboratory test identified *C. difficile* infection	Laboratory test identified MRSA bloodstream infection
Denominator	100 cases performed	1000 or 10,000 patient days. Infant units are excluded	1000 patient days
Case finding	Microbiology cultures. Readmissions, operating room schedule review, MD notes with wound descriptions. Calls to patients post discharge	Microbiology lab testing	Blood cultures
Risk adjustment	Variables depend on case type and include length of surgery, presence of diabetes, American Society of Anesthesiologists score, wound class, age, gender, emergency, trauma, body mass index	Community prevalence, *C. difficile* test method, medical school affiliation, number of ICU beds, hospital type, ED case	Community prevalence, average length of stay, medical school affiliation, number of ICU beds, hospital type
Defining infection	Complex definitions at 3 levels: superficial incisional, deep incisional, and organ space	A positive *C. difficile* test after hospital day 3. Do not report if a repeat test is positive within 14 days from the same location	MRSA in the blood after hospital day 3, do not report if a repeat test is positive within 14 days from the same location
Recent changes	NHSN collaborates with surgical specialties to improve clinical congruence	No clinical interpretation is allowed. SIRs are provided for whole hospital only, not by unit	No clinical interpretation is allowed. SIRs are provided for whole hospital only, not by unit
DHHS 2020 goal (set in 2015)	30% reduction	30% reduction	50% reduction
2016 progress (1 year)	6% reduction in select procedures	8% reduction	7% reduction
Evidence-based interventions	Close attention to sterile technique Limiting foot traffic in operating rooms Focus on environmental disinfection Protocolized pre-operative antibiotics	Minimize the use of antibiotics that have a high propensity to cause *C. difficile* infection Close attention to environmental disinfection using a sporicidal agent Use of contact precautions Diagnostic stewardship (send tests only when clinical suspicion for *C. difficile* infection exists without other causes for loose stool)	Use of contact precautions Emphasis on hand hygiene Reduce CLABSI

Adapted from Mu, et al., Hospital Compare and National Healthcare Safety Network [20, 33, 35, 40–42]

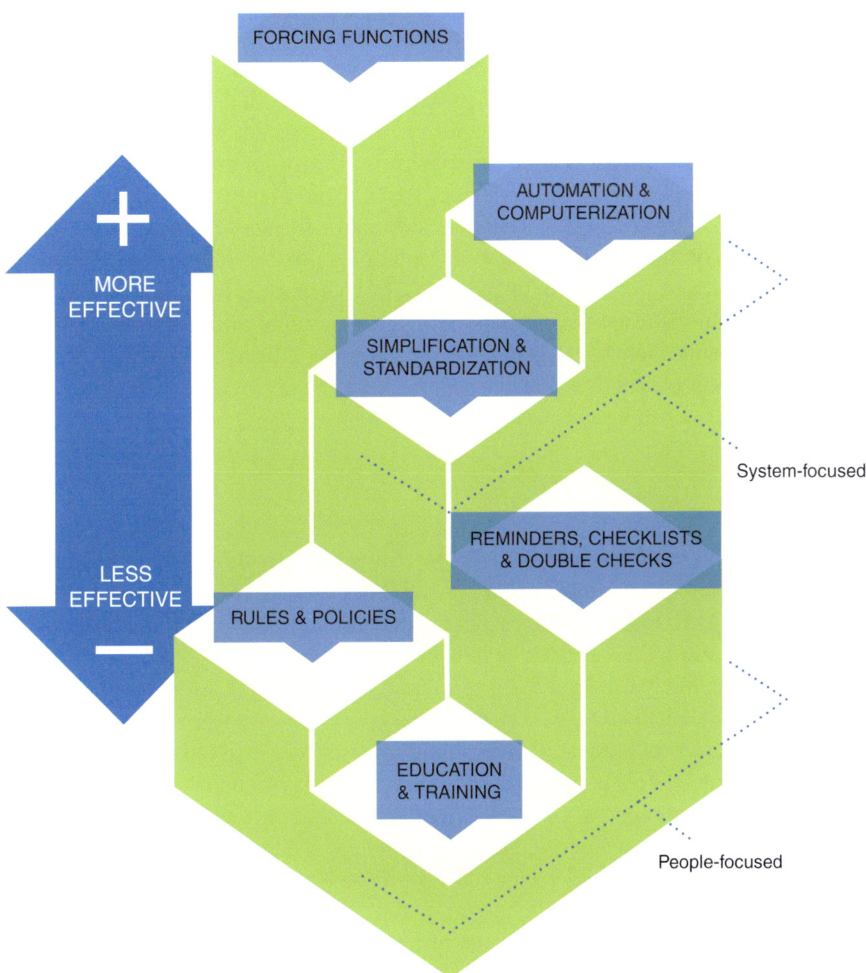

Fig. 4.1 The hierarchy of intervention effectiveness [38]

less effective [38]. Sustainable change requires systems-focused interventions with automated or forced functions when possible [38]. Examples of such interventions that have been shown to reduce healthcare-associated infections include: computer-assisted forced functionality for ordering, safety needles, standardized pre-operative antibiotics, laboratory rejection of inappropriate specimens, and the use of ultraviolet light–emitting disinfecting robots.

In an AHRQ publication soliciting thought leaders' predictions for patient safety in 2025, Lucian Leape, internationally recognized as a leader of the patient safety movement, predicted that through accountability and professional training that incorporates safety science training, HAIs will be nearly eliminated to the point that when one does occur, members of the healthcare system will wonder how this could happen and promptly commit to "this will never happen again" [39]. Kirk Hamilton, an architect specializing in design of healthcare facilities, describes an ideal, well-designed physical environment that is designed for ease of surface disinfection, optimal air handling, and enhanced compliance with hand hygiene [39]. David W. Bates, an expert in health information technology, describes the integration of smart devices that can aid in prevention through identifying patients at risk [39]. Susan Sheridan, former Director of Patient Engagement for the Patient-Centered Outcomes Research Institute (PCORI), describes an environment where patients are true partners in care and patient safety research will explore the depths of the emotional and economic toll that arise when events such as HAIs occur [39]. As these advances hopefully become reality, infection prevention metrics will be here to stay, evolving to better indicate our success or failure.

Controlling healthcare-associated infections to control healthcare costs? The Catheter-Associated Urinary Tract Infection (CAUTI) example
According to Calderon, there are an estimated 290,000 CAUTIs annually in the US, resulting in excess healthcare costs totaling $290 million [19]. Calculations like these have been used to justify the increasing dedication of resources to healthcare-associated infection prevention efforts. But are the costs associated with these efforts actually offset by the avoidance of infections? The most effective method to reduce CAUTI is thought to be reduction of indwelling urinary catheter use. However, eliminating the use of these catheters comes at a cost. Equipment such as bladder scanners and external urine collection devices is required for successful implementation [19]. Healthcare worker staffing may need to be increased to care for patients without indwelling catheters, as they are more likely to need intermittent catheterization, assistance ambulating to the bathroom, and/or frequent changes of wet bed linens [19]. To avoid a relatively small number of infections in a given hospital each month, a much larger number of patients must be treated with these expensive interventions. Even with extensive nationwide efforts to decrease CAUTIs, national healthcare-associated infection rates have declined only modestly, with some recent years actually experiencing increased infection rates in a number of US states [20]. Because of the extensive resources that have been poured into the CAUTI initiative thus far, with minimal benefit seen, CAUTI remains controversial as an appropriate indicator of overall quality of care.

References

1. HAI Data [Internet]. CDC.gov. 2018 [cited 1/22/19]. Available from: https://www.cdc.gov/hai/data/index.html.
2. Currie K, Melone L, Stewart S, King C, Holopainen A, Clark A, et al. Understanding the patient experience of health care–associated infection: a qualitative systematic review. Am J Infect Control. 2018;46(8):936–42.
3. Semmelweis I. Etiology, concept and prophylaxis of childbed fever. Madison: University of Wisconsin Press; 1983.
4. Dixon RE. Control of health-care-associated infections, 1961—2011. Morb Mortal Wkly Rep (MMWR). 2011;60:58–63.
5. Wise RI, Ossman EA, Littlefield DR. Personal reflections on nosocomial staphylococcal infections and the development of hospital surveillance. Med J Aust. 1978;12:543–6.
6. Finland M, McGowan JE Jr. Nosocomial infections in surgical patients. Observations on effects of prophylactic antibiotics. Arch Surg. 1976;111:143–5.
7. McGowan JE Jr, Barnes MW, Finland M. Bacteremia at Boston City Hospital: occurrence and mortality during 12 selected years (1935–1972), with special reference to hospital-acquired cases. J Infect Dis. 1975;132:316–35.
8. Haley RW, Quade D, Freeman HE, et al. The SENIC project: study on the efficacy of nosocomial infection control (SENIC PROJECT): summary of study design. Am J Epidemiol. 1980;111:472–85.
9. Haley RW, Culver DH, White JW, et al. The efficacy of infection surveillance and control programs in preventing nosocomial infections in US hospitals. Am J Epidemiol. 1985;121:182–205.
10. Weinstein RA. Nosocomial infection update. Emerg Infect Dis. 1998;4:416–20.
11. Berens M. Infection epidemic carves deadly path [Internet]. Chicago Tribune. 2002 [cited 22 January, 2019]. Available at: http://www.chicagotribune.com/news/chi-0207210272jul21-story.html.
12. Institute of Medicine. To err is human: building a safer health system. Washington, DC: National Academies Press; 2000.
13. McKibben L, Horan T, Tokars JI. Guidance on public reporting of healthcare-associated infections: recommendations of the Healthcare Infection Control Practices Advisory Committee. Am J Infect Control. 2005;33:217–26.
14. HHS Family of Agencies [Internet]. HHS.gov. 2016 [cited 24 January 2019]. Available from: https://www.hhs.gov/about/agencies/index.html.
15. National Action Plan to prevent HAI: roadmap to elimination [Internet]. Health.gov. 2013 [cited 23 November 2018]. Available from: https://health.gov/hcq/pdfs/hai-action-plan-executive-summary.pdf.
16. Longitudinal program evaluation of the HHS action plan to prevent healthcare-associated infections [Internet]. Health.gov. 2011 [cited 22 November 2018]. Available at https://health.gov/hcq/pdfs/hhs-action-plan-eval-report.pdf.
17. Summary of progress toward the 2013 national targets for elimination of health care-associated infections [Internet]. Health.gov [cited 24 January 2019]. Available from: https://health.gov/hcq/prevent-hai-previous-targets.asp.
18. The hospital value-based purchasing (VBP) program [Internet]. 2018 [cited 22 January 2019]. Available from: https://www.cms.gov/Medicare/Quality-Initiatives-Patient-Assessment-Instruments/Value-Based-Programs/HVBP/Hospital-Value-Based-Purchasing.html.
19. Calderon L, Kavanagh K, Rice M. Questionable validity of the catheter-associated urinary tract infection metric used for value-based purchasing. Am J Infect Control. 2015;43(10):1050–2.

20. 2016 national and state health-care associated infections report [Internet]. www.cdc.gov. 2018 [cited 20 January 2019]. Available from: https://www.cdc.gov/hai/data/portal/progress-report.html.
21. Bartles R, Dickson A, Babade O. A systematic approach to quantifying infection prevention staffing and coverage needs. Am J Infect Control. 2018;46(5):487–91.
22. Hazamy P, Van Antwerpen C, Tserenpuntsag B, Haley V, Tsivitis M, Doughty D, et al. Mandatory reporting of Hip replacement procedures: validating accuracy, New York State 2008. Am J Infect Control. 2010;38(5):E99.
23. Tsivitis M, Van Antwerpen C, Haley V, Tserenpuntsag B, Doughty D, Hazamy P. New York State Department of Health: mandatory public reporting – validation of CABG data. Am J Infect Control. 2011;39(5):E127.
24. Hazamy P, Van Antwerpen C, Tserenpuntsag B, Haley V, Tsivitis M, Doughty D, et al. Trends in validity of central line–associated bloodstream infection surveillance data, New York State, 2007–2010. Am J Infect Control. 2013;41(12):1200–4.
25. Bagchi S, Watkins J, Pollock D, Edwards J, Allen-Bridson K. State health department validations of central line–associated bloodstream infection events reported via the National Healthcare Safety Network. Am J Infect Control. 2018;46(11):1290–5.
26. Backman L, Carusillo E, D'aquila L, Melchreit R, Fekieta R. Validation of surgical site infection surveillance data in colon procedures reported to the Connecticut department of public health. Am J Infect Control. 2017;45(6):690–1.
27. Levinson D. CMS validated hospital inpatient quality reporting program data but should use additional tools to identify gaming [Internet]. Oig.hhs.gov. 2017 [cited 18 January 2019]. Available from: https://oig.hhs.gov/oei/reports/oei-01-15-00320.pdf/.
28. Madden GR, Weinstein RA, Sifri CD. Diagnostic stewardship for healthcare-associated infections: opportunities and challenges to safely reduce test use. Infect Control Hosp Epidemiol. 2018;39(2):214–8.
29. Centers for Medicare and Medicaid Services. Medicare program: revisions to payment policies under the physician fee schedule and other revisions to Part B for CY 2016. Final rule with comment period. Fed Regist. 2015;80:70885–1386.
30. Morgan DJ, Malani P, Diekema DJ. Diagnostic stewardship leveraging the laboratory to improve antimicrobial use. JAMA. 2017;318:607–8.
31. Durand DJ, Lewin JS, Berkowitz SA. Medical-imaging stewardship in the accountable care era. N Engl J Med. 2015;373(18):1691–3.
32. McDonald EG, Saleh RR, Lee TC. Mindfulness-based laboratory reduction: reducing utilization through trainee-led daily 'time outs. Am J Med. 2017;130:e241–4.
33. CDC/NHSN surveillance definitions for specific types of infections [Internet]. CDC.gov. 2017 [cited 26 April 2017]. Available at: https://www.cdc.gov/nhsn/pdfs/pscmanual/17pscnosinfdef_current.pdf.
34. Cohen SH, Gerding DN, Johnson S, et al. Clinical practice guidelines for Clostridium difficile infection in adults: 2010 update by the Society for Healthcare Epidemiology of America (SHEA) and the Infectious Diseases Society of America (IDSA). Infect Control Hosp Epidemiol. 2010;31:431–55.
35. The NHSN standardized infection ratio (SIR): a guide to the SIR [Internet]. CDC.gov/NHSN. 2018 [cited 11 November 2018]. Available from: https://www.cdc.gov/nhsn/pdfs/ps-analysis-resources/nhsn-sir-guide.pdf.
36. The targeted assessment for prevention (TAP) strategy: HAI: CDC [Internet]. CDC.gov/HAI. 2018. Available from: https://www.cdc.gov/hai/prevent/tap.html.
37. Doron S, Nasraway S. The trouble with studying bundles. Crit Care Med. 2011;39(10):2355–7.
38. Cafazzo J, St-Cyr O. From discovery to design: the evolution of human factors in healthcare. Healthc Q. 2012;15(sp):24–9.
39. Henriksen K, Oppenheimer C. Envisioning patient safety in the year 2025: eight perspectives [Internet]. AHRQ.gov. ND. Available from: https://www.ahrq.gov/downloads/pub/advances2/vol1/Advances-Henriksen_104.pdf.

40. Tracking infections in acute care hospitals/facilities | NHSN | CDC [Internet]. Cdc.gov. 2018 [cited 21 December 2018]. Available from: https://www.cdc.gov/nhsn/acute-care-hospital/index.html.
41. Mu Y, Edwards J, Horan T, Berrios-Torres S, Fridkin S. Improving risk-adjusted measures of surgical site infection for the National Healthcare Safely Network. Infect Control Hosp Epidemiol. 2011;32(10):970–86.
42. Hospital compare data [Internet]. Data.Medicare.gov. [cited 21 December 2018]. Available from: https://data.medicare.gov/data/hospital-compare.

Chapter 5
Evolution of Modern Cardiovascular Quality Metrics

Ifeany David Chinedozi and Benjamin Wessler

Introduction: What Is Good Cardiac Care?

It is the winter of 1990 and a 68-year-old woman with a history of hypertension presents with a syndrome of stuttering chest pain and associated dyspnea. She was working at the time and was encouraged by her coworkers to go to the emergency room. Ultimately, she was admitted to her local hospital and treated for a non-ST elevation myocardial infarction and discharged home. She was told—and believed—that the care she received was excellent.

At the time, there was a growing body of evidence to inform the treatment of patients with acute coronary syndromes (ACS) and there was clear evidence that aspirin therapy was associated with clinically meaningful decreases in the risk of recurrent vascular events and death [1]. Surprisingly though, at the time, there was no guarantee that she would receive aspirin. In fact there was a one in six chance that our patient would not receive this lifesaving medication during her hospitalization despite the compelling data available at the time [2]. Quality measures in cardiovascular medicine aim to close this disconnect—between the care that is delivered and care that is known to be effective. This chapter describes the evolution of these metrics with attention to limitations and a look toward what the future holds.

We explore the major themes that led to the growth and maturation of quality measures in cardiovascular medicine and explore whether these efforts have achieved their primary goal of improving the clinical outcomes that matter to

I. D. Chinedozi
Tufts University School of Medicine, Boston, MA, USA

B. Wessler (✉)
Division of Cardiology, Tufts Medical Center, Boston, MA, USA

Predictive Analytic sand Comparative Effectiveness (PACE) Center, Tufts Medical Center, Boston, MA, USA
e-mail: bwessler@tuftsmedicalcenter.org

© Springer Nature Switzerland AG 2020
D. N. Salem (ed.), *Quality Measures*, https://doi.org/10.1007/978-3-030-37145-6_5

patients. There have been unintended consequences and even possible harm resulting from these measures, and we must appreciate these lessons as we look forward toward the future of this maturing science.

In the Beginnings: Nightingale's Impact on Healthcare Quality Measures

The very backbone of medicine has always been deeply rooted in the tenet that clinicians, and particularly physicians, do good and minimize harm. However, this end has not always been met. In many instances throughout the history of medicine, it appears that much harm was done often because outcomes were not systematically assessed. How exactly physicians measured their performance was largely unknown until Florence Nightingale left her mark. Her insistence on measuring the outcomes associated with the treatments she provided as a nurse to wounded soldiers during the Crimean War led to what has been described as a revolution in understanding the quality of care [3, 4].

If the premise is true that the bedrock of medicine is grounded in the pursuit of good, and the veracity of the dictum "primum non nocere" is established, then the question of measuring outcomes becomes central to understanding the role of treatments. Common sense might dictate that patient-centered outcomes should matter and should be an important benchmark in the practice of medicine. However, the evolution of medicine itself from a primarily paternalistic framework in some ways has contradicted the universal adoption of patient-centered outcomes-based practice. This can help explain why it took until the late 1850s for a credibly recorded account of outcomes-centered medicine.

Good Cardiovascular Health: Not Just the Absence of Outcomes?

To begin understanding quality metrics in cardiovascular medicine, we must look first with a wide lens to see how cardiac health is defined. The American Heart Association (AHA) has outlined three broad targets and ideas that guide how cardiovascular health is pursued, measured, and achieved: (1) primordial prevention, (2) childhood roots of cardiovascular diseases, and (3) balancing population-wide prevention with individualized approaches [5]. Cardiac health exists on a continuum, and while interventions may have as an ultimate goal reducing the absolute risk of experiencing adverse events during one's lifetime, it is clear that both good and poor cardiovascular health exist early in life. In cardiovascular medicine, metrics have largely focused on late clinical events and largely ignore the longitudinal view of these diseases (Table 5.1).

Table 5.1 Identifying cardiac health metrics beginning early in life. Metrics exist across primordial, primary, and secondary prevention astrata

Goal/ Metric	Poor health		Intermediate health		Ideal health	
	Definition	Prevalence, %	Definition	Prevalence, %	Definition	Prevalence, %
Current smoking						
Adults >20 y of age	Yes	24	Former ≤12 mo	3	Never or quit >12 mo	73 (51 ncver; 22 former >12 mo)
Children 12–19 y of age	Tried prior 30 days	17			Never tried; never smoked whole cigarette	83
Body mass index						
Adults >20 y of age	≥30 kg/m2	34	25–29.9 kg/m2	33	<25 kg/m2	33
Children 2–19 y of age	>95th percentile	17	85th–95th percentile	15	<85th percentile	69
Physical activity						
Adults >20 y of age	None	32	1–149 min/wk. moderate intensity or 1–74 min/wk. vigorous intensity or 1–149 min/wk. moderate + vigorous	24	≥150 min/wk. moderate intensity or ≥75 min/wk. vigorous intensity or ≥150 min/wk. moderate + vigorous	45
Children 12–19 y of age	None	10	>0 and <60 min of moderate or vigorous activity every day	46	≥60 min of moderate or vigorous activity every day	44
Healthy diet score						
Adults >20 y of age	0–1 components	76	2–3 components	24	4–5 components	<0.5
Children 5–19 y of age	0–1 components	91	2–3 components	9	4–5 components	<0.5
Total cholesterol						
Adults >20 y of age	≥240 mg/dL	16	200–239 mg/dL or treated to goal	38 (27; 12 treated to goal)	<200 mg/dL	45

(continued)

Table 5.1 (continued)

	Poor health		Intermediate health		Ideal health	
Goal/ Metric	Definition	Prevalence, %	Definition	Prevalence, %	Definition	Prevalence, %
Children 6–19 y of age	≥200 mg/ dL	9	170–199 mg/ dL	25	<170 mg/dL	67
Blood pressure						
Adults >20 y of age	SBP ≥140 or DBP	17	SBP 120–139 or DBP 80–89 mm hg or treated to goal	41 (28; 13 treated to goal)	<120/<80 mm hg	42
Children 8–19 y of age	>95th percentile	5	90th–95th percentile or SBP ≥120 or DBP ≥80 mm hg	13	<90th percentile	82
Fasting plasma glucose						
Adults >20 y of age	≥126 mg/ dL	8	100–125 mg/ dL or treated to goal	34 (32; 3 treated to goal)	<100 mg/dL	58
Children 12–19 y of age	≥126 mg/ dL	0.5[a]	100–125 mg/ dL	18	<100 mg/dL	81

Poor Heath Metrics are common at young ages, long before clinic events occur. (Ref. Lloyd-Jones et al. [5])

Some percentages do not appear to add up because of rounding

SBP indicates systolic blood pressure: DBP diastolic blood pressure

[a]Estimate not reliable

Primordial prevention efforts focus on minimizing the development of risk factors for cardiovascular disease [6, 7]. Good care within this preventive framework should start early in life *before* the development of established (traditional) cardiovascular risk factors and is distinct from the primary and secondary prevention concepts that focus on the risk factors themselves. Primordial prevention generally focuses at the population level through education and public health initiatives to prevent development of cardiovascular risk factors (e.g., deterring cigarette smoking or advocating for restricted sodium content in commercially available processed foods). These efforts often overlap with primary prevention interventions focused on patients who possess these risk factors though have not had events (e.g., statin therapy in patients with a 10-year predicted risk of atherosclerotic cardiovascular disease (ASCVD) >7.5%) and secondary prevention efforts focused on minimizing disease recurrence (e.g., dual antiplatelet therapy following acute myocardial infarction) [5].

Cardiovascular disease often begins early in adolescence or young adulthood. This recognition has shifted the focus of preventive strategies and the target for defining "good health" since many people come into middle adulthood with adverse risk profiles that place them at a higher risk for adverse cardiac events. Increasingly it is recognized that when an initial cardiac presentation is in the setting of an acute event, there were a series of missed opportunities for interventions to improve an individual's cardiac status. These early markers of cardiovascular risk have been come central to our understanding of how to improve cardiovascular health [5, 8] though they remain largely absent from the standard quality measures that are currently used in cardiovascular medicine.

As quality metrics mature, a third concept that guides measurement is the importance of balancing population-wide measurement strategies with individual measurement strategies. There is a population/risk paradox in cardiovascular medicine where the majority of events affect patients who are not in high-risk categories. This is because most of the population lies below average risk. Patients with high individual risk (e.g., prior MI) are unlikely to benefit from strategies focused on lower-risk patients (increasing appropriate primary prevention statin prescriptions). At the same time, various screening strategies for hypercholesterolemia, diabetes, and hypertension utilized in adolescents and young adults that have led to marked reduction in cardiac events do little for patients with known disease who are already being treated. Appropriately balancing quality metrics for these different target populations (few high-risk individuals vs many low-risk individuals) is a central (and unresolved) tension in the contemporary era [5].

With cardiac care focused across these broad domains, the central questions that emerge are whether providers and health systems deliver (and patients receive) the care that is known to be effective and appropriate. To address these unknowns, public and private entities have created systems to measure and broadly assess the quality of delivered cardiovascular care.

Genesis of Cardiovascular Health Quality Measures

Given the diversity of ways to improve cardiovascular outcomes, improvements in health were long assumed. In fact there were many examples where patients were not made to feel better or live longer—and treatments were not having the intended effects. The scope of these contemporary issues became widely apparent only after the Institute of Medicine published their groundbreaking report of widespread healthcare-associated patient injuries [9]. With the publication of *To Err is Human* in November 1999, the public had to face these issues for the first time. There was intense media coverage and public discourse about the variety of ways patients are harmed through misuse, overuse, and underuse of medical resources. There was also substantial focus on iatrogenic injuries. Following this public engagement, the IOM produced a subsequent report aimed at highlighting what the pillars of healthcare should be in twenty-first-century America. The 2001 published report of *Crossing the Quality Chasm: A New Health System for the 21st Century* was far less user-friendly and did not receive as much attention [10]. However, the IOM identified the six aims of healthcare that are applicable across practice settings and specialties. These are:

1. *Safety:* patients and communities should be safe when they encounter the healthcare system as much as they could in their own homes
2. *Effectiveness:* the evidence for medicine should be grounded in science and should be based on treatments that have been shown to be working well
3. *Patient centricity:* the patient's autonomy and cultural and social contexts should be integral to the interaction with and treatment of the patients.
4. *Timeliness of care:* prompt administration of care should be implemented, reducing long waiting times and unnecessary delays to healthcare
5. *Efficiency:* getting serious about maximizing available resources, reducing waste, and minimizing the total cost of healthcare to patients, insurers, and the government
6. *Equity:* identifying and actively working to bridge the racial and ethnic divide in the health status of populations/communities [10, 11].

The public response to these reports were profound—evidenced by a 20% increase in the number of Americans who were dissatisfied with the quality of healthcare in general [12]. Although the IOM's assessments were stark, the undeniable conclusion was that systematic changes were needed. Following these groundbreaking reports, myriad efforts to standardize outcome measurement across many domains of patient care started to crystalize [11].

Evaluating Health Services

Donabedian models are often used to examine health services and quality of care. In this framework, cardiovascular health quality assessment is classified into (1) structure, (2) process, and (3) outcomes quality evaluations. According to the Agency for Healthcare Research and Quality (AHRQ), structural measures relate to the capacity of various healthcare systems to deliver high-quality care [13]. Examples of structural measures range from whether a cardiology group uses electronic medical records, to cardiologist to patient ratios. Process measures on the other hand address concerns such as the ability of cardiologists to deliver care that is deemed appropriate for a given condition (i.e., aspirin therapy following acute myocardial infarction). Of note, a vast majority of current reportable quality measures are based on process measures and are often described as helping patients know what to expect for specific cardiovascular problems. Outcome measures in cardiovascular care represent measuring concepts that are indisputably more important to patients, for instance, the rate of bleeding or mortality after percutaneous coronary intervention in a given healthcare setting. Although outcome evaluation is currently considered the gold standard in the hierarchical order of quality evaluation, many variables, if not well adjusted for, can lead to misleading information (at best) and erroneous conclusions (at worst). Without robust guards against these potential errors, quality measurement might not accomplish the broad goals of improving outcomes that matter.

Historical Perspectives of Outcome Versus Process-Based Quality Evaluation

Cardiovascular medicine was one of the first fields to implement standardized quality assessment metrics on a national level in the United States. Starting with Joint Commission on Accreditation of Healthcare Organizations (JCAHO) through to current efforts guided by the Hospital Readmission Reduction Program (HRRP) and beyond, there have been many attempts to measure the quality of care. Many lessons have been learned through these experiences as the field has moved toward understanding and effectively implementing quality evaluation (Fig. 5.1).

1918–1980s: Early Experience

Leveraging ideas championed by Dr. Ernest Codman, the American College of Surgeons (ACS) developed a set of Minimum Standards for Hospitals in 1918 and initiated on-site hospital inspections. In 1950, the American College of Physicians,

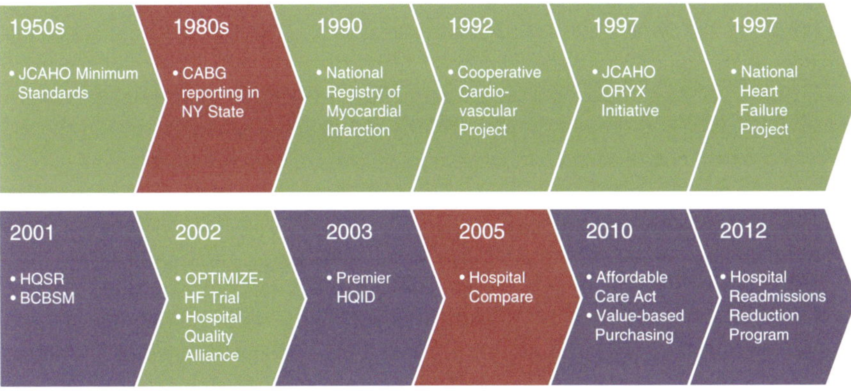

Fig. 5.1 Timeline of quality improvement programs in cardiovascular care. Green: quality measurement programs; red: public reporting; purple: pay-for-performance programs. BCBSM indicates Blue Cross Blue Shield of Michigan Participating Hospital Agreement Incentive Program, CABG coronary artery bypass graft, HQID hospital quality incentives demonstration, HQSR Hawaii Medical Service Association Hospital Quality Service and Recognition Pay-for-Performance Program, JCAHO Joint Commission on Accreditation of Healthcare Organizations, OPTIMIZE-HF Organized Program to Initiate Lifesaving Treatment in Hospitalized Patients With Heart Failure. (From Chatterjee and Joynt [14])

American Hospital Association, American Medical Association, and the Canadian Medical Association joined the ACS to form the Joint Commission (formerly the Joint Commission on Accreditation of Hospitals (JCAH)). This umbrella organization was, by design, an independent, nonprofit with the goal of providing voluntary hospital accreditation. The JCAH introduced a set of "minimum standards" of quality in the 1950s. This was the first codified attempt at systematic hospital health quality assessment and set the stage for quality evaluation. Data and methods from this program were later incorporated into the process for hospital accreditation under the ORYX initiative with the goal of identifying specific areas of improvement.

Approximately 30 years later, the state of New York took part in the first systematic evaluation of cardiac outcomes. Beginning in 1989, through a novel data collection program, the Cardiac Surgery Reporting System (CSRS) started to prospectively collect information on all patients who underwent open heart surgery. CSRS collected performance information for individual surgeons that was ultimately made public through a *Newsday* Freedom of Information Act request and published in 1991 [15].

Using aggregate data from this program, surgical outcomes were assessed across 30 hospitals in New York, and coronary artery bypass grafting (CABG) outcomes took center stage [16]. CSRS looked at patients who had undergone surgical revascularization without any other major cardiac surgery between 1989 and 1992. 12,269 operations were performed in 1989, 13,946 in 1990, 14,944 in 1991, and 15,733 in 1992 for a total of 56,892 CABG procedures. During the years under study, there was a 30.6% increase in cases and a decrease in mortality (from 3.53% to 2.78% over 4 years) despite an increase in disease severity (predicted in-hospital mortality rose from 2.62% to 3.54% over the same timeframe). This outcome trend was presented as evidence that quality improvement efforts were effectively reducing mortality following open-heart surgery (Table 5.2). This conclusion was challenged almost immediately.

A follow-up analysis tested a separate hypothesis that over these monitored years high-risk cases were treated elsewhere. Omoigui and colleagues looked at CABG cases performed at Cleveland Clinic from 1989 to 1993 and evaluated where patient referrals originated [17].

Their analysis showed that patients from New York ($n = 482$) were more often re-do procedures compared to patients from Ohio ($n = 6036$) [44% vs 22%, $P < 0.001$]. New York patients treated at Cleveland Clinic were also more likely to be NYHA functional class III or IV (48% vs 42%, $P = 0.04$). These observations resulted in higher predicted mortality for New York patients treated in Cleveland

Table 5.2 Volume, observed mortality, expected mortality, and risk-adjusted mortality in New York 1989 through 1992

	1989	1990	1991	1992	Total*
Volume	12,269	13,946	14,944	16,028	57,187
Actual mortality rate, %	3.52	3.14	3.08	2.78	3.11
Expected mortality rate, %	2.62	2.97	3.16	3.54	…
Risk-adjusted mortality rate, %	4.17	3.28	3.03	2.45	…

Reproduced from Ref. [16]

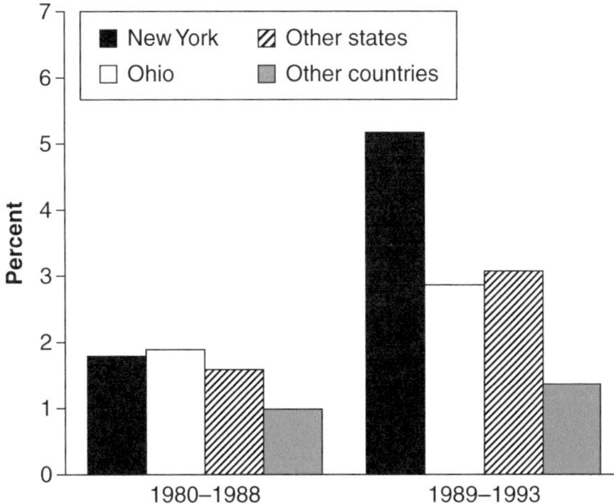

Fig. 5.2 Observed CABG mortality rates at the Cleveland Clinic from before (1980–1988) and during (1989–1993) periods of public reporting in New York. Data are presented by referral source. (Reproduced from Ref. [17])

Table 5.3 Threats to interpreting outcomes in cardiology [17–20]

Action	Effect	Remedy
Discourage treatment of high-risk patients [17]	Lower observed mortality	Exclude high-risk groups from public reporting [18]
Avoid patients with unmeasured risk factors [19]	Lower observed mortality	Optimize risk adjustment methods with updating
Upcoding of risk factors [20]	Raise predicted risk	Standardize definitions

compared to patients from Ohio (Fig. 5.2). Since these differences were not observed during the decade prior to the institution of the CSRS program, the authors claimed that the observed decrease in mortality in New York State may be related, at least in part, to outmigration of high-risk cases to other centers.

Through insights gained from this early experience, it became clear that there are numerous threats to accurate measurement and interpretation of cardiovascular metrics (Table 5.3). Providers and health systems can act to improve measurement objectives without actually improving the clinical outcomes that matter to patients. Operators can avoid treating high-risk patients, and hospitals/health systems can discourage treatment (referral or intervention) for patients who are likely to die [17]. This is especially troubling when high-risk patients are often the patients most likely to benefit from treatment [21]. Providers can also avoid treating patients when actual risk is perceived to be higher than predicted risk [19]. Such behaviors have the broad effect of "gaming" the measurement system to improve metrics without actually improving outcomes. In a more insidious way, these efforts undermine the trustworthiness of these measurement efforts.

This early experience underscores the challenges that accompany efforts to measure quality in cardiovascular medicine. While there is broad interest from a number of stakeholders—including patients, physicians, payers, and health systems—in doing this well and understanding how effective care is, there are important downstream consequences of these efforts that must be fully understood. Ultimately, outcome differences are only meaningful if appropriate (and accurate) risk adjustment can be done and if differences in hospital case-mix are incorporated into risk adjustment models. State-of-the-art risk adjustment techniques often ignore important cardiovascular risk predictors such as multimorbidity [22] and frailty [19], and existing databases pose limitations that continue to plague measurement efforts [15].

Attempts to Evaluate Process Measures

National Myocardial Infarction Registry (NMIR)

In 1990, 1073 hospitals across the United States joined what would become the National Myocardial Infarction Registry (NMIR) [23]. The express purpose of this registry was to collect data on the treatment of patients with acute myocardial infarction (AMI). The registry was conceived as a phase IV, observational registry and was sponsored by Genentech. Between 1990 and 1993, 240,989 patients with AMI were enrolled. Process measures fell far short of what would have been deemed appropriate care based on the evidence available at the time [24, 25]. Only 35.1% of appropriate patients received thrombolytic treatment and the time from ED presentation to tPA treatment averaged 99 minutes. There was also overuse of calcium channel blockers and the underutilization of beta blocker and aspirin therapy.

The Minnesota Heart Survey (MHS) Registry

This prospective registry started in 1990 as a component of the Minnesota Heart Survey [26]. The registry enrolled patients with symptoms suggestive of AMI. The use of thrombolytic therapy, symptoms time onset, medical history and risk factors, and demographic information were assessed while patients were admitted in coronary care units. During this 3-year follow-up, and similar to the NMIR, it was found that only 34% of eligible patients received thrombolytic therapy. Among the patients who received thrombolysis, men were more likely to have been treated within 12 hours (45%) compared to 33% for women (adjusted male/female odds ratio was 1.33 at 95% CI, 0.94–1.87).

The Cooperative Cardiovascular Project

The Health Care Quality Improvement (HCQI) initiative launched the Cooperative Cardiovascular Project (CCP) as a pilot in four states: Alabama, Connecticut, Iowa, and Wisconsin in 1992 [2, 27]. The aim of this study was to assess whether Medicare patients were receiving appropriate care in the setting of AMI. By the time the main initiative concluded in 1995, it was reported that among "ideal candidates" for specific interventions, only 83% received aspirin therapy, 69% received thrombolytics, and 70% received heparin. At discharge, only 77% received aspirin therapy and 45% received beta blockers. Adherence to these quality indicators was better in states participating in the CCP pilot compared to those that were not participating, and care in the CCP states was associated with lower mortality [28].

National Heart Failure (NHF) Project

The Centers for Medicaid and Medicare Services (formerly the Health Care Financing Administration) formulated the National Heart Failure (NHF) project in 1999 [29]. The purpose of this initiative was to define and measure compliance with a set of quality metrics in patients with heart failure (HF). For example, the project emphasized the measurement of left ventricular (LV) systolic function in HF patients and the administration of ACE inhibitors to patients with diagnosed LV systolic dysfunction. The study found inconsistent assessment of LV systolic function across hospitals (21–66%) and underutilization of ACE inhibitors in patients who clearly qualified (51–93%).

Associations with Clinical Outcomes

The first attempt to quantify the relationship between process measures and clinical outcomes took place in New Zealand [30]. Investigators sought to understand whether adhering to the Royal College of Physicians Stroke Audit Package (RCPSAP) was associated with clinical outcomes including disability and mortality. A total of 181 stroke patients were enrolled at 1 of 4 hospitals and followed for 12 months or until death. There was a modest relationship between some of the RCPSAP process measures and short-term outcomes. For example, having a swallow assessment recorded before feeding was associated with better short-term outcomes. It was noted, however, that none of the process measures were significantly associated with outcomes at 12 months and that hospitals with the best process measure scores had the worst risk-adjusted outcomes. While this small trial offered clues to the process measure/outcome relationship, many questions remained.

As in the setting of stroke, the relationship for AMI appears similarly complex. Data from the Can Rapid Risk Stratification of Unstable Angina Patients Suppress Adverse Outcomes with Early Implementation of the American College of Cardiology/American Heart Association Guidelines (CRUSADE) trial showed that a 10% increase in adherence to process measures was associated with a 10% decrease in in-hospital mortality [31]. However a subsequent evaluation of process measures for a cohort of Medicare suggested that the observed association with process measures and short-term outcomes was weak at best (process measures explain only 6% of hospital-level variation in risk-adjusted 30-day mortality rates) [32].

Heart failure studies have shown a similarly sobering relationship between process measures and the morbidity and mortality outcomes that matter to patients. In the acute setting, the Organized Program to Initiate Lifesaving Treatment in Hospitalized Patients With Heart Failure (OPTIMIZE-HF) Registry was used to assess whether adherence to guideline-based care was associated with improved outcomes. This evaluation showed that process measures were not associated with lower mortality at 60 or 90 days though use of ACE inhibitors/ARBs at the time of discharge was associated with a lower rate of the composite of rehospitalization or mortality at 60 or 90 days [33]. Interestingly, beta-blocker use at the time of discharge, which was not one of the original ACC/AHA quality metrics for patients with HF, was one of the few process measures associated with reduced morbidity and mortality at discharge.

Similar observations were made in the American Heart Association's Get With The Guidelines Program for heart failure (GWTG-HF) [34]. Among 4460 hospitals that report data to Centers for Medicare and Medicaid (CMS), there were 215 hospitals (5%) enrolled in the GWTG-HF program. These participating hospitals had higher rates of four HF process measures (Table 5.4) when compared to hospitals that did not participate in the program. There was no difference in 30-day mortality rates between participating hospitals and nonparticipating hospitals though 30-day readmission rates were lower in GWTG-HF hospital. These data taken together suggest a weak (at best) relationship between process measures and outcomes for patients hospitalized for heart failure. Clearly more reliable ways to understand and measure quality were needed.

These early assessments of process measures demonstrated clear and consistent underutilization of therapies that were known to be effective at the time. These observations cut across demographic strata and clinical syndromes and strongly suggested that there were major opportunities to improve delivered care and clinical outcomes. Unfortunately the relationship between improving process measures and improving patient-centered outcomes was much less clear (Table 5.4). While process measures remain simple to measure and relatively easy to improve (especially when adherence is quite low), it does not necessarily follow that patients will feel better or live longer. In fact there are examples in AMI [32] and ADHF [33] care where clinical outcomes were relatively insensitive to improvements in process measures. As the relationships between process measures and improved clinical outcomes emerged, it became evident that the definition of "quality care" was not straightforward.

Trying to Define and Encourage Quality

President Clinton and the National Quality Forum

In 1999, President Clinton's Advisory Commission on Consumer Protection and Quality in the Health Care Industry recommended formation of the National Quality Forum [35] to improve quality measurement and assessment. The NQF was conceived as a nonprofit, public-private *voluntary consensus standards setting body* charged with developing a national strategy for healthcare quality measurement and reporting. It was believed that the NQF could function as a forum where various

Table 5.4 Associations between improving process measures and clinical outcomes

Citation	Condition	Process quality metric	Clinical outcome	Association
[30]	Stroke	Head CT, swallow study prior to feeding, multidisciplinary team meeting[a]	Survival to hospital discharge	Process measures were associated with improved survival at the hospital level
[31]	Myocardial infarction	Nine individual ACC/AHA class I guideline-recommended therapies[b]	In-hospital mortality	10% increase in process adherence associated with 10% decrease in mortality
[32]	Myocardial infarction	Receipt of beta blockers and aspirin at discharge	Risk-standardized 30-day mortality	Process measures explain only 6% of hospital-level variation in 30-day mortality rates
[33]	Acute heart failure	Discharge instructions, evaluation of LVEF, ACE-I or ARB use for low LVEF, smoking cessation advice, anticoagulation at discharge for atrial fibrillation	60- or 90-day mortality and readmission	Process measures not associated with 60- or 90-day mortality. ACE inhibitor or ARB at discharge associated with lower readmission
[34]	Acute heart failure	Evaluation of LVEF, ACE-I or ARB use for low LVEF, discharge instructions, smoking cessation advice	Risk-adjusted 30-day readmission and mortality	Process measures were not associated with decrease in 30-day mortality and were associated with reduction in 30-day readmission

From Refs. [30–34]

LVEF is left ventricular ejection fraction, *ACE-I* is angiotensin converting enzyme inhibitor, *ARB* is angiotensin receptor blocker.

[a]Center effect was noted where the hospitals with the lowest process score had the best case mix adjusted survival status at hospital discharge.

[b]These therapies were aspirin, beta blocker, heparin, IV IIbIIIa use within 24 hours and discharge on aspirin, beta-blocker, clopridogrel, ACE-I, lipid lowering mediations

healthcare stakeholders (from across public and private entities) could work together to craft a vision of American healthcare quality. Using a formal Consensus Development Progress, the NFQ worked to define quality metrics that could be used for both public reporting and internal assessment. The forum also worked to optimize data collection and reporting. The work of the NFQ ultimately led to standards of quality later adopted by Centers for Medicare and Medicaid [35].

Ten years out, the NQF announced the Cardiovascular Consensus Standards Endorsement and Maintenance 2010 project [36]. The goal was to identify cardiovascular measures for reporting and quality improvement that are specific to cardiac conditions. Disease groups include coronary artery disease, atrial fibrillation, implantable cardioverter defibrillators (ICD), heart failure, and hypertension. While a list of 39 measures has been assembled and endorsed [36] and is being used by numerous federal agencies (including CMS), questions remain about the evidence showing a robust association between measurement and improved clinical outcomes.

The Emerging Reality of Pay for Performance

One of the most important national trends in cardiovascular quality measurement and improvement is Pay for Performance (P4P). This framework holds that when financial incentives are aligned with delivery of appropriate care, there is motivation to improve performance. There is an associated benefit for policymakers and hospital administrators in that improved quality is aligned with lower costs.

The initial experience with this model took place in Hawaii through the Hospital Quality Service and Recognition program [37]. This program was started in 2001 and rewarded high-quality care as assessed using claims data and hospital-reported data. Outcomes including in-hospital complications, length of stay, patient satisfaction, and process of care metrics were assessed. During the 4-year implementation period, P4P was associated with decreases in complication rates and LOS. Blue Cross and Blue Shield undertook a similar study of incentives for cardiovascular care in 85 Michigan hospitals [38]. This program awarded direct financial incentives to hospitals that increased adherence to guideline-based process metrics (aspirin on discharge for AMI, beta blocker on discharge for AMI, ACE-I on discharge for CHF). This study found that P4P in this setting increased adherence to cardiovascular process measures and could be cost effective (cost per QALY was between $12,967 and $30,081).

The nationwide hospital level P4P experiment started in 2003 with the Premier Hospital Quality Incentive Demonstration (HQID). This program paid bonuses to hospitals based on achieving improvements to disease-specific process measures. In a comparison to nonparticipating hospitals, this program demonstrated improvements in achieving guideline-based process measures [39] though among hospitals participating in the CRUSADE imitative [31] there was no clear signal that P4P decreased in-hospital mortality for patients with AMI [40].

Despite the murky relationship between P4P efforts and improved clinical outcomes, these programs have been broadly embraced by policymakers and are central to Medicare's Value-Based Purchasing Program [41]. As these incentive programs have matured (phase I included rewards only for high achievement, phase II rewards were given for high achievement, top performers, and significant improvement), there was evidence that these tools did not incentivize the lowest-performing hospitals as originally designed. Instead P4P resulted in the strongest incentives for hospitals that had quality metrics just above the median, and questions still remain about whether these models of improving care quality can improve care for those who need quality improvement most [42].

P4P efforts to measure and assess quality are plagued by some of the same process of care and public reporting issues that troubled earlier efforts. Neither a good score (nor more money) can serve as a reliable surrogate for appropriate care [43]. Although the current P4P system had as a goal optimizing transparency by fostering publicly disclosed quality scores, there is growing concern that providers have lost faith in these tools. If all that providers must do to be reimbursed better is to report great "quality" numbers, then surely the system can be "gamed." This method of quality assessment will only remain relevant if P4P incentives can reliably tied to outcomes that matter.

Value-Based Purchasing

P4P became a major policy focus of the Affordable Care Act (ACA) through the Hospital Value-Based Purchasing (HVBP) program introduced by CMS in 2011. With passage of the ACA in 2010, the federal government made a major shift toward value-based medical care. This program reimburses hospitals based on performance on multiple domains of care (including both process outcomes and clinical outcomes) and patient experience and cost efficiency [36]. Early results of this program were underwhelming (though perhaps not surprising) given the history of P4P. After 3 years, it was noted that 30-day risk-adjusted mortality for incentivized conditions dropped by a similar amount in hospitals participating in HVBP and nonparticipating hospitals during the post-intervention period (difference in trends −0.03% point difference for each quarter, 95% confidence interval −0.08% to 0.13% point difference, $P = 0.35$) [44]. A similar lack of benefit was seen in patient experience outcome (another express goal of the program) [45]. There are many potential reasons for this failure, including the fact that at inception, HVBP ignored critical design features that were believed necessary for success: Incentives were not large enough to motivate significant hospital-based investments in improving care, the focus on multiple conditions and outcomes was too broad for pointed change efforts, and there was no easy way for providers and organizations to know how they were doing [46]. In contrast to the HVBP, another ACA-based experiment in P4P aimed at decreasing hospital readmissions showed initial promise.

The Hospital Readmissions Reduction Program (HRRP)

Launched as part of the ACA, the main objective of the HRRP initiative was to improve the quality of care given to patients with heart failure, acute myocardial infarction, and pneumonia by tying reimbursement to readmissions. The central tenet driving this program is that quality care is associated with lower readmission rates [36]. The tool used to benchmark hospital readmission rates for HF had moderate discrimination but was deemed appropriate for this task [47]. Immediately after implementation, national data began to show a significant decrease in 30-day readmissions across these domains [48]. However, very early on there were concerns that this measured outcome that was defined by an arbitrary timeframe and did not account for the competing risk of death [49]. The most recent study to evaluate this program included a cohort of 8.3 million hospitalizations for HF, AMI, and pneumonia (mean age 79.6 [8.7] years and 53.4% female of which 7.9 million were alive at the time of hospital discharge (3.2 million HF patients, 1.8 million AMI, and three million pneumonia patients) [50]. Within the 30-day period following hospitalization, there were 270,517 deaths among the HF patients, 128,088 for AMI, and 246,154 deaths among the pneumonia subset. Mortality trends were established before and after the HRRP announcement. The assessment looked at periods: Periods 1 and 2 spanned the timeframe before the announcement of HRRP (April 2005 to September 2007 and October 2007 to March 2010), and Periods 3 and 4 extended from the time the HRRP was announced (April 2010 to September 2012) and its implementation (October 2012 to March 2015). During the period after HRRP was announced (Periods 2–3), there was a greater increase in post-discharge 30-day mortality (0.49 with a 0.22% difference in change, $p = 0.01$) when compared to baseline. This change was also evident during HRRP implementation [Periods 3–4 (0.52% increase with a difference in change of 0.25%, $p = 0.001$)]. These data suggest that though readmissions have decreased, post-hospitalization mortality for heart failure has in fact increased while post-hospitalization mortality for acute myocardial infarction has declined [50, 51]. Of note, when the timeframe for analysis was extended to 45 days post-hospitalization, there was no observed increase in mortality following hospitalization for HF seen (Fig. 5.3).

These observations raise important concerns about the 30-day rehospitalization outcome (in particular) and simple yet easily defined outcomes (in general) and call urgently for more study. It is reasonable to think that in the setting of complex disease states such as heart failure or AMI, not all readmissions within 30 days represent low-quality care—and thus not all readmissions should be avoided. Additionally, when benchmarking expected rehospitalization rates, the limitations of current approaches to risk adjustment must be considered [47, 52]. A key criticism of HRRP is that the financial incentives aimed at reducing readmissions are substantially greater than the incentives aimed at reducing mortality [39, 46]. Since these penalties disproportionately affect providers serving socioeconomically disadvantaged populations [53] and safety-net hospitals operate in resource-constrained environments, most provider networks face difficult choices about which performance metrics to prioritize [54].

Merit-Based Incentive Program

The most recent experiment in measuring quality comes full circle looking again to the performance of individual providers. Borne as part of the Medicare Access and CHIP Reauthorization Act (MACRA), the Merit-Based Incentive Program (MIPS) replaced the sustainable growth rate (SGR) formula (and necessary Congressional action to avoid fee cuts). In broad terms the MIPS program rewards clinicians for providing high-value care [55]. The program works by converting provider performance (submitted either as an individual or as a group) into a

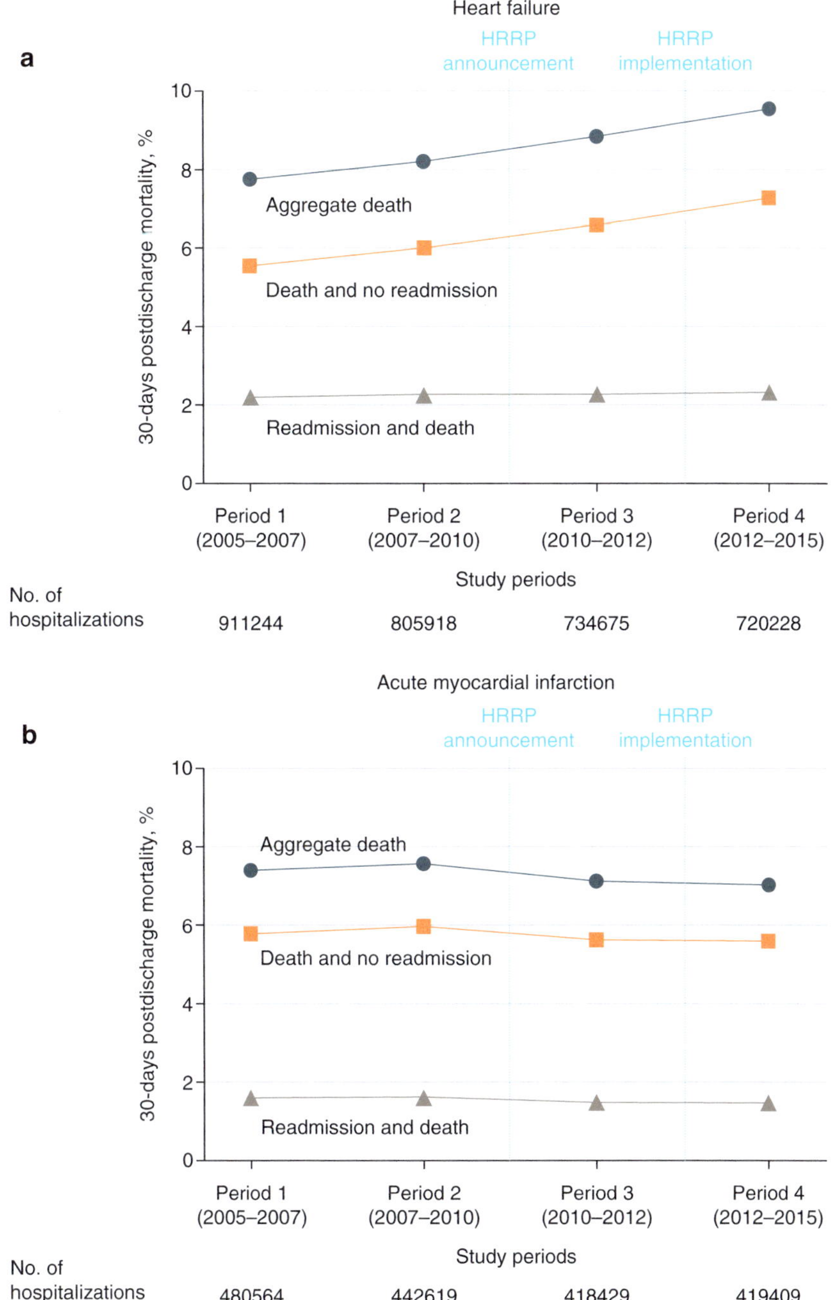

Fig. 5.3 Adapted from [50] showing trends in observed 30 day post-discharge mortality for patients admitted to the hospital with heart failure (**a**) or acute myocardial infarction (**b**) before and during HRRP

quality score using the six measures that clinicians score highest on. There is substantial heterogeneity on metric selection and data submission and quality metrics sometimes lack clinical relevance resulting in concerns about interpretability and applicability [56]. While initial results are not yet available, surely there will be challenges to understanding the results and what they mean to the outcomes of patients.

Risk Adjustment: Achilles' Heel of Quality Assessment

When performance is benchmarked against predicted event rates, it is worth considering some of the uncertainty that underlies the risk-adjustment tools that are currently being tested and used [47, 52, 57]. With current methods it will always be true that major dimensions of risk will be excluded from risk-adjustment tools either because of difficulties with definitions or measurement or model building techniques. While there is substantial interest the C-statistic of predictive models, there has been relatively little attention paid to issues of calibration—how well-predicted outcomes match observed outcome rates [58, 59]. Calibration is relatively insensitive to changes in discrimination and poor calibration must be guarded against in the setting of quality assessment so that provider performance is not compared to an inaccurate baseline event rate. Perhaps more importantly, as treatment eras change recalibration and updating of risk-adjustment tools is necessary [60] to ensure there is no loss in performance over time. These issues represent challenges to our current tools, and without clear and rigorous quality control and honest reconciliation of limitations, provider and public trust in these risk-adjustment systems will erode.

Conclusion

The history of quality assessment in cardiovascular medicine shows us that despite many attempts at measuring care, there are few clear successes as assessed by improved patient-centered outcomes. Unfortunately, much of the measurement in cardiology happens at a clinically advanced stage and thus misses early opportunities to improve cardiac health. Public reporting of outcomes has had unintended consequences, and improvements in process measures may not be worthwhile if they are not closely linked to improvements in clinical outcomes. Risk adjustment, which has assumed a central role in contemporary quality assessment in cardiology, is also limited, and accurate (and updated) risk adjustment tools remain understudied. These uncertainties will continue to threaten the validity of these efforts and leave open questions about the quality of delivered care. If there can be transparency and fidelity in the measurement of cardiovascular quality, then there will be high confidence in these performance metrics. Without direct evidence of improved clinical outcomes, faith in these attempts at measuring quality will erode—and ultimately will be lost.

References

1. Anon. Secondary prevention of vascular disease by prolonged antiplatelet treatment. Antiplatelet Trialists' Collaboration. Br Med J (Clin Res Ed). 1988;296:320–31.
2. Ellerbeck EF, Jencks SF, Radford MJ, et al. Quality of care for Medicare patients with acute myocardial infarction. A four-state pilot study from the Cooperative Cardiovascular Project. JAMA. 1995;273:1509–14.
3. Tooley SA. The life of Florence Nightingale. London: S.H. Bousfield & Co., Ltd.; 1905. ISBN-13: 978-1104449629.
4. Higginson IJ, Carr AJ. Measuring quality of life: using quality of life measures in the clinical setting. BMJ. 2001;322:1297–300.
5. Lloyd-Jones DM. Cardiovascular risk prediction: basic concepts, current status, and future directions. Circulation. 2010;121:1768–77.
6. Strasser T. Reflections on cardiovascular diseases. Interdiscip Sci Rev. 1978;3:225–30.
7. Gillman MW. Primordial prevention of cardiovascular disease. Circulation. 2015;131:599–601.
8. Ford ES, Ajani UA, Croft JB, et al. Explaining the decrease in U.S. deaths from coronary disease, 1980–2000. N Engl J Med. 2007;356:2388–98.
9. Anon. To err is human. Washington, D.C.: National Academies Press; 2000.
10. Anon. Crossing the quality chasm. Washington, D.C.: National Academies Press; 2001.
11. Berwick DM. A user's manual for the IOM's 'quality chasm' report. Health Aff. 2002;21:80–90.
12. Blendon RJ, Altman DE, Benson JM, Brodie M. Health care in the 2004 presidential election. N Engl J Med. 2004;351:1314–22.
13. Anon. No title. Available at: http://www.ahrq.gov/talkingquality/measures/types.html.
14. Chatterjee P, Joynt KE. Do cardiology quality measures actually improve patient outcomes? J Am Heart Assoc. 2014;3:e000404.
15. Wasfy JH, Borden WB, Secemsky EA, McCabe JM, Yeh RW. Public reporting in cardiovascular medicine: accountability, unintended consequences, and promise for improvement. Circulation. 2015;131:1518–27.
16. Hannan EL, Kilburn H, Racz M, Shields E, Chassin MR. Improving the outcomes of coronary artery bypass surgery in New York State. JAMA. 1994;271:761–6.
17. Omoigui NA, Miller DP, Brown KJ, et al. Outmigration for coronary bypass surgery in an era of public dissemination of clinical outcomes. Circulation. 1996;93:27–33.
18. Peberdy MA, Donnino MW, Callaway CW, et al. Impact of percutaneous coronary intervention performance reporting on cardiac resuscitation centers: a scientific statement from the American Heart Association. Circulation. 2013;128:762–73.
19. Rowe R, Iqbal J, Murali-krishnan R, et al. Role of frailty assessment in patients undergoing cardiac interventions. Open Heart. 2014;1:e000033–e000033.
20. Green J, Wintfeld N. Report cards on cardiac surgeons. Assessing New York State's approach. N Engl J Med. 1995;332:1229–32.
21. Kent DM, Hayward RA. Limitations of applying summary results of clinical trials to individual patients: the need for risk stratification. JAMA. 2007;298:1209–12.
22. Forman DE, Maurer MS, Boyd C, et al. Multimorbidity in older adults with cardiovascular disease. J Am Coll Cardiol. 2018;71:2149–61.
23. Rogers WJ, Bowlby LJ, Chandra NC, et al. Treatment of myocardial infarction in the United States (1990 to 1993). Observations from the National Registry of Myocardial Infarction. Circulation. 1994;90:2103–14.
24. Yusuf S, Sleight P, Held P, McMahon S. Routine medical management of acute myocardial infarction. Lessons from overviews of recent randomized controlled trials. Circulation. 1990;82:II117–34.
25. Gunnar RM, Bourdillon PD, Dixon DW, et al. ACC/AHA guidelines for the early management of patients with acute myocardial infarction. A report of the American College of Cardiology/American Heart Association Task Force on Assessment of Diagnostic and Therapeutic Cardiovascular Procedures (subcommit). Circulation. 1990;82:664–707.

26. Rosamond WD, Shahar E, McGovern PG, Sides TL, Luepker RV. Trends in coronary thrombolytic therapy for acute myocardial infarction (the Minnesota Heart Survey Registry, 1990 to 1993). Am J Cardiol. 1996;78:271–7.
27. Gunter N, Moore L, Odom P. Cooperative cardiovascular project. J S C Med Assoc. 1997;93:177–9.
28. Marciniak TA, Ellerbeck EF, Radford MJ, et al. Improving the quality of care for Medicare patients with acute myocardial infarction: results from the Cooperative Cardiovascular Project. JAMA. 1998;279:1351–7.
29. Masoudi FA, Ralston DL, Wolfe P, et al. Baseline quality indicator rates from the National Heart Failure Project: a HCFA initiative to improve the care of medicare beneficiaries with heart failure. Congest Heart Fail. 7:53–6.
30. McNaughton H, McPherson K, Taylor W, Weatherall M. Relationship between process and outcome in stroke care. Stroke. 2003;34:713–7.
31. Peterson ED, Roe MT, Mulgund J, et al. Association between hospital process performance and outcomes among patients with acute coronary syndromes. JAMA. 2006;295:1912–20.
32. Bradley EH, Herrin J, Elbel B, et al. Hospital quality for acute myocardial infarction: correlation among process measures and relationship with short-term mortality. JAMA. 2006;296:72–8.
33. Fonarow GC, Abraham WT, Albert NM, et al. Association between performance measures and clinical outcomes for patients hospitalized with heart failure. JAMA. 2007;297:61–70.
34. Heidenreich PA, Hernandez AF, Yancy CW, Liang L, Peterson ED, Fonarow GC. Get with the guidelines program participation, process of care, and outcome for medicare patients hospitalized with heart failure. Circ Cardiovasc Qual Outcomes. 2012;5:37–43.
35. Anon. No title. Available at: http://www.qualityforum.org/Measures_List.aspx.
36. National Quality Forum. NQF-Endorsed® Standards. 1999. Available at: http://www.qualityforum.org/Measures_List.aspx.
37. Berthiaume JT, Chung RS, Ryskina KL, Walsh J, Legorreta AP. Aligning financial incentives with quality of care in the hospital setting. J Healthc Qual. 2006;28:36–44, 51.
38. Nahra TA, Reiter KL, Hirth RA, Shermer JE, Wheeler JRC. Cost-effectiveness of hospital pay-for-performance incentives. Med Care Res Rev. 2006;63:49S–72S.
39. Lindenauer PK, Remus D, Roman S, et al. Public reporting and pay for performance in hospital quality improvement. N Engl J Med. 2007;356:486–96.
40. Glickman SW, Ou F-S, DeLong ER, et al. Pay for performance, quality of care, and outcomes in acute myocardial infarction. JAMA. 2007;297:2373–80.
41. Centers for Medicare & Medicaid Services (CMS) H. Medicare program; hospital inpatient value-based purchasing program. Final rule. Fed Regist. 2011;76:26490–547.
42. Ryan AM, Blustein J, Casalino LP. Medicare's flagship test of pay-for-performance did not spur more rapid quality improvement among low-performing hospitals. Health Aff. 2012;31:797–805.
43. Hayward RA. Kent DM. 6 EZ steps to improving your performance: (or how to make P4P pay 4U!). JAMA. 2008;300:255–6.
44. Figueroa JF, Tsugawa Y, Zheng J, Orav EJ, Jha AK. Association between the Value-Based Purchasing pay for performance program and patient mortality in US hospitals: observational study. BMJ. 2016;353:i2214.
45. Papanicolas I, Figueroa JF, Orav EJ, Jha AK. Patient hospital experience improved modestly, but no evidence medicare incentives promoted meaningful gains. Health Aff (Millwood). 2017;36:133–40.
46. Jha AK. Time to get serious about pay for performance. JAMA. 2013;309:347.
47. Keenan PS, Normand ST, Lin Z, et al. An administrative claims measure suitable for profiling hospital performance on the basis of 30-day all-cause readmission rates among patients with heart failure. Circ Cardiovasc Qual Outcomes. 2008;1:29–37.
48. Zuckerman RB, Sheingold SH, Orav EJ, Ruhter J, Epstein AM. Readmissions, observation, and the hospital readmissions reduction program. N Engl J Med. 2016;374:1543–51.
49. Konstam MA. Heart failure in the lifetime of Musca Domestica (the common housefly). JACC Heart Fail. 2013;1:178–80.

50. Wadhera RK, Joynt Maddox KE, Wasfy JH, Haneuse S, Shen C, Yeh RW. Association of the hospital readmissions reduction program with mortality among medicare beneficiaries hospitalized for heart failure, acute myocardial infarction, and pneumonia. JAMA – J Am Med Assoc. 2018;320:2542–52.
51. Gupta A, Allen LA, Bhatt DL, et al. Association of the hospital readmissions reduction program implementation with readmission and mortality outcomes in heart failure. JAMA Cardiol. 2018;3:44.
52. Krumholz HM, Chaudhry SI, Spertus JA, Mattera JA, Hodshon B, Herrin J. Do non-clinical factors improve prediction of readmission risk? JACC Heart Fail. 2016;4:12–20.
53. Joynt KE, Jha AK. Characteristics of hospitals receiving penalties under the hospital readmissions reduction program. JAMA. 2013;309:342.
54. Figueroa JF, Joynt KE, Zhou X, Orav EJ, Jha AK. Safety-net hospitals face more barriers yet use fewer strategies to reduce readmissions. Med Care. 2017;55:229–35.
55. Rathi VK, McWilliams JM. First-year report cards from the Merit-Based Incentive Payment System (MIPS). JAMA. 2019;321:1157.
56. MacLean CH, Kerr EA, Qaseem A. Time out — charting a path for improving performance measurement. N Engl J Med. 2018;378:1757–61.
57. O'Brien SM, Shahian DM, Filardo G, et al. The society of thoracic surgeons 2008 cardiac surgery risk models: part 2—isolated valve surgery. Ann Thorac Surg. 2009;88:S23–42.
58. Van Calster B, Nieboer D, Vergouwe Y, De Cock B, Pencina MJ, Steyerberg EW. A calibration hierarchy for risk models was defined: from utopia to empirical data. J Clin Epidemiol. 2016;74:167–76.
59. Cook NR. Use and misuse of the receiver operating characteristic curve in risk prediction. Circulation. 2007;115:928–35.
60. Steyerberg EW, Borsboom GJJM, van Houwelingen HC, Eijkemans MJC, Habbema JDF. Validation and updating of predictive logistic regression models: a study on sample size and shrinkage. Stat Med. 2004;23:2567–86.

Chapter 6
Along the Road to Quality in Cancer Care

Joshua Dower, Fei Song, Diane Y. Sun, and Rachel J. Buchsbaum

Introduction: Framing the Problem

Cancer remains one of the leading causes of death in the United States despite significant strides made in cancer care. While approximately 600,000 cancer deaths are projected to occur in the United States in 2019, improvements in cancer prevention, treatment, and surveillance have contributed to a combined cancer death rate decline of 27% in the past 2 decades [1]. Recognition of the growing contribution of cancer to the national death rate and the importance of setting standards for cancer care stem as far back as 1922, when the American College of Surgeons established the Commission on Cancer, a consortium of professional organizations, with the mandate to improve life for cancer patients through provision and oversight of comprehensive quality care (https://www.facs.org/quality-programs/cancer/coc). The Commission on Cancer sponsors a number of initiatives through its member organizations and collaborators, including the American Joint Committee on Cancer, accreditation for various cancer care programs with regard to care, and the National Cancer Database.

Cancer care has also had remarkable impact on US healthcare spending. With estimates of 18 million cancer survivors in 2020, the total cost of cancer care in the

---

Joshua Dower, Fei Song and Diane Y. Sun contributed equally to this chapter.

J. Dower · F. Song · D. Y. Sun
Department of Medicine, Tufts Medical Center, Tufts University School of Medicine, Boston, MA, USA

R. J. Buchsbaum (✉)
Department of Medicine, Tufts Cancer Center, Tufts Medical Center, Tufts University School of Medicine, Boston, MA, USA
e-mail: rbuchsbaum@tuftsmedicalcenter.org

© Springer Nature Switzerland AG 2020
D. N. Salem (ed.), *Quality Measures*, https://doi.org/10.1007/978-3-030-37145-6_6

United States is projected to be \$173 billion in 2020, a 39% increase in merely 10 years [2]. As part of the Cancer Control Blueprint series, Yabroff and others pointed out many factors associated with increased costs, including population growth, increasing intensity of treatments, and cost of antineoplastic and palliative medications [3–5]. Rising costs in the complex setting of the US healthcare system lead to significant financial burden on cancer patients and their families. Growing awareness of the need to determine the value of the healthcare being delivered led to initiation of the Quality of Health Care in America project by the Institute of Medicine (IOM) [6, 7]. Concurrent focus on the quality of cancer care specifically led the National Cancer Institute and the National Academy of Sciences to form the National Cancer Policy Board, which determined both an ideal state for cancer care delivery as well as an assessment of the current state at the time. The articulated differences between ideal and reality and resulting recommendations led to a seminal report (*Ensuring Quality Cancer Care* [8]) by the IOM in 1999, framed by five key questions:

1. *What is the state of the cancer care "system?"*
2. *What is quality cancer care and how is it measured?*
3. *What problems are evident in the quality of cancer care and what steps can be taken to improve care?*
4. *How can we improve what we know about the quality of cancer care?*
5. *What steps can be taken to overcome barriers of access to quality cancer care?*

The IOM defined quality as "the degree to which health services for individuals and populations increase the likelihood of desired health outcomes and are consistent with current professional knowledge," and specified that poor quality can mean too much or too little care, or the wrong care.

The ten resulting recommendations in the IOM report were organized around questions 3–5 above. With regard to evident problems and steps to take, recommendations included ensuring that cancer management is done by experienced professionals in high-volume settings, that care is delivered in line with systematically developed evidence-based guidelines, that quality of care is monitored using a core set of quality metrics, that initial treatment plans are developed with a full complement of resources necessary to implement the care plan, and that quality of care at the end of life is ensured with the incorporation of palliative and hospice care. With regard to advancing knowledge about the quality of cancer care, recommendations included the need for investment in clinical trials to address questions about cancer care management, a cancer data system to provide quality benchmarks for use by care systems, and national studies of patients with cancer assessing patterns of cancer care and factors associated with good care. With regard to overcoming barriers in access to quality care, recommendations included enhanced services for under-insured and uninsured individuals to assure healthcare equity and the need for studies to determine underlying factors leading to the lack of quality cancer care for some populations.

How Is Quality Measured?

It remains clear that quality care is essential for the appropriate and effective management of cancer patients. However, as cancer therapy has evolved to include increasingly complex and specialized therapies, the assessment of what is quality care in cancer has become similarly complex. Quality of care is perceived differently depending on who is making the assessment. From the patient perspective, responsiveness to patient concerns and a strong connection with a provider can define high-quality care. From the provider perspective, a physician may perceive quality in terms of availability of therapies targeted to the disease in question and the associated outcomes. From the payer and system perspectives, quality may be perceived in terms of patient satisfaction scores, access to care, and cost measures.

Since the 1990s, the Institute of Medicine (IOM) has proposed different approaches to measure quality in cancer care [9]. These included analyzing Structural Quality, Process Quality and Outcomes Quality. Structural Quality focuses on the infrastructure in place for providing cancer care, including qualified physicians and the ability to carry out diagnostic and therapeutic procedures involved in cancer treatment. While necessary to provide good care, Structural Quality was felt to be an inadequate measure of quality. Similarly, Outcomes Quality, which monitors patient clinical and functional status as well as other statistical measurements like morbidity and mortality, was not felt to be appropriate in measuring quality due to the dependence of outcomes on factors outside medical care itself.

Ultimately, the IOM felt that Process Quality was the best approximation of quality care. This method examines exactly what providers are doing for their patient and whether they are doing it well. An example of this in cancer care would be appropriately synthesizing the latest research regarding a specific malignancy and applying the results of that research appropriately to patients. Essential to this is utilizing evidence-based professional practices, and evaluating practitioners against themselves and their peers to assess performance. This method can also account for overuse, underuse, and accurate use of therapy, all of which significantly impact patients' quality of life.

A result of the articulated focus on quality in cancer care has been the development of a number of organized initiatives that seek to understand and improve quality in cancer care across different tiers of healthcare delivery, including the National Initiative for Cancer Care Quality, the Oncology Demonstration Projects, and the Quality Oncology Practice Initiative.

National Initiative for Cancer Care Quality

The National Initiative for Cancer Care Quality (NICCQ) was developed in efforts to monitor care quality after it was discovered that many cancer patients were not receiving state-of-the-art care. The system focused on breast and colorectal cancer care in five major metropolitan areas, and factored in four key features: valid measures of care quality, privacy of individuals, a representative patient population, and multiple data sources [10].

The NICCQ defined quality measures by both performance of care as well as patient outcomes. Clinicians and hospitals were reviewed on whether they recommended or performed a particular type of care, such as diagnostic testing, surgery, or treatment, based on guidelines. Quality was investigated within five domains: diagnostic evaluation, surgery, adjuvant therapy, management of treatment toxicity, and post-treatment surveillance. For example, if a patient were to undergo emetogenic chemotherapy, then the patient should also receive anti-emetic medication as part of management of treatment toxicity. If appropriate supportive treatments were not received by a patient, then quality care was not adequately obtained. Within each of the five domains, factors such as timing, referral, testing, pathology, technical quality, and patient respect were evaluated as well.

In performing these quality measurements, it was necessary to obtain a patient sample size representative of the overall population. The NICCQ gathered participants from the American College of Surgeons' National Cancer Database, all of whom were newly diagnosed patients, regardless of other comorbidities. Over 400 patients with either breast or colorectal cancer from Atlanta, Cleveland, Houston, Kansas City, and Los Angeles were recruited. Data collection was completed via patient surveys and medical records.

The study found that on average, breast cancer patients received 85% of recommended care while colorectal cancer patients received 78% of recommended care [10]. There was no significant difference between different urban cities. While these overall statistics were better than expected, adherence to individual components of care was variable. For example, referral within the five domains of breast cancer care was only 13%, while testing reached up to 96% adherence. Post-treatment surveillance for colorectal cancer was only 50%, while adherence to pathology was 93%. This data suggests that while a large proportion of patients receive recommended care, patients are not receiving consistent care within all factors and domains recognized by the NICCQ.

This study is important in various ways. First, the study exemplifies one method for quantifying cancer care quality. In addition, the five domains of care recognized by the NICCQ can be assessed across different metropolitan areas to evaluate differences and trends on a larger scale. Such data collection enables analysis as to whether quality oncologic care varies based on socioeconomic factors, which then facilitates equal delivery of quality cancer care across populations.

Oncology Demonstration Projects

The need for greater quality care in oncology has also been recognized at a national level. The Centers for Medicare and Medicaid Services (CMS) developed a number of demonstration projects to improve early detection and treatment of cancer, known as the Oncology Demonstration Projects [11]. All projects were designed to provide additional care for cancer patients and also to collect data to see if these additional measures improve quality of life.

The first project, running from January to December 2006, was a voluntary study that focused on analyzing care provided by office-based oncologists [12]. The goal was to promote evidence-based clinical practices that were proven to lead to better outcomes, as well as to determine whether practices were following well-established guidelines. More than 5600 physicians participated in the study. It was well received because of its focus on quality of life, rather than treatment outcomes and life expectancy. Medicare and Medicaid reimbursed physicians every time s/he inquired about common adverse effects from chemotherapy treatments, such as nausea, vomiting, pain, or fatigue. Rather than treating the cancer, this project by the CMS emphasized the importance of treating the patient.

The project was not without controversy. By addressing issues such as pain, fatigue, and vomiting, the project gave incentives for physicians to treat the patient holistically, from cancer diagnosis to treatment to post-treatment care. Almost three million claims were submitted from the project, resulting in one of the most costly projects ever funded by the CMS [13]. In a review article by Doherty et al., multiple oncologists had noted difficulty using the billing system and difficulty in understanding the adherence guidelines. In addition, the time it took to look up the project's guidelines was also a variable factor in the study [14]. Concerns were raised about the requirement for coinsurance imposed on patients and about the fact that oncologists practicing in academic medical centers were not included. When the project deadline passed, the CMS Inspector General noted that the Medicare Payment Advisory Commission, having visited oncologists in five states in review of the demonstration project, found that "most oncologists did not believe it would lead to quality improvements for patients or produce any useful research findings" [13]. Centers for Medicaid and Medicare Services, as well as American Society of Clinical Oncology (ASCO), defended the costly initiative. Physician leaders within both CMS and ASCO noted that the project was a milestone in itself given that the government was taking action toward measuring and improving quality and that the initiative was the first step to measuring quality as a basis for reimbursement. Overall, the CMS and ASCO found this project to be pivotal in transitioning the focus of healthcare delivery systems toward higher quality and service toward cancer patients.

The Oncology Care Model (OCM) is an ongoing study by the CMS that focuses on effectiveness and efficiency of specialty care. This project began in June 2016, designed as a five-year model to focus on "better care, smarter spending, and healthier people" [15, 16]. In this model, physicians enter into payment arrangements that include financial and performance accountability for episodes of care surrounding chemotherapy administration. Essentially, the model tests whether additional funding for enhanced services and financial incentives for oncologists ultimately leads to decreased Medicare spending while also improving quality. There are currently 176 practices and 11 payers participating in his model. The goal is to use financial incentives to increase care coordination, appropriateness of care, and access of care for patients who have Medicare and are also undergoing chemotherapy. OCM hopes to create a model that comprehensively addresses the complex healthcare needs of chemotherapy patients [17].

The payment model starts when a patient receives chemotherapy. Medicare receives that claim and then continues to follow for a 6-month period. Practices participating in the OCM are required to undergo "practice redesign activities," which include enhanced services to the patients, such as 24/7 access to a clinician, a documented care plan for each patient, and treatment plans that are consistent with evidence-based medicine. Every practice must also use a certified electronic health record and utilize data for continuous monitoring over time. The financial incentives to providing higher quality of care include monthly enhanced financial resources to help manage and coordinate care for Medicare beneficiaries, as well as performance-based payment (PBP). The PBP is calculated based on whether the practice is providing high-quality care and reduced expenditures below a certain price. For example, if a practice were to create a plan of care for pain, the practice would be financially rewarded based on the PBP. Other services that result in financial reward include timely care, palliative/end of life care, and patient experience measures around symptom management and psychosocial care. As noted above, the goal for this oncology care model is to reduce cost while maintaining quality care.

Quality Oncology Practice Initiative

The need for expanding quality measures within oncology at the level of individual practices and practitioners has also been recognized. While physicians practicing in large practices may have had access to data about the quality of care they provided, small practice groups lacked resources for this. In 2002, ASCO launched a feasibility study among a small group of selected oncologists that focused on assessing and sharing the quality of the care they delivered by providing tools and resources needed to measure, compare, and improve their practices on an individual level. The group produced a set of criteria representing ideals that define a high-quality level of cancer care, formulated from evidence-based medical literature, as well as evidence-based standards deemed important by the group [18]. Oncologists were invited to participate in the pilot between 2002 and 2004. Data was collected by data abstractors within the practices (many of whom were research nurses). Practices generated a list of patients for chart review, including patients who had died within the previous 6 months in order to measure end-of-life quality care. Abstractors entered data into an on-line data entry system for analysis and comparison with other practices [19]. Overall, nearly 10,000 patient records were submitted.

In this initiative, certain aspects that define quality cancer care were acknowledged. For example, factors such as whether pain was addressed, whether evidence-based treatment was applied, and whether patient safety measures such as the use of flow sheets recording chemotherapy doses and blood counts were incorporated into the data for measuring quality. The study found multiple discrepancies in the way certain providers treated patients. Participants in this pilot initiative found the results universally helpful. Overall, physicians saw statistically significant variation among practices. There were differences in assessing pain in patients close to death, documentation of informed chemotherapy, and utilizing granulocytic and erythroid growth factor administration guidelines. Awareness of the variations between and within practice groups led to specific changes in practice standards and processes in individual practice groups [20].

The results of this work became the Quality Oncology Practice Initiative (QOPI) in 2006, a voluntary initiative open to all ASCO members [19]. This initiative provides resources to practice groups that enable them to use their practice data for targeted ongoing improvement in the context of a framework of national practice standards. The QOPI Certification Program for individual practices as well as consortia applying QOPI certification standards across various practice groups is the next step in the evolution of this initiative. By seeking to improve cancer patient care and provide tools to respond to evolving workplace changes, this program facilitates the goal of high-quality out-patient care for the greater oncologic population by giving individual practices standardized goals and metrics for quality cancer care [21, 22].

Recent Developments

In recent years, other groups have worked both to reevaluate the existing data on quality and to define it further. Spinks et al. set out to reevaluate the results from the 1999 IOM recommendations in their 2012 review article [23]. They found that progress had been made on all of the proposed recommendations, such as the implementation of process-oriented quality measurements of cancer care and redirecting patients to larger cancer treatment centers with more robust infrastructures for treatments. However, the group highlighted persistent gaps compared to the ideal state, in particular noting the need for stronger systems to collect and record data on care quality and outcomes in order to make further advancements in quality care. They also noted continued growth in the uninsured population at that time without sufficient growth in a supporting medical system, preventing improvement in quality care for these patients.

Certain patient-specific factors such as race, socioeconomic status, and age affect the quality of care, in part due to variable access to care. Health equity is a key component for improving quality of cancer care. The racial gap in cancer mortality is well known. Black patients have lower survival rates than white patients for every cancer type. After adjusting for sex, age, and stage at diagnosis, the relative risk of death after a cancer diagnosis is 33% higher in black patients and 51% higher in American Indians/Alaska Native patients than in white patients [1, 24]. Socioeconomic inequalities are widening, with higher mortality rates of cervical, lung, and liver cancers in poorer countries compared with affluent nations, with differences in diet, smoking rates, and health literacy as contributing factors [1]. The

1999 IOM report acknowledged the barriers to access to care and recommended focus on screening and early detection in order to obtain the greatest improvements in outcome in early stages of disease. National and state-wide programs such as the Centers for Disease Control and Prevention's National Breast and Cervical Cancer Early Detection Program seek to provide screening to the poor and uninsured. Lack of health insurance is a persistent barrier to access to cancer care, including preventive care (Agency for Healthcare Research and Quality. National Healthcare Disparities Report 2010. https://www.ahrq.gov/research/findings/nhqrdr/index.html). Progress in this area in particular has been limited, with poor access to care remaining a barrier to improvement in quality cancer care. In 2017, a joint position statement by the American Association for Cancer Research, the American Cancer Society, ASCO, and the National Cancer Institute articulated a framework for research in cancer health disparities, prioritizing focus on defining data measurement in disparities research, disparities in cancer incidence, disparities in cancer survival, improving community engagement, and disparities in cancer clinical trials [25].

Kenneth Kehl and his group explored quality from the perspective of the patient in 2015 [26]. They surveyed the patient's perceived role in treatment decision-making regarding chemotherapy, radiation, and surgery. They first determined the preferred role of the patient (whether the patient preferred to make a medical decision independently of the physician, with the physician's advice, or allow the physician to make the decision without the patient's input) and then determined what actually transpired (whether or not the patient was involved in the decision-making process). They then examined how the above preferences dictated the patient's perceived overall quality of cancer care based on a five-point rating scale. They found that patients perceived higher quality of care when the patients were included in the decision-making with the physician. This conclusion emphasizes the important role of shared decision-making in perceived quality from a patient perspective.

Multidisciplinary care teams working in patient-centered approaches have been shown to significantly influence clinical decision-making, though studies showing consequent improvement in patient outcomes such as survival are limited [23, 27, 28]. Due to lack of standard research criteria as well as variable endpoints and follow-up periods, more formal study is needed to validate the commonly held view of the value of multidisciplinary care teams. There have also been significant challenges regarding delivery of multidisciplinary care, including patient-centered factors such as health literacy, and physician limitations such as lack of resources or staffing for careful coordination of care [29, 30]. Proposed solutions include providing education to patients and providers, changing the culture of the field to incorporate more support services, and incorporating technology to aid in the coordination of care.

In 2017, Ramsdale et al. explored the concept of Process Quality in a vulnerable population further when examining the growing geriatric oncologic population [31]. They underscored the importance of perceived quality of life from the perspective of the older adult, who at baseline lives with numerous additional comorbidities and non-medical concerns that can impact the perceived quality of cancer care.

Additionally, these authors highlighted the fact that many elderly adults are excluded from clinical trials due to their comorbidities, making conclusions around quality from the existing literature difficult to apply to this population [32, 33]. Elderly patients are also more vulnerable to complications resulting from polypharmacy and often require more extended psychosocial support. Thus the elderly cancer patient population require a different standard of quality assessment compared to younger patients, a challenge the RAND Corporation responded to with the Assessing Care of Vulnerable Elders (ACOVE) project [33, 34]. While these authors continued to emphasize the importance of Process Quality, they also felt Structural Quality to be equally important and proposed the advent of the patient-centered medical home to help improve quality of cancer care for this specific population. This more robust delivery system would include multidisciplinary providers communicating together and with the patient, allowing for a stronger support and decision-making system, and increasing the overall quality of care for a medically and socioeconomically complex patient.

What Are the Mechanisms for Measuring, Reporting, and Responding to Errors and Quality Concerns in Cancer Care?

While it is important to quantify quality in cancer therapy, it is just as important to understand and report medical errors when they happen. This enables further growth and development of the medical field as well as individual practitioners, that is, a learning system. Along with measuring quality, accurate reporting and responding to medical errors is a top priority for providing the best care to cancer patients.

The Joint Commission is an independent, non-profit national organization providing voluntary accreditation programs for hospitals and healthcare providers (https://www.jointcommission.org). As such, their standards and guidelines serve as foundational measures of quality and safety in patient care throughout the United States. Their guidelines emphasize such goals as appropriately identifying patients, properly labeling all medications, and avoiding infection through adequate handwashing. While these guidelines apply to all branches of medicine rather than specifically to the cancer population, they have become the basis for quality and safety performance assessment of and by healthcare providers and institutions in a number of disease-specific areas, including cancer.

In 2018, Weingart et al. presented data on chemotherapy errors and how those errors are reported [35]. They found medical errors to occur in all parts of the care process from prescribing to administering chemotherapy, at an approximate rate of one to four per 1000 orders and affecting at least 1–3% of oncology patients. Many errors were corrected before reaching a patient, such as fixing errors in written chemotherapy orders prior to the chemotherapy being dispensed. Quantifying these medication errors became challenging due to the current reporting systems in place.

National incident reporting systems provide a larger database of organizations from which to base analysis of the most error-prone steps in the process of care [35, 36]. Individual hospitals rely on voluntary reporting systems that collect individual incidents to catalog the signal events, without clear standardized national or specialty-directed systems in place for collecting and assessing medical errors. Many institutions have utilized electronic health record (EHR) systems to aid in this reporting process, seeking to capture EHR data to support quality measurement such as errors or patient satisfaction [37]. However technical difficulties and associated cost and labor have made application in this area challenging, as these systems have been developed to support administrative and billing data needs rather than quality metrics and health outcomes [38]. Many errors thus go underreported on the national scale, while institutions that emphasize safety culture may have a proportionately higher volume of incidents reported. Finally, this review also highlighted the growing risk with oral chemotherapy taken at home, as this introduces opportunities for patient errors such as missed or wrong doses, wrong drug, poor adherence, or over-adherence. Proposed safeguards against these types of errors include involving patients and families with education and empowerment to recognize and prevent errors [35, 39].

Responding to these errors has been a top priority for many. In recent years, the American Society of Oncology (ASCO) and Oncology Nursing Society (ONS) have jointly set standards for safe chemotherapy administration [40]. Originally published in 2009 and updated semi-annually, these recommendations emphasize the importance of packaging of chemotherapies in a clear way, standardization of prescribing including electronic orders without the use of confusing abbreviations, and confirmation between physicians. These also encourage patient participation in their own care both to prevent errors and to report errors if they occur. These strategies provide a framework by which organizations can improve their practice, though many institutions have yet to fully adopt these recommendations.

Discussion

Since the original call to action by the IOM in 1999, there has been significant progress in understanding and measuring quality care for cancer patients. Areas in which most progress is evident are those that can be driven by professional societies and/or independent practice groups. We have seen such groups as ASCO develop strategies to safely administer chemotherapy; their propositions are slowly becoming standard of care for hospitals and infusion centers. The NICCQ has proposed clear strategies on how to quantify high-quality cancer care by narrowing the focus of study to concrete outcomes in evaluation and treatment of specific malignancies. Physician practices have evolved as professional society guidelines have emphasized the study and improvement of quality of cancer care. Establishing practice metrics and incentivizing practitioners to measure quality, such as in the Oncology Demonstration Projects, has led to data collection and reporting on the quality of treatment and harms to patients. Recognition of the importance of shared decision-making has led to inclusion of patient perceptions as a component in determining quality metrics. As a whole, the field of oncology is shifting toward understanding and delivering quality care based on clear guidelines, with individual practitioners at the frontline.

Even with all the available data and strong intentions of practitioners to provide only quality care, it remains clear that there is still much progress to be made. One clear weakness that remains central to the issue of quality is the lack of a national database and organized collection system that could assist hospitals to efficiently document gaps in quality care. Such a system would allow for physicians and other providers to self-audit and improve the quality of their care. In addition, research in the field of quality has remained a difficult challenge due to the lack of uniform guidelines and standards for research in quality cancer care. The Quality Oncology Practice Initiative is a first step in that direction by setting specific quality-defining criteria for reporting and analysis, highlighting discrepancies in multiple aspects of practice. However, this initiative needs further development with increased data input and cooperation across oncology societies to create multi-disciplinary feedback and guidelines for practitioners delivering complex cancer care. Many of the studies reviewed in this chapter indicate that some guidelines are not yet being consistently utilized in direct patient care. Developing an internal system with the aim of designing thoughtful and practical studies would help develop an effective learning database for the practitioners and those who study the field.

Much of the challenge to advancing the study of quality of cancer care lies in the complex system in which cancer care is delivered. Our healthcare system is largely fragmented in a number of respects including care access and care delivery. We continue to see alarming inequity of care between racial and socioeconomic groups, with patients in certain groups receiving inferior care. Health equity is a complex topic made even more controversial when considered in the setting of larger socio-economic forces affecting our society, of which healthcare is only one portion. Multiple factors, including but not limited to education and literacy, availability and access to care, and language and cultural barriers, need to be considered when treating patients across socioeconomic and demographic boundaries. Currently there are no guidelines in place for improving the disparities in cancer care. In addition, work reviewed in this chapter indicates that patients need to partake in shared decision-making in order to perceive higher quality of care. This can only occur if patients can understand the basics on their care from the beginning of diagnosis. Understanding social disparities and the knowledge gaps of patients is crucial for providing high-quality care. In contrast to the focus of this chapter, the current national spotlight is still on the efficacy of care rather than the quality of care delivered or whether there is equipoise of health determinants. Nevertheless, the striking mortality differences between socioeconomic groups highlight the importance as well as the challenge of addressing health equity in our society.

While progress has been made, there is still much to be learned regarding both the study of the quality of cancer care and the actual delivery of quality cancer care. Many groups have developed theories and ideas on what constitutes high-quality care, some of which are already in effect in the healthcare system. Many patients continue to experience inferior care. Ensuring quality care for cancer patients remains a significant challenge even in the setting of good intentions and hard work. With further research and resources, we will continue to see forward progress along the road to the time when all patients receive the same high quality of care as they face the life-changing challenge of cancer.

References

1. Siegel RL, Miller KD, Jemal A. Cancer statistics, 2019. CA Cancer J Clin. 2019;69:7–34. https://doi.org/10.3322/caac.21551.
2. Mariotto AB, Yabroff KR, Shao Y, Feuer EJ, Brown ML. Projections of the cost of cancer care in the United States: 2010–2020. J Natl Cancer Inst. 2011;103:117–28. https://doi.org/10.1093/jnci/djq495.
3. Bradley CJ, et al. Antineoplastic treatment of advanced-stage non-small-cell lung cancer: treatment, survival, and spending (2000 to 2011). J Clin Oncol. 2017;35:529–35. https://doi.org/10.1200/jco.2016.69.4166.
4. Bradley CJ, et al. Trends in the treatment of metastatic colon and rectal cancer in elderly patients. Med Care. 2016;54:490–7. https://doi.org/10.1097/mlr.0000000000000510.
5. Yabroff KR, Gansler T, Wender RC, Cullen KJ, Brawley OW. Minimizing the burden of cancer in the United States: goals for a high-performing health care system. CA Cancer J Clin. 2019; https://doi.org/10.3322/caac.21556.
6. Kohn LT, Corrigan JM, Donaldson MS, editors. To err is human: building a safer health system. Washington DC: National Academies Press (US); 2000.
7. Institute of Medicine (US) Committe on Quality of Health Care in America. Crossing the quality chasm: a new health system for the twenty-first century. Washington (DC): National Academies Press (US); 2001.
8. Hewitt M, Simone JV, editors. Ensuring quality cancer care. Washington DC: National Academies Press (US); 1999.
9. Moulton G. IOM report on quality of cancer care highlights need for research, data expansion. Institute of Medicine. J Natl Cancer Inst. 1999;91:761–2.
10. Malin JL, et al. Results of the National Initiative for Cancer Care Quality: how can we improve the quality of cancer care in the United States? J Clin Oncol. 2006;24:626–34. https://doi.org/10.1200/jco.2005.03.3365.
11. Twombly R. Medicare demonstration projects acknowledge evidence-based medicine in cancer care. J Natl Cancer Inst. 2005;97:6–7. https://doi.org/10.1093/jnci/97.1.6.
12. Announces CMS. Medicare oncology demonstration project. J Oncol Pract. 2006;2:25.
13. Erickson J. Chemotherapy demonstration project: CMS & ASCO defend 'critical first step'. Oncol Times. 2006;28:10–2. https://doi.org/10.1097/01.COT.0000303881.00250.f9.
14. Doherty J, Tanamor M, Feigert J, Goldberg-Dey J. Oncologists' experience in reporting cancer staging and guideline adherence: lessons from the 2006 medicare oncology demonstration. J Oncol Pract. 2010;6:56–9. https://doi.org/10.1200/jop.091083.
15. Associates A. First Annual Report from the Evaluation of the Oncology Care Model: Baseline Period; 2018.
16. Oncology Care Model. Center for Medicare & Medicaid Services.
17. Oncology Care Model. Center for Medicare & Medicaid Services Newsroom-Fact Sheets.
18. Neuss MN, et al. A process for measuring the quality of cancer care: the Quality Oncology Practice Initiative. J Clin Oncol. 2005;23:6233–9. https://doi.org/10.1200/jco.2005.05.948.

19. McNiff K. The quality oncology practice initiative: assessing and improving care within the medical oncology practice. J Oncol Pract. 2006;2:26–30. https://doi.org/10.1200/jop.2006.2.1.26.
20. Jacobson JO, et al. Improvement in oncology practice performance through voluntary participation in the Quality Oncology Practice Initiative. J Clin Oncol. 2008;26:1893–8. https://doi.org/10.1200/jco.2007.14.2992.
21. McNiff KK, Bonelli KR, Jacobson JO. Quality oncology practice initiative certification program: overview, measure scoring methodology, and site assessment standards. J Oncol Pract. 2009;5:270–6. https://doi.org/10.1200/jop.091045.
22. Blayney DW, et al. Development and future of the American Society of Clinical Oncology's Quality Oncology Practice Initiative. J Clin Oncol. 2014;32:3907–13. https://doi.org/10.1200/jco.2014.56.8899.
23. Spinks T, et al. Ensuring quality cancer care: a follow-up review of the Institute of Medicine's 10 recommendations for improving the quality of cancer care in America. Cancer. 2012;118:2571–82. https://doi.org/10.1002/cncr.26536.
24. DeSantis CE, Miller KD, Goding Sauer A, Jemal A, Siegel RL. Cancer statistics for African Americans, 2019. CA Cancer J Clin. 2019;69(3):211–33. https://doi.org/10.3322/caac.21555.
25. Polite BN, et al. Charting the Future of Cancer Health Disparities Research: A Position Statement from the American Association for Cancer Research, the American Cancer Society, the American Society of Clinical Oncology, and the National Cancer Institute. Cancer Res. 2017;77:4548–55. https://doi.org/10.1158/0008-5472.can-17-0623.
26. Kehl KL, et al. Association of actual and preferred decision roles with patient-reported quality of care: shared decision making in cancer care. JAMA Oncol. 2015;1:50–8. https://doi.org/10.1001/jamaoncol.2014.112.
27. Taylor C, et al. Multidisciplinary team working in cancer: what is the evidence? Br Med J. 2010;340:c951. https://doi.org/10.1136/bmj.c951.
28. Croke JM, El-Sayed S. Multidisciplinary management of cancer patients: chasing a shadow or real value? an overview of the literature. Curr Oncol (Toronto, ON). 2012;19:e232–8. https://doi.org/10.3747/co.19.944.
29. Balogh EP, et al. Patient-centered cancer treatment planning: improving the quality of oncology care. Summary of an Institute of Medicine workshop. Oncologist. 2011;16:1800–5. https://doi.org/10.1634/theoncologist.2011-0252.
30. Levit L, Smith AP, Benz EJ, Ferrell B. Ensuring quality cancer care through the oncology workforce. J Oncol Pract. 2010;6:7–11. https://doi.org/10.1200/jop.091067.
31. Ramsdale EE, Csik V, Chapman AE, Naeim A, Canin B. Improving quality and value of cancer care for older adults. Am Soc Clin Oncol Educ Book. American Society of Clinical Oncology. Annual Meeting. 2017;37:383–93. https://doi.org/10.14694/edbk_175442.
32. Wenger NS, Shekelle PG. Assessing care of vulnerable elders: ACOVE project overview. Ann Intern Med. 2001;135:642–6.
33. Wenger NS, Roth CP, Shekelle P. Introduction to the assessing care of vulnerable elders-3 quality indicator measurement set. J Am Geriatr Soc. 2007;55 Suppl 2:S247–52. https://doi.org/10.1111/j.1532-5415.2007.01328.x.
34. Shekelle PG, MacLean CH, Morton SC, Wenger NS. Acove quality indicators. Ann Intern Med. 2001;135:653–67.
35. Weingart SN, Zhang L, Sweeney M, Hassett M. Chemotherapy medication errors. Lancet Oncol. 2018;19:e191–9. https://doi.org/10.1016/s1470-2045(18)30094-9.
36. Rinke ML, Shore AD, Morlock L, Hicks RW, Miller MR. Characteristics of pediatric chemotherapy medication errors in a national error reporting database. Cancer. 2007;110:186–95. https://doi.org/10.1002/cncr.22742.
37. Spinks T, et al. Delivering high-quality Cancer care: the critical role of quality measurement. Healthcare (Amsterdam, Netherlands). 2014;2:53–62. https://doi.org/10.1016/j.hjdsi.2013.11.003.

38. Spinks TE, et al. Improving cancer care through public reporting of meaningful quality measures. Health Affairs (Project Hope). 2011;30:664–72. https://doi.org/10.1377/hlthaff.2011.0089.
39. Schwappach DL, Wernli M. Medication errors in chemotherapy: incidence, types and involvement of patients in prevention. A review of the literature. Eur J Cancer Care. 2010;19:285–92. https://doi.org/10.1111/j.1365-2354.2009.01127.x.
40. Neuss MN, et al. 2016 Updated American Society of Clinical Oncology/Oncology Nursing Society Chemotherapy Administration Safety Standards, Including Standards for Pediatric Oncology. J Oncol Pract. 2016;12:1262–71. https://doi.org/10.1200/jop.2016.017905.

Chapter 7
Quality Measures for Palliative Care

Tamara Vesel and Jatin Dave

Importance

Measuring quality is critical for evaluating and improving health and health care delivery. This is especially important in care of patients at end of life due to ongoing variability in care [1, 2]. Up to 27% of Medicare budget in the United States is being spent in the last 12 months of beneficiary's lives [3]. Due to advances in health care and public health, more people are living and dying with chronic diseases. This change requires proactive exploration of patient preferences and priorities, careful care planning and decision making, and a comprehensive approach to care to meet the needs of patients with progressive chronic illness. Despite significant efforts and recent improvements, studies have demonstrated ongoing gaps in the quality of care with avoidable physical and emotional suffering and variability in the care of patients with chronic illness [4]. Recent research supports that early palliative care interventions improve the patient's outcomes [5].

Quality measurement compares the care provided with the consistent and current professional standards in order to increase the likelihood of desired outcomes. Meaningful measurement of quality is the foundation of an accountable and high-performing health care system. This is not only essential for improving care but also for public reporting (with benchmarking for comparison), incentive payment alignment, as well as the accreditation/certification process of health care systems. Valid (supported by evidence), clinically meaningful (measuring what matters), actionable (under the control of clinicians), reliable (reproducible from center to center),

T. Vesel (✉)
Division of Palliative Care, Department of Medicine, Tufts Medical Center, Tufts University School of Medicine, Boston, MA, USA
e-mail: tvesel@tuftsmedicalcenter.org

J. Dave
Division of Palliative Care, Department of Medicine, Tufts Medical Center, Tufts University School of Medicine, New England Quality Care Alliance, Boston, MA, USA

D. N. Salem (ed.), *Quality Measures*, https://doi.org/10.1007/978-3-030-37145-6_7

feasible (easily measurable), aligned (across payers), and comparable (for benchmarking) quality measures are at the center of performance improvement efforts. Quality measurement is important from three perspectives:

1. To provide optimal clinical care
2. For continuous performance improvement
3. Clinical research

With recent health care reform in United States, there is growing awareness of the need to balance triple aim (better care, better health, and lower cost) for optimal health care [6]. Recently this framework has been expanded to a quadruple aim with the addition of fourth aim focusing on clinical satisfaction to incorporate improving the work life of those who deliver this care [7]. Palliative care improves care and health and has the potential to lower cost, as well as improve work–life balance of health care professionals [8, 9]. Health care organizations are increasingly measuring their success by benchmarking their performance on these quadruple aims and therefore it is important to review quality measures related to palliative and hospice care in this context [10].

The field of quality measurement is rapidly evolving with focus on what matters from patients' perspective in addition to what matters from health care system and policy standpoint [11–13]. The challenge is measuring changes of the patient's health over time as well as looking at the whole person while measuring quality [14]. We are increasingly realizing that patient care, especially palliative care (and good care in general), often demands clinicians to focus on outcomes beyond usual focus on survival and health [15]. Therefore it is imperative to keep a balanced perspective especially when measuring quality of palliative care so we find equilibrium between measuring what matters vs. measuring accurately how we influence the human aspect of the process of dying persons and their families.

Despite multiple studies showing significant gaps in performance and higher costs associated with end-of-life care, until recently there was paucity of concise portfolio of valid and clinically relevant (applicable across all ages, settings of care, disciplines/ diseases, and capturing multiple domain of suffering) quality measures [16–25].

In this chapter, we describe the challenges and opportunities for quality measurement for palliative care, list of high-value quality measures in palliative care, and efforts to operationalize the measurement via registries.

Challenges and Opportunities for Quality Measurement in EOLC

Challenges

There is lack of consensus regarding the operational definition of palliative care, there are several terms used to describe this approach to care such as serious illness care, hospice (and end-of-life care), supportive care, and advanced illness care [26, 27].

A major challenge for measuring quality of palliative care is defining the denominator for each indicator/measure (i.e., the group of patients to which the indicator is applicable) [27].

National Quality Forum (NQF) states: "Palliative care generally refers to patient and family-centered care that optimizes quality of life by anticipating, preventing, and alleviating suffering across the continuum of patient's illness" [28]. Palliative care accomplishes these goals by

1. Expert assessment and management of symptoms
2. Psychosocial and spiritual support of patient and caregivers and
3. Careful exploration of patients' goals/preferences. This is achieved by alignment of care plan with careful decision support and coordination of care.

Hospice is another term with many different meanings globally, but in the United States, hospice is often used as a benefit/program caring for patients who are in the last 6 months of their terminal illness.

We are going to use the term "palliative care" to cover all these concepts broadly for the remaining of this chapter. This is based on the assumption that although hospice and palliative are distinct types of care, they have similar foundational attributes, such as the interdisciplinary team-based care focusing on the whole person, on quality of life, and on dignified death. From the measurement standpoint, valid outcome measures in palliative care require adjustment of patient characteristics and preferences.

Defining the population who benefits from palliative care is also challenging. Recently "serious illness" is proposed as a common phrase to describe this population. Serious illness is defined as "a health condition that carries a high risk of mortality and either negatively impacts a person's daily function or quality of life or excessively strains their caregiver" [24]. Seriously ill patients need care that is proactive, seamless and aligned with patient preferences especially with change in health status/needs.

Opportunities

Recent efforts to define "gold standard" measures of palliative care will advance the field with consensus on quality measures with acceptable sensitivity and specificity and balance between quality measures across all settings/population vs. more specific measures for specific groups.

Recent evidence suggests that the current system of quality measurement in the United States (in general – not specific to palliative care) is unnecessarily costly [29]. An average US physician spends 785 hours annually on quality measurement activities, and collectively the health care system is spending more than $15.4 billion reporting quality measures to various organizations [30]. There has been growing awareness and urgency to align measures, use valid/standard measures, and make them easier to report [31, 32]. Integrated palliative care registries, national use of standard measures and benchmarking are all significant opportunities to improve quality measurement for patients in need for palliative care [33, 34].

List of High-Value Quality Measures (See Table 7.1)

In 2001, health care leaders from across the country met to develop consensus on standards of palliative care and practice guidelines. This initiative resulted in the first edition of National Consensus Project's Clinical Practice (NCP) Guidelines in 2004 [35]. This effort formalized available evidence-based processes and practices and described core concepts, structures, and processes necessary for quality care. Eight domains of practice were identified, and key elements/recommendations within each domain for the provision of safe and reliable high-quality palliative care were agreed upon. The NCP guidelines set expectations for excellence among clinicians providing palliative care. These guidelines have been updated several times with the fourth edition published in 2018 [36]. Several systematic reviews have also summarized about 20 sets or frameworks with more than 350 quality measures for palliative care [37].

In 2006, National Quality Forum (NQF) identified palliative care and hospice as a national priority area for health care quality improvement, adopted the NCP Clinical Practice Guidelines for Quality Palliative Care, and created 38 preferred practices within the domains described in NCP guidelines [38]. In 2012, NQF endorsed 14 quality measures for palliative and end-of-life care [39].

American Academy of Hospice and Palliative Medicine (AAHPM) and Hospice and Palliative Nurses Association (HPNA) partnered on a sequential consensus project on Measuring What Matters (MWM) and assembled a list of 10 consensus indicators for internal measurement of quality in the settings serving hospice and palliative patients [40]. The MWM team identified existing indicators (about 75 measures) available in the public domain as of October 2013 and tested them for reliability and validity. The Technical Advisory Panel (TAP) rated these indicators on their scientific soundness and referred a set of 34 indicators for review by the Clinical User Panel (CUP). The CUP rated those indicators based on three dimensions:

1. How meaningful is this for patients/families?
2. How actionable is this for providers/organizations?
3. How large is the potential impact?

The CUP achieved consensus on the top 12 indicators for further input. With feedback from AAHPM and HPNA members and advocacy groups the final set of 10 indicators across 6 domains was finalized [41]. There were no measures selected for social or cultural aspects of care or care of the imminently dying patients.

Several international frameworks have also informed the quality improvement movement such as United Kingdom's Department of Health recommended 34

Table 7.1 Evolution of quality measures focusing on palliative care

2014 NCP's domains	2012 NQF endorsed quality measures	2015 AAHPM and HPNA measuring what matters measures
1. *Structure and Processes of Care* – interdisciplinary team assessment based on patient/family goals of care; prognosis; disposition (level of care – Inpatient unit, home); safety		*Comprehensive assessment* 1. Hospice: Percentage of patients enrolled for more than 7 days for whom a comprehensive assessment was completed within 5 days of admission (documentation of prognosis, functional assessment, screening for physical and psychological symptoms, and assessment of social and spiritual concerns). 2. Seriously ill patients receiving specialty palliative care in an acute hospital setting: Percent of all patients admitted for more than 1 day who had comprehensive assessment (screening for physical symptoms and discussion of the patient/family's emotional or psychological needs) completed within 24 hours of admission.
2. *Physical Aspects of Care* – pain, dyspnea, nausea/vomiting, fatigue, constipation, performance status, medical diagnoses, medications (add/wean/titrate)	1. 1634: Hospice and Palliative Care – Pain Screening (UNC) (paired with measure 1637) 2. 1637: Hospice and Palliative Care – Pain Assessment (UNC) (paired with measure 1634) 3. 1617: Patients treated with an opioid who are given a bowel regimen (RAND) 4. 1628: Patients with advanced cancer assessed for pain at outpatient visits (RAND) 5. 1638: Hospice and Palliative Care- Dyspnea Treatment (UNC) (paired with measure 1639) 6. 1639: Hospice and Palliative Care – Dyspnea Screening (UNC) (paired with measure 1638) 7. 1625: Hospitalized patients who die an expected death with an ICD that has been deactivated (RAND)	*Screening for Physical Symptoms* 3. Percentage of seriously ill patients receiving specialty palliative care in an acute hospital setting for more than 1 day or patients enrolled in hospice for more than 7 days who had a screening for physical symptoms (pain, dyspnea, nausea, and constipation) during the admission visit. *Pain Treatment* 4. For seriously ill patients receiving specialty palliative care in an acute hospital setting for more than 1 day or patients enrolled in hospice for more than 7 days who screened positive for moderate-to-severe pain on admission, the percent with medication or non-medication treatment, within 24 hours of screening. *Dyspnea Screening and Management* 5. Percentage of patients with advanced chronic or serious life-threatening illnesses who are screened for dyspnea. For those who are diagnosed with moderate or severe dyspnea, a documented plan of care to manage dyspnea exists (ambulatory physician care)

(continued)

Table 7.1 (continued)

2004 NCP's eight domains	2012 NQF endorsed quality measures	
3. *Psychological Aspects of Care* – anxiety, depression, delirium, cognitive impairment; stress, anticipatory grief, coping strategies; pharm/non-pharm treatment; patient/family grief/bereavement		*Discussion of Emotional or Psychological Needs* 6. Percentage of seriously ill patients receiving specialty palliative care in an acute hospital setting for more than 1 day or patients enrolled in hospice for more than 7 days with chart documentation of a discussion of emotional or psychological needs.
4. *Social Aspects of Care* – family/friend communication/interaction/ support; caregiver crisis	8. 0208: Family Evaluation of Hospice Care (NHPCO) (maintenance) 9. 1632: CARE – Consumer Assessments and Reports of End of Life (Center for Gerontology and Health Care Research) 10. 1623: Bereaved Family Survey (PROMISE Center)	No Indicator
5. *Spiritual Aspects of Care* – spiritual/religious/ existential; hopes/fears; forgiveness	12. 1647: Percentage of hospice patients with documentation in the clinical record of a discussion of spiritual/religious concerns or documentation that the patient/caregiver did not want to discuss (Deyta)	*Discussion of Spiritual/Religious Concerns* 7. Percentage of hospice patients with documentation of a discussion of spiritual/ religious concerns or documentation that the patient/ caregiver/family did not want to discuss
6. *Cultural Aspects of Care* – language, ritual, dietary, other		No Indicator

7. *Care of the Imminently Dying (reworded as Care of the Patient at the End of Life)* – presence; recognition and communication to patient/family education/ normalization; prognosis (e.g., hours to days, very few days, etc.)	13. 0209: Comfortable dying (NHPCO) (maintenance)	No Indicator
8. *Ethical and Legal Aspects of Care* – decision maker; advance directives	14. 1626: Patients admitted to the ICU who have care preferences documented (RAND) 15. 1641: Hospice and Palliative Care – Treatment Preferences (UNC)	*Documentation of Surrogate* 8. Percentage of seriously ill patients receiving specialty palliative care in an acute hospital setting for more than 1 day or patients enrolled in hospice for more than 2 days with name and contact information for surrogate decision maker in the chart or documentation that there is no surrogate. *Treatment Preferences* 9. Percentage of seriously ill patients receiving specialty palliative care in an acute hospital setting for more than 1 day or patients enrolled in hospice for more than 7 days with chart documentation of preferences for life-sustaining treatments. *Care Consistency with Documented Care Preferences* 10. If a vulnerable elder has specific treatment preferences (e.g., a DNR order, no tube feeding, or no hospital transfer) documented in a medical record, then these treatment preferences should be followed.

indicators as well as additional frameworks/measurement sets from Australia, Denmark, and the Netherlands among others [42–46]. The majority of these quality indicator frameworks were developed through an iterative process with literature review and expert consensus. There is need for balancing generic measures for measurement across the settings and conditions vs. having more specific quality measures for particular settings/conditions.

Hospice Quality Reporting Program (HQRP) in the US: Section 3004 of the Patient Protection and Affordable Care Act authorized the Secretary of the Department of Health and Human Services to establish a quality reporting program for hospices [47]. On July 1, 2014, hospices nationwide began submitting the Hospice Item Set (HIS), a standardized patient-level data collection instrument used to collect the data needed for the calculation of the seven quality measures [48]. These measures focus on important patient care processes around hospice admission that are clinically recommended or required in the hospice conditions of participation including discussion of patient preferences regarding life-sustaining treatments; care for spiritual and existential concerns; and management of pain (including opioid-induced constipation) and dyspnea. CMS also implemented the Consumer Assessment of Healthcare Providers and Systems (CAHPS) Hospice Survey in 2015, which addresses additional aspects of care that consumers and other stakeholders find important [49]. The information includes data on communication, coordination, and whether care provided was concordant with patient and family wishes in a culturally appropriate way. In 2017, CMS implemented Hospice and Palliative Care Composite Process Measure – *Comprehensive Assessment at Admission*, this measure combines all care processes captured by the seven HIS measures and reflects how many patients receive all the screening and assessment in a timely manner after admission to hospice [50]. The national average on this measure for the period from April 1, 2017, to March 31, 2018, was 84.2%. On August 16, 2017, CMS unveiled the new *Hospice Compare* website [51]. The goal of Hospice Compare is to help consumers compare hospice providers on their performance and assist consumers in making decisions that are right for them.

The National Quality Forum (NQF)–endorsed seven Hospice Item Set (HIS) quality measures initially displayed on Hospice Compare are:

1. Hospice and Palliative Care – Treatment Preferences – NQF #1641
2. Hospice and Palliative Care – Beliefs/Values Addressed – NQF #1647
3. Hospice and Palliative Care – Pain Screening – NQF #1634
4. Hospice and Palliative Care – Pain Assessment – NQF #1637
5. Hospice and Palliative Care – Dyspnea Screening – NQF #1639
6. Hospice and Palliative Care – Dyspnea Treatment – NQF #1638
7. Hospice and Palliative Care – Patients treated with opioids who are given a bowel regimen – NQF #1617

National and International Organizational Efforts in Operationalizing Measurement Via Registries

Gliklich et al. define registry as "an organized system that uses observational study methods to collect uniform data (clinical and other) to evaluate specific outcomes for a population defined by a particular disease, condition, or exposure, and that serves one or more predetermined scientific, clinical, and/or policy purposes" [52].

There have been multiple registries in the US and internationally to measure outcomes of palliative care (see Table 7.2) [44, 46, 53–62]. Registries' goal is to assess the quality of care with appropriate benchmarks and help to develop collaborative improvements in quality of care. With the growth of these registries, there is a growing need and opportunity to integrate information into a more coordinated system while still maintaining the ability to capture the local context of various subsystems.

We would like to review two registries in details – one in the US and one in Australia. To our knowledge, there is no global comprehensive palliative care registry comparing palliative and end-of-life data from all over the world.

CAPC Registry

Center for Advanced Palliative Care (CAPC) registry was established in 1999 as a national program office of the Robert Wood Johnson Foundation in order to improve the care of patients within the health care system in the US.

CAPC's mission is to increase availability of quality palliative care services for people living with serious illness. CAPC is the only repository of the data on hospital-based palliative care team characteristics and best practices in the US.

The registry uses three key metrics:

1. Palliative care service penetration – that is initial palliative care consults as a percentage of annual hospital admissions (mean penetration rate changed from 2.5% in 2008 to 5.3% in 2017).
2. Staffing levels/Interdisciplinary teams – the mean FTE (full-time equivalent for palliative care members) per palliative care team in 2017 was 8.3.

    CAPC also provides information on funding source for staffing – example in 2017 – 90% of physicians, APRNs, RNs, and social workers were funded through the palliative care budget while nearly 30% of chaplains were paid from other budgets or were volunteers.
3. Length of Stay and Time to Consult: in 2017 – average length of stay for patients who were discharged alive was 11.4 days with mean time from admission to palliative consult was 5.5 days; for patients who died the mean length of stay was 10.9 with time from admission to consult being 6 days.

CAPC registry helps individual programs to establish and grow in their institution while their data are being compared with national benchmarks. The use of this registry data and national comparisons can be helpful to advocate for the program

Table 7.2 Example of palliative care registries

Registry name	Countries covered	Population/settings of care focused	Website	In existence since
National Palliative Care Registry	US	US palliative care programs across the continuum of care (membership not required)	https://registry.capc.org	1999
Palliative Care Quality Network (PCQN)	US	Member organizations: Hospital programs	https://www.pcqn.org/	2013
Quality Data Collection Tool for Palliative Care (QDACT-PC)	US	Member organizations: US palliative care programs across the continuum of care	http://www.gpcqa.org/qdact	2016
Coalition of Hospices Organized to Investigate Comparative Effectiveness (CHOICE)	US	R21 Grant involving 12 hospices in 11 states	Report is published and not ongoing. https://healthit.ahrq.gov/ahrq-funded-projects/choice-coalition-hospices-organized-investigate-comparative-effectiveness/final-report	2012 (ended in 2014)
Palliative Care Quality Registry The Swedish Register of Palliative Care (SRPC)	Sweden	Palliative care program in Sweden	http://palliativ.se/	2005
National Hospice and Palliative Care Registry	Germany	Outpatient and inpatient hospice and palliative care in Germany	http://www.hospiz-palliativ-register.de	2009
Palliative Care Registry	Winnipeg	All palliative care patients in Winnipeg	http://mchp-appserv.cpe.umanitoba.ca/viewConcept.php?conceptID=1414	2000
The European Sentinel GP Networks Monitoring End-of-Life Care (EURO SENTIMELC)	Belgium, Netherlands, Italy, and Spain	Covering 2–4% of the general population in each country	http://www.endoflifecare.be/project/euro-sentimelc	2009–2010
Australian Palliative Care Outcomes Collaborative (PCOC)	Australia	Hospitals and Primary care network in Australia	https://ahsri.uow.edu.au/pcoc/about/index.html	2009
Danish Palliative Care Database (DPD)	Denmark	All patients who received palliative care in Denmark	http://www.dmcgpal.dk/	2010

on the business/administrative level: to tie operational metrics and quality improvement, diversify palliative care team, and track operational metrics over time. The other incentive for the programs to collect data is their contribution to growing field of research and being profiled in a national registry.

Recent effort to integrate all the organizations involved in quality registries in palliative care in the US led to the development of Palliative Care Quality Collaborative (PCQC) [63]. With the support of a grant from the Gordon and Betty Moore Foundation, five organizations (American Academy of Hospice and Palliative Care Medicine (AAHPM), Center to Advance Palliative Care (CAPC) and affiliated National Palliative Care Research Center (NPCRC), Global Palliative Care Quality Alliance (GPCQA), and Palliative Care Quality Network (PCQN)) convened to develop a quality improvement organization (the Palliative Care Quality Collaborative) with a unified registry to capture both program- and patient-level quality data, to improve the care of patients with serious illness, including those receiving palliative care.

Australian Palliative Care Outcomes Collaboration (PCOC) Registry

The Palliative Care Outcomes Collaboration (PCOC) is an Australian national registry that implements standardized clinical assessment tools to measure and benchmark patient outcomes in palliative care in Australia. Participation in PCOC is voluntary and it provides assistance to palliative care providers in their effort to improve their clinical practice. This is achieved via the PCOC patient outcome improvement framework which is designed to:

- Provide clinicians with the tools to systematically assess individual patient experiences using validated clinical assessment tools
- Define a common clinical language between palliative care providers to support assessment and care planning
- Facilitate the routine collection of national palliative care data to drive quality improvement through reporting and benchmarking
- Provide regular patient outcome reports and workshops to facilitate service-to-service benchmarking, and support research using the PCOC longitudinal database

Australian registry is funded by the Australian government and Department of Health and was initiated in 2009. Their assessment framework incorporates five validated clinical assessment tools:

- Palliative Care Phase
- Palliative Care Problem Severity Score (PCPSS)
- Symptom Assessment Scale (SAS)
- Australia-Modified Karnofsky Performance Status (AKPS) Scale
- Resource Utilisation Groups – Activities of Daily Living (RUG-ADL)

These are not only robust detailed data, these efforts represent real-life outcomes of over 40,000 Australians who die an expected death every year. Individual data are compared with benchmark data and reported on annual bases to the participating organization.

Participation in PCOC provides evidence for organizations and palliative care services to meet core actions in the standards of care for patients requiring palliative care in Australia and beyond.

Future Research and Directions

Despite the inevitable nature of death and growing use of hospice and palliative care services, measuring performance for palliative care is complex as the care is frequently delivered at a number of sites including home, clinic, hospital, and long-term care facilities.

Measures to assess quality of palliative care and hospice must capture key aspects important to patients and families and reflect comprehensive multidisciplinary outcomes of care. To fill this gap, Patient and Family Reported Outcome Measures (PROM) are often used via standardized questionnaires given to patients or families. PROMs are emerging as the gold standard of identifying subjective experience in palliative care. PROMs are increasingly used in palliative care and likely will become the future of quality measures of the patient's and family's subjective experiences.

In 2018, Centers for Medicare and Medicaid Services (CMS) awarded $5.5 Million grant over 3 years to AAHPM, the National Coalition for Hospice and Palliative Care, and RAND to develop Patient-Reported Measures for Community-Based Palliative Care [64]. These measures will be used for CMS's Quality Payment Programs (QPP). Along with this new measures development project, the unification of palliative care quality registries, new testing methodologies to identify the population with serious illness for inclusion in quality measures, and growing alternative payment models for palliative care have potential to enhance the field of quality measurement for palliative care. Center for Advance Palliative Care (CAPC) in partnership with National Quality Forum (NQF) is coordinating efforts to develop a national strategic plan to incentivize and/or require delivery of high-quality care for people with serious illness and their families via the Serious Illness Quality Alignment Hub ("the Hub").

The Hub has four tracks, each focused on developing requirements and/or incentives for access to high-quality palliative care for appropriate patient populations: Needs Assessment, Accountability Committee, Quality Measurement Committee, and National Serious Illness Projects. The hub is focusing on how to help health care organizations better align between what they are currently held accountable for and what consistent palliative care approaches can deliver. The Hub will be finalizing a set of recommended metrics that can be used by purchasers, health insurers, and ACOs to hold themselves and their palliative care teams accountable for high-quality care consistent with national guidelines.

Despite the tremendous progress made in the field of quality measurement of palliative care, there are still significant gaps in holistically measuring palliative care. For example, there is known gap due to not having validated measures in social or cultural aspects of care or care of the imminently dying patients. With growing and emerging field of quality measurement in palliative care, we expect to see more uniform integration of these measures into standard quality measure sets used by all payers [65–70].

References

1. Dying in America. Improving quality and honoring individual preferences near the end-of-life. Washington, DC: National Academy of Sciences; 2015.
2. NIH State-of-the-Science Conference Statement on improving end-of-life care. NIH Consens State Sci Statements. 2004;21(3):1–26.
3. Riley GF, Lubitz JD. Long-term trends in medicare payments in the last year of life. Health Serv Res. 2010;45(2):565–76.
4. Barnato AE, Herndon MB, Anthony DL, Gallagher PM, Skinner JS, Bynum JP, Fisher ES. Are regional variations in end-of-life care intensity explained by patient preferences? A Study of the US Medicare Population. Med Care. 2007;45(5):386–93.
5. Kavalieratos D, Corbelli J, Zhang D, et al. Association between palliative care and patient and caregiver outcomes: a systematic review and meta-analysis. JAWA. 2016;316(20):2104–14.
6. Whittington JW, Nolan K, Lewis N, Torres T. Pursuing the triple aim: the first 7 years. Milbank Q. 2015;93(2):263–300.
7. Bodenheimer T, Sinsky C. From triple to quadruple aim: care of the patient requires care of the provider. Ann Fam Med. 2014;12(6):573–6.
8. Yosick Y, Crook RE, Gatto M, Maxwell TL, Duncan I, Ahmed T, Mackenzie A. Effects of a population health community-based palliative care program on cost and utilization. J Palliat Med. 22(9):1075–81. https://doi.org/10.1089/jpm.2018.0489.
9. Gaertner J, Siemens W, Meerpohl JJ, et al. Effect of specialist palliative care services on quality of life in adults with advanced incurable illness in hospital, hospice, or community settings: systematic review and meta-analysis. BMJ. 2017;357:j2925.
10. Morrow E, Call M, Marcus R, Locke A. Focus on the quadruple aim: development of a resiliency center to promote faculty and staff wellness initiatives. Jt Comm J Qual Patient Saf. 2018;44(5):293–8.
11. Patient Reported Outcomes (PROs) in Performance Measurement. National Quality Form. 2013. https://www.qualityforum.org/Publications/2012/12/Patient-Reported_Outcomes_in_Performance_Measurement.aspx. Accessed 17 Apr 2019.
12. Lendon JP, Ahluwalia SC, Walling AM, et al. Measuring experience with end-of-life care: a systematic literature review. J Pain Symptom Manage. 2015;49(5):904–15 e1–3.
13. Antunes B, Harding R, Higginson IJ. Implementing patient-reported outcome measures in palliative care clinical practice: a systematic review of facilitators and barriers. Palliat Med. 2014;28(2):158–75.
14. Shippee ND, Shippee TP, Mobley PD, Fernstrom KM, Britt HR. Effect of a whole-person model of care on patient experience in patients with complex chronic illness in late life. Am J Hosp Palliat Care. 2017;35(1):104–9.
15. Gawande A. Being mortal: medicine and what matters in the end. New York: Metropolitan Books, Henry Holt and Company; 2014.

16. National Consensus Project for Quality Palliative Care. Clinical practice guidelines for quality palliative care. 4th ed. 2018. https://www.nationalcoalitionhpc.org/ncp/ Accessed 17 Apr 2019.
17. Agency for Healthcare Research and Quality. National quality measures clearinghouse. http://www.qualitymeasures.ahrq.gov/tutorial/varieties.aspx. Accessed 17 Apr 2019.
18. Teno J. Toolkit of Instruments to Measure End-of-Life Care (TIME) Center for Gerontology and Health Care Research. Brown Medical School; 2001.
19. Lorenz K, Lynn J, Morton S, et al. End-of-life care and outcomes. Evidence Report/Technology Assessment No. 110. AHRQ Publication No. 05-E004-2 Agency for Healthcare Research and Quality. Rockville, MD; 2004.
20. Mularski RA, Dy SM, Shugarman LR, et al. A systematic review of measures of end-of-life care and its outcomes. Health Serv Res. 2007;42(5):1848–70.
21. Dy SM, Shugarman LR, Lorenz KA, et al. A systematic review of satisfaction with care at the end- of-life. J Am Geriatr Soc. 2008;56(1):124–9.
22. Hanson LC, Scheunemann LP, Zimmerman S, et al. The PEACE project review of clinical instruments for hospice and palliative care. J Palliat Med. 2010;13(10):1253–60. https://doi.org/10.1089/jpm.2010.0194.
23. Systematic Reviews of Instruments Relevant to Palliative Care. Palliative care research cooperative. 2016. https://pcrc.app.box.com/v/instrument-reviews. Accessed 11 Nov 2018.
24. Albers G, Echteld MA, de Vet HC, et al. Evaluation of quality-of-life measures for use in palliative care: a systematic review. Palliat Med. 2010;24(1):17–37.
25. De Roo ML, Leemans K, Claessen SJ, et al. Quality indicators for palliative care: update of a systematic review. J Pain Symptom Manag. 2013;46(4):556–72.
26. Hui D, De La Cruz M, Mori M, et al. Concepts and definitions for "supportive care," "best supportive care," "palliative care," and "hospice care" in the published literature, dictionaries, and textbooks. Support Care Cancer. 2012;21(3):659–85.
27. Kelley AS, Bollens-Lund E. Identifying the population with serious illness: the "denominator" challenge. J Palliat Med. 2018;21(S2):S7–S16.
28. National Quality Forum. Palliative care and end-of-life care—A consensus report. Washington, DC: National Quality Forum; 2012. http://www.qualityforum.org/. Accessed 17 Apr 2019.
29. Schuster MA, Onorato SE, Meltzer DO. Measuring the cost of quality measurement: a missing link in quality strategy. JAMA. 2017;318(13):1219–20.
30. Casalino LP, Gans D, Weber R, et al. US physician practices spend more than $15.4 billion annually to report quality measures. Health Aff (Millwood). 2016;35(3):401–6.
31. Meyer GS, Nelson EC, Pryor DB, et al. More quality measures versus measuring what matters: a call for balance and parsimony. BMJ Qual Saf. 2012;21(11):964–968.32.
32. Saver BG, Martin SA, Adler RN, et al. Care that matters: quality measurement and health care. PLoS Med. 2015;12(11):e1001902.
33. Registries in Hospice and Palliative Medicine. http://aahpm.org/quality/registries-in-hpm. Accessed 17 Apr 2019.
34. Virdun C, Luckett T, Lorenz KA, et al. National quality indicators and policies from 15 countries leading in adult end-of-life care: a systematic environmental scan. BMJ Support Palliat Care. 2018;8:145–54.
35. From the national consensus project for quality palliative care (a consortium of the american academy of hospice and palliative Medicine, the center to advance palliative care, hospice and Palliative nurses association, last acts partnership, and national Hospice and palliative care organization). J Palliat Med. 2004;7(5):611–27.
36. Ferrell BR, Twaddle ML, Melnick A, Meier DE. J Palliat Med. 2018;21(12):1684–9.
37. Pasman HR, Brandt HE, Deliens L, Francke AL. Quality indicators for palliative care: a systematic review. J Pain Symptom Manag. 2009;38(1):145–56.
38. NQF (National Quality Forum) A National Framework and Preferred Practices for Palliative and Hospice Care Quality. 2006. Available at http://www.qualityforum.org/Publications/2006/12/A_National_Framework_and_Preferred_Practices_for_Palliative_and_Hospice_Care_Quality.aspx. Accessed 17 Apr 2019.

39. NQF Endorses Palliative and End-of-Life Care Measures. https://www.qualityforum.org/News_And_Resources/Press_Releases/2012/NQF_Endorses_Palliative_and_End-of-Life_Care_Measures.aspx. Accessed 17 Apr 2019.
40. Dy SM, Kiley KB, Ast K, Lupu D, Norton SA, McMillan SC, Herr K, Rotella JD, Casarett DJ. Measuring what matters: top-ranked quality indicators for hospice and palliative care from the American Academy of Hospice and Palliative Medicine and Hospice and Palliative Nurses Association. J Pain Symp Manag. 49(4):773–81.
41. Measuring What Matters. http://aahpm.org/quality/measuring-what-matters. Accessed 17 Apr 2019.
42. Ko W, Deliens L, Miccinesi G, et al. Care provided and care setting transitions in the last three months of life of cancer patients: a nationwide monitoring study in four European countries. BMC Cancer. 2014;14:960.
43. Block LVD, Onwuteaka-Philipsen B, Koen Meeussen K, et al. Nationwide continuous monitoring of end-of-life care via representative networks of general practitioners in Europe. BMC Fam Pract. 2013;14:73.
44. Currow D, Allingham S, Yates P, et al. Improving national hospice/palliative care service symptom outcomes systematically through point-of-care data collection, structured feedback and benchmarking. Support Care Cancer. 2015;23:307–15.
45. Casarett DJ, Harrold J, Oldanie B, et al. Advancing the science of hospice care: coalition of hospices organized to investigate comparative effectiveness. Curr Opin Support Palliat Care. 2012;6:459–64.
46. Groenvold M, Adsersen M, Danish Palliative MB. Care database. Clin Epidemiol. 2016;8:637–43.
47. Zheng NT, Li Q, Hanson LC, Wessell KL, Chong N, Sherif N, Broyles IH, Frank J, Kirk MA, Schwartz CR, Levitt AF, Rokoske F. Nationwide quality of hospice care: findings from the Centers for Medicare & Medicaid Services Hospice Quality Reporting Program. J Pain Symptom Manag. 2018;55(2):427–32.
48. Fact Sheet: Hospice Item Set. https://www.cms.gov/medicare/quality-initiatives-patient-assessment-instruments/hospice-quality-reporting/downloads/his-fact-sheet.pdf. Last Accessed 17 Apr 2019.
49. CAHPS Hospice Survey. https://hospicecahpssurvey.org/. Last Accessed 17 Apr 2019.
50. Hospice and Palliative Care Composite Process Measure – Comprehensive Assessment at Admission. Last Accessed 17 Apr 2019.
51. Medicare Hospice Compare. https://www.medicare.gov/hospicecompare/#search. Last Accessed 17 Apr 2019.
52. Gliklich RE, Dreyer NA, editors. Registries for evaluating patient outcomes: a user's guide. 2nd ed. Agency for Healthcare Research and Quality (US): Rockville, MD; 2010.
53. The National Palliative Care Registry; The Palliative Care Quality Network; The Global Palliative Care Quality Alliance: Quality Measurement Collaboratives and Registries. In: The National Palliative Care Registry; The Palliative Care Quality Network; The Global Palliative Care Quality Alliance, 2016.
54. The Center to Advance Palliative Care. https://www.capc.org/. Last Accessed 17 Apr 2019.
55. Pantilat SZ, Marks AK, Bischoff KE, Bragg AR, O'Riordan DL. The Palliative care quality network: improving the quality of caring. J Palliat Med. 2017;20(8):862–8.
56. Kamal AH, Bull J, Kavalieratos D, et al. Development of the quality data collection tool for prospective quality assessment and reporting in Palliative care. J Palliat Med. 2016;19(11):1148–55.
57. Kamal AH, Kirkland KB, Meier DE, Morgan TS, Nelson EC, Pantilat SZ. A person-centered, registry-based learning health system for palliative care: a path to coproducing better outcomes, experience, value, and science. J Palliat Med. 2018;21(S2):S61.
58. Casarett D. CHOICE: Coalition of Hospices Organized to Investigate Comparative Effectiveness – Final Report. (Prepared by the University of Pennsylvania under Grant No. R21 HS021780). Rockville, MD: Agency for Healthcare Research and Quality; 2014.

59. Martinsson L, Heedman PA, Lundström S, Axelsson B. Improved data validity in the Swedish Register of Palliative Care. PLoS One. 2017;12(10):e0186804.
60. Bausewein C, Schildmann E, Rosenbruch J, Haberland B, Tänzler S, Ramsenthaler C. Starting from scratch: implementing outcome measurement in clinical practice. Ann Palliat Med. 2018;7(Suppl 3):S253–61.
61. Van den Block L, Onwuteaka-Philipsen B, Meeussen K, et al. Nationwide continuous monitoring of end-of-life care via representative networks of general practitioners in Europe. BMC Fam Pract. 2013;14:73.
62. Menec V, Lix L, Steinbach C, Ekuma O, Sirski M, Dahl M, Soodeen R. Patterns of health care use and cost at the end of life. Winnipeg, MB: Manitoba Centre for Health Policy; 2004.
63. Going Further Together –Update on Formation of the Palliative Care Quality Collaborative. http://aahpm.org/uploads/Palliative_Care_Quality_Collaborative_Panel_Discussion_v6.pdf. Accessed 17 Apr 2019.
64. MACRA Funding Opportunity: Measure Development Awardees for the Quality Payment Program. https://www.cms.gov/Medicare/Quality-Initiatives-Patient-Assessment-Instruments/Value-Based-Programs/MACRA-MIPS-and-APMs/9-21-18-QPP-Measures-Cooperative-Agreement-Awardees.pdf. Last Accessed 17 Apr 2019.
65. Dumont S, Fillion L, Gagnon P, et al. A new tool to assess family caregivers' burden during end-of-life care. J Palliat Care. 2008;24(3):151–61.
66. Cooper B, Kinsella GJ, Picton C. Development and initial validation of a family appraisal of caregiving questionnaire for palliative care. Psychooncology. 2006;15(7):613–22.
67. Cohen R, Leis AM, Kuhl D, et al. QOLLTI-F: measuring family carer quality of life. Palliat Med. 2006;20(8):755–67.
68. Prigerson HG, Jacobs SC. Traumatic grief as a distinct disorder: a rationale, consensus criteria, and a preliminary empirical test. In: Stroebe MS, Hansson RO, Stroebe W, et al., editors. Handbook of bereavement research: consequences, coping, and care. Washington, DC: American Psychological Association; 2001.
69. Department of Health. End-of-life care strategy: quality markers and measures for end-of-life care. London: Department of Health; 2009.
70. Henry M, Hudson Scholle S, Briefer FJ. Accountability for the quality of care provided to people with serious illness. J Palliat Med. 2018;21(S2):S68–73.

Chapter 8
Developing a Hospital Quality Metrics System and Dashboard

Alexander Pavoll, Catherine Feleppa Camenga, and Saul N. Weingart

Introduction: The Quality Conundrum

Measurement Overload

Hospitals and health systems are responsible for reporting at least 400 distinct quality measures to regulatory and accreditation agencies including the Centers for Medicare and Medicaid Services, state health departments, boards of registration in medicine, state Medicaid agencies, the US Occupational Safety and Health Administration, the Joint Commission, and others. Additionally, hospitals may elect to participate in disease management registries which offer reliable, risk-adjusted data sets that provide clinicians with information to guide quality improvement efforts.

Quality measures track a variety of care-related structures. Processes and outcomes include compliance with effective, evidence-based practices for the care of patients with conditions such as stroke, heart failure, or myocardial infarction (based on chart abstraction), patient experience (based on consumer surveys), and resource utilization (drawn from hospital administrative systems) such as hospitalized patients' lengths of stay, readmission rates, and emergency department boarder time.

A. Pavoll · C. F. Camenga
Department of Quality and Patient Safety, Tufts Medical Center, Boston, MA, USA

S. N. Weingart (✉)
Department of Medicine, Tufts Medical Center, Tufts University School of Medicine, Boston, MA, USA
e-mail: sweingart@tuftsmedicalcenter.org

© Springer Nature Switzerland AG 2020
D. N. Salem (ed.), *Quality Measures*, https://doi.org/10.1007/978-3-030-37145-6_8

Measurement Burden

Many metrics, including reports of infectious diseases, require sophisticated screening tools to flag candidate cases for expert internal review and are subject to external validation audits. Other metrics, including those designed to capture surgical complications, rely on the quality of physician documentation, medical record coding, and the validity of the underlying algorithms and their inclusion and exclusion criteria. All in all, hospital and health systems spend enormous time and treasure recruiting and training staff to collect and report a complex array of quality metrics, manage electronic data capture and submission, and conduct validation studies. Quality measurement imposes a major responsibility, challenge, and burden on healthcare organizations.

Inconsistent Scoring and Validity

While the value of quality measurement is undisputed, the value of specific measures has come under increasing attention and scrutiny [1–6]. In a recent review, Salem and colleagues describe multiple measures that are antiquated or ill-informed, measures that are overly specified, and measures that lack validation [7]. And yet, hospital and healthcare systems continue to be accountable for many of these quality measures – measures that result in publicly reported ratings that may be misleading to consumers and that result in arbitrary financial rewards and penalties [8]. The Patient Safety Indicators (PSIs), for example, contain surgical complication algorithms derived from discharge diagnoses codes. Many PSIs are incorporated into Medicare's value-based payment program, large insurers' pay-for-performance programs, US News and Leapfrog Group quality ratings, and other proprietary ranking systems [9–13]. They have been endorsed by the National Quality Forum [14]. However, of 17 commonly used PSI measures, a single measure had evidence of validity in a systematic review performed by Johns Hopkins University researchers [15].

Navigating the Measurement Imperative

Clearly, quality measurement is important. Quality measures help organizations set priorities and goals, shape organizational improvement projects designed to enhance (and measure) key processes and outcomes, and provide accountability to internal stakeholders such as the board of trustees as well as external stakeholders such as government overseers, accreditation bodies, payers, and consumers. However, given the proliferation of quality metrics and the high stakes associated with performance on these measures, how can hospitals and medical centers artfully negotiate the multiple demands placed upon them? We posit that it is impossible to optimize performance for all of the various quality measures that hospitals and health systems must report and track. They are difficult enough to report and track, especially given the fact that various programs use subtly different definitions, time frames, and risk adjusters. Understanding the array of performance measures exceeds the expertise of many highly sophisticated hospital leaders, their governing bodies, and knowledgeable consumers. Health quality measurement is the ultimate "inside baseball" and, as a result, may detract from its goal of driving improved performance.

To make sense of the proliferation of quality measures and to guide our organizational performance goals, our organization selected a subset of high-value measures to monitor and manage. We believe that focusing on "measures that matter" is a productive way to bring some degree of order and coherence to an increasingly incoherent measurement and regulatory environment. We describe below how we have approached this challenge, how we selected, tracked and reported on key metrics, and how we set up an infrastructure to manage this process. While this formulation is derived from the experience of a single healthcare organization, we believe that our approach and recommendations are broadly replicable.

What's an Organization to Do?

Setting

Tufts Medical Center and Floating Hospital for Children is a 415-bed academic medical center in downtown Boston, serving adults and children in metropolitan Boston and southern New England. Tufts has a high case mix index, serves Chinatown and South Boston neighborhoods as well as an urban safety net population, and is known for its tertiary care programs in cardiac and neurosurgery, trauma, and high-risk obstetrics.

Getting Started

With a change in the leadership of the Quality Department at Tufts Medical Center in 2013, we undertook a review of the measurement requirements of the hospital and shared that information with senior leadership and the Board of Trustees' Quality of Care Committee. Recognizing the challenges of improvement, the risk of a scattershot approach, and the benefit of a narrowly focused effort, the Board tasked leadership to select a manageable set of key quality metrics that were well-validated, that represented processes and outcomes important to our patients, and that were potentially actionable with adequate resources and attention. The Board was particularly interested in measures that, if improved, would have a significant impact on quality of care, support a culture of safety and transparency, and support the goal of implementing high reliability processes across the organization.

The Quality Dashboard

In an iterative fashion, with input from a variety of clinical stakeholders, the department leadership team proposed a set of metrics that were aligned with the five of six quality domains identified in the Institute of Medicine's *Quality Chasm* report: safety, effectiveness, efficiency, patient centeredness, timeliness, and equity (STEEP) [16]. (The equity domain was initially deferred given the absence of sound metrics.) These items were incorporated in a dashboard.

Proposed measures satisfied several criteria. They were generalizable to multiple clinical areas and reportable internally without reliance on external (often lagged) government or insurer reports. They met specified definitions and codes. Some of the dashboard metrics are also used by public agencies, such as the PSI measures developed by the US Agency for Healthcare Research and Quality (AHRQ) [17]. PSI measures are used by Medicare and reported publicly by some insurer pay-for-performance programs and by hospital rating programs like the Leapfrog Group. We also included important and potentially preventable infection measures including central line-associated bloodstream infections (CLABSIs), catheter-associated urinary tract infections (CAUTIs), and surgical site infections. Infections are reported as both rates (e.g., infections per patient or line days) and standardized infection ratios (SIRs). SIRs are risk-adjusted to allow for comparison across hospitals and to improve the value of benchmarking. In assembling the dashboard, the team sought to utilize measures drawn from existing dashboards and reports whenever possible. The end result was a three-page display of trended data with monthly results in tabular and graphic fashion, a rolling 12-month average, and a year-over-year comparison. The dashboard was created in Microsoft Excel and used a color scheme that displayed results in three shades:

- Values that met or exceeded the goal were shaded light green.
- Values that were 95% of the goal or greater were shaded a light orange.
- Values less than 95% of the goal were shaded a darker orange.

The dashboard metrics are presented in Table 8.1.

We set goals for each measure based on national benchmarks whenever possible, generally aiming for the top tenth percentile of academic medical centers. We set a goal of zero for specific patient-harm event categories (an aspirational goal). We revisited each goal every fiscal year and considered adding new, relevant metrics or removing those that had "topped out." "Topped out" measures had near-perfect scores for an extended period of time, indicating that the practice had become ingrained in daily clinical practice.

We also selected among competing measures. For example, we dropped a convoluted Medicare sepsis measure (whose validity had not been demonstrated to

Table 8.1 Tufts Medical Center's quality dashboard

Safe	Preventable harm rollup (sum of all Harm Bubble items)
	Workplace injuries
	Workplace injury events
	Days lost due to workplace injuries
	Workplace assaults
	Falls
	Falls # total/with injury (excluding NICU)
	Falls rate/1000 patient-days
	Falls with injury rate/1000 patient-days
	Medication errors
	Serious medication errors reaching the patient (count)
	Serious medication error (rate/1000 patient-days)
	Central line-associated bloodstream infections (CLABSI count)
	CLABSI overall rate/1000 line-days across all inpatient units)
	CLABSI pediatric rate/1000 line-days (includes all pediatric units)
	Catheter-associated urinary tract infections (CAUTI count)
	CAUTI ICU rate/1000 line-days (excluding NICU)
	CAUTI adult med-surg units rate/1000 line-days (including Neuroscience intermediate care unit)
	CAUTI pediatric units rate/1000 line-days (excluding NICU)
	Pressure injuries (PI) (total PI incidence from observations)
	PIs (stages 3, 4, and unstageable PIs from billing codes)
	PIs in adult ICU (rate/1000 patient-days)
	PIs in adult med-surg units (rate/1000 patient-days)
	PIs in pediatrics (rate/1000 patient-days)
	Serious reportable events (count)
	AHRQ PSI-90 Composite (observed/expected)
	AHRQ PSI-90 Composite (count of cases)
	Hand hygiene performance (compliance rate)
Effective	Acute myocardial infarction mortality index (IQI-32)
	Heart failure mortality index (IQI-16)
	Pneumonia mortality index (IQI-20)
	Sepsis mortality index
	Vizient mortality index (severity adjusted)
Efficient	Vizient mean length of stay (LOS)
	Vizient LOS index (severity adjusted)
	Vizient all-cause unplanned 30-day readmission rate
	Vizient direct cost index (severity adjusted)
Patient centered	Overall rating – adult inpatient (HCAHPS)
	Overall MD rating – adult outpatient (CGCAHPS)
	Overall rating – pediatric inpatient (Child CAHPS)
	Overall rating – emergency department (Press Ganey)
	Overall rating – ambulatory surgery (OASCAHPS)

(continued)

Table 8.1 (continued)

Timely	Emergency Department wait time in minutes, from arrival to provider
	Emergency Department wait time in minutes, from disposition to floor
	Lag time for new patients to obtain appointment
	Percentage of new patients scheduled within 25 days
	Call abandonment rate (adult clinics, non-Call Center)
	Call abandonment rate (adult Call Center)
	Call abandonment rate (pediatric clinics, non-Call Center)
General	Discharges
	Clinic volume
	Medicare case mix index (CMI)
	Total case mix index (CMI)

improve outcomes) in favor of a risk-adjusted sepsis mortality measure that compares observed-to-expected mortality. Decision-makers balanced the fact that the Medicare measure was publicly reported against the risk-adjusted outcome measure, concluding that the risk-adjusted measure was both easier to understand and more meaningful to clinicians and consumers.

A process was established for updating the monthly dashboard using email reminders to departmental measure "owners," automated feeds from existing measure scorecards, and abstractions from the monthly reports provided by various vendor sites such as Press Ganey (patient experience data) and Vizient (risk-adjusted benchmarking of academic medical center performance). Enlisting support from various departments in the development and review of the quality dashboard promoted alignment across the organization. The dashboard is displayed on the Medical Center's internal website and is accessible to all employees.

The Board of Trustees' Quality of Care Committee's lay trustees also requested a simplified, rolled-up summary of the full dashboard (Fig. 8.1). This single-page scorecard presented the last 2 months' performance across the following metrics key performance metrics and bucketed it into a modified version of the STEEP format.

- Safety

  - Serious reportable events
  - Mortality observed/expected ratio
  - Workplace injuries resulting in lost days

- High-risk processes

  - Central line-associated bloodstream infections
  - Catheter-associated urinary tract infections
  - Medication errors reaching the patient
  - Patient safety composite (PSI-90) [17]

- Patient experience

  - Inpatient experience (overall rating 0–10 from HCAHPS survey) [18]
  - Ambulatory experience (overall rating 0–10 from CGCAHPS survey)

Tufts Medical Center	QUALITY DASHBOARD - January 2019			
Measure	Goal	Dec	Jan	FY18 Total
Safety				
Serious Reportable Events	0	6	3	40
Mortality Index	0.73	1.12	0.90	0.80
Workplace Injuries	0	4	3	63
High-Risk Processes				
Central Line Infections	0	3	3	15
Urinary Catheter Infections	0	5	2	36
Medication Errors Reaching Patient	0	3	3	40
Patient Safety Composite	5	8	9	83
Patient Experience				
Inpatient Experience	83.0%	83.7%	90.5%	77.3%
Ambulatory Experience	86.7%	87.1%	86.6%	87.2%
Care Transitions				
Length of Stay Index	0.88	0.97	0.95	0.90
Readmission Rate	12.0%	9.8%	10.2%	12.6
ED Wait Time: Discharge to Floor	120	186	194	141

Fig. 8.1 Tufts Medical Center's summary quality dashboard

- Care transitions

  - Length of stay observed/expected ratio
  - Time from Emergency Department discharge to floor (for admissions, in minutes)

Each metric on this list was accompanied with a colored arrow to show stable performance, improvement, or decline. We used the traditional red/yellow/green stoplight-colored arrows as intuitive visual indicators. An "Insights" section was added to the bottom of the page to explain the metrics qualitatively. This section summarized how many measures met or exceeded the goal, the types of serious events reported to the state Public Health Department, and other relevant commentary. The Insights section focused on exceptions, provided updates when a measure had a marked change, or indicated when a relevant quality improvement project was started.

The Harm Bubble

The lay members of the Board of Trustees' Quality of Care Committee also requested a simplified presentation of quality data, one that helped them to better understand how many patients were harmed in the course of their care. Rather than presenting infection or adverse drug event rates, the new document presented monthly harm counts. In this way, board members could directly appreciate whether the organization was progressing in our goal of achieving zero harm.

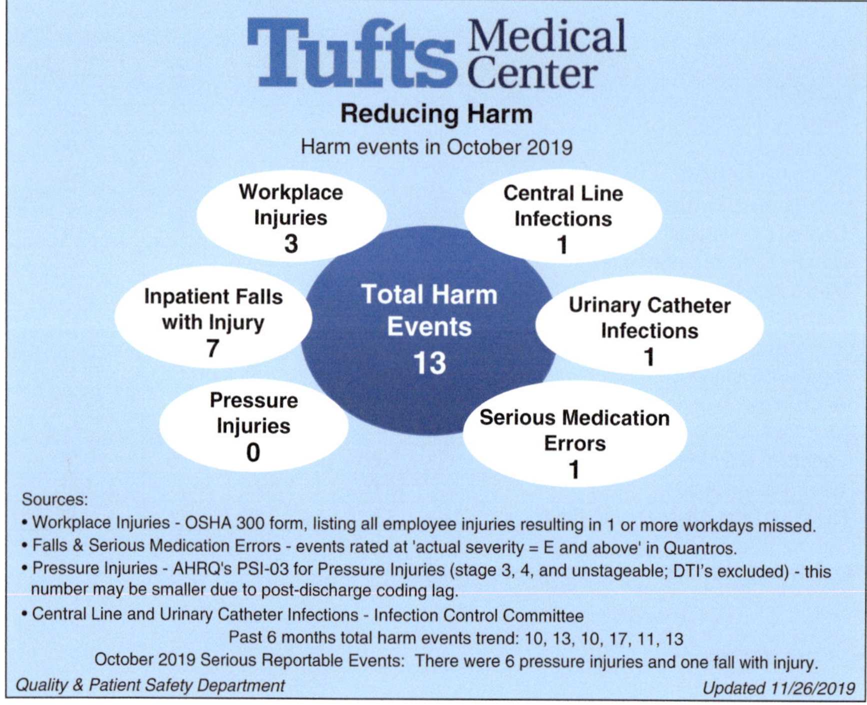

Fig. 8.2 Tufts Medical Center's Harm Bubble

To display harm as counts, we adopted a visualization tool called the Harm Bubble (Fig. 8.2). Each bubble represented a different type of care-associated injury, along with a central bubble with the total number of harm events. We selected well-established indicators of care-associated harm including CAUTIs, CLABSIs, falls with injury, serious medication events, and pressure injuries (ascertained by the hospital wound care team). A count of workplace employee injuries was added later to demonstrate the commitment to harm prevention for both patients and staff. Although the initial version of the Harm Bubble included a count of "serious reportable events" (SREs) that required reporting to the state Department of Public Health, this item was later included as a footnote to avoid double-counting other event types (such as falls with injury) that were also SREs.

Using Measures to Drive Quality

Setting Priorities

Hospital quality leaders are responsible for reviewing, updating, and recommending quality measures to the Board each year. Leaders attempt to incorporate performance measures that require consistently high levels of performance for public reporting as well as measures that reflect organizational priorities for continuous quality improvement. This balance requires a consensus approach across multiple stakeholders. Each year, we follow a goal-setting methodology that begins with an "environmental scan" of quality and patient safety hazards, novel improvement strategies, and a gap analysis. We identified and quantified quality and safety hazards by asking internal experts and stakeholders – including representatives from the Patient Family Advisory Council – to participate in a risk-stratification exercise. The annual gap analysis and quality goals were reviewed and approved by the Quality Committees and ultimately the Board of Trustees. Goals are operationalized and incorporated into an annual quality work plan. Many of the dashboard measures are associated with specific projects in the annual work plan, as the projects are intended to drive these measures to higher levels of performance.

Monitoring Progress and Driving Improvement

Quality leaders review the dashboard each month in advance of the Board of Trustees' Quality Committee to allow for a "deep dive" into selected measures, to understand proposed modifications to various measures, to discuss revisions and enhancements to the dashboard, and to keep up to date with measure development and reporting.

Monthly reporting up through the Quality Committee structure ensures for program oversight and accountability. Education of the members is ongoing as new measures or changes in measures are reported. Over time, the dashboard has helped quality leaders and board members to identify areas that require or have benefitted from focused improvement efforts. We have paid special attention to the Emergency Department throughput metrics, ambulatory access measures, and infection rates. An important principle is to avoid major year-to-year changes. Quality improvement takes time: time to establish the right measures, to put the right interventions in place, and to sustain the gains.

Summary and Conclusion

Policy makers need to recognize that the proliferation of quality metrics has become burdensome and unmanageable. As a result, hospital and health systems need to focus on the subset of measures that are tied to meaningful clinical outcomes. In our experience, it was not difficult to select a set of measures that were relevant and actionable – recognizing that it may take multiple interventions over several years to make a meaningful and sustained improvement.

We found no perfect solution to the dashboard challenge. While some audiences prefer counts to rates, or graphs to tables, others like it the other way around. There was an ongoing tension between showing rolled-up summaries (e.g., of infection rates) and the request for more granular information on service-specific performance (e.g., in the intensive care unit compared to the medical-surgical floor).

We learned that it is important to report and display key measures in a way that quality experts can use and that lay board members can understand and interpret. This remains a work in progress. We found that less is more, that simple is better, and that measures that represent the harm to individual patients and staff create the opportunity for an informed and transparent conversation about those areas where we excel as an organization and those where we may fall short.

References

1. Jha AK. Value-based purchasing: time for reboot or time to move on? JAMA. 2017;317(11):1107–8.
2. Jha AK. Seeking rational approaches to fixing hospital readmissions. JAMA. 2015;314(16):1681–2.
3. Joynt KE, Jha AK. Thirty-day readmissions – truth and consequences. N Engl J Med. 2012;366(15):1366–9.
4. Zuckerman RB, Joynt Maddox KE, Sheingold SH, Chen LM, Epstein AM. Effect of a hospital-wide measure on the readmissions reduction program. N Engl J Med. 2017;377(16):1551–8.
5. Wadhera RK, Joynt Maddox KE, Wasfy JH, Haneuse S, Shen C, Yeh RW. Association of the hospital readmissions reduction program with mortality among Medicare beneficiaries hospitalized for heart failure, acute myocardial infarction, and pneumonia. JAMA. 2018;320(24):2542–52.
6. Health Affairs Blog. Measures that matter – but to whom? 2016. Available at: https://www.healthaffairs.org/do/10.1377/hblog20160310.053833/full/. Last accessed 7 Mar 2019.
7. Esposito ML, Selker HP, Salem DN. Quality over quantity: how the rise in quality measures is not producing quality results. J Gen Intern Med. 2015;30(8):1204–7.
8. CMS. Hospital value-based purchasing. 2017. Available at: https://www.cms.gov/Outreach-and-Education/Medicare-Learning-Network-MLN/MLNProducts/downloads/Hospital_VBPurchasing_Fact_Sheet_ICN907664.pdf. Last accessed 7 Mar 2019.
9. Agency for Healthcare Research and Quality. Patient safety indicators overview. Available at: https://www.qualityindicators.ahrq.gov/modules/psi_overview.aspx. Last accessed 7 Mar 2019.
10. CMS. Medicare learning network hospital value-based purchasing booklet. 2017. Available at: https://www.cms.gov/Outreach-and-Education/Medicare-Learning-Network-MLN/MLNProducts/downloads/Hospital_VBPurchasing_Fact_Sheet_ICN907664.pdf. Last accessed 7 Mar 2019.
11. US News & World Report. FAQ: how and why we rank and rate hospitals. 2018. Available at: https://health.usnews.com/health-care/best-hospitals/articles/faq-how-and-why-we-rank-and-rate-hospitals. Last accessed 7 Mar 2019.
12. US News & World Report. 2018–2019 best hospitals procedures & condition ratings. 2018. Available at: https://www.usnews.com/static/documents/health/best-hospitals/BHPC_Methodology_2018-19.pdf. Last accessed 7 Mar 2019.
13. Leapfrog hospital safety grade scoring methodology. 2018. Available at: https://www.hospitalsafetygrade.org/media/file/HospitalSafetyGrade_ScoringMethodology_Fall2018_Final.pdf. Last accessed 7 Mar 2019.
14. National Quality Forum. Patient safety indicators: complications. Available at: https://www.qualityforum.org/Projects/n-r/Patient_Safety_Measures_Complications/Patient_Safety_Measures_Complications.aspx. Last accessed 7 Mar 2019.

15. Winters BD, Bharmal A, Wilson RF, et al. Validity of the agency for health care research and quality patient safety indicators and the centers for medicare and medicaid hospital-acquired conditions: a systematic review and meta-analysis. Med Care. 2016;54(12):1105–11.
16. Committee on Quality Health Care in America, Institute of Medicine. Crossing the quality chasm: a new health system for the 21st century. Washington, DC: National Academy Press, 2001.
17. Agency for Healthcare Research and Quality. Agency for Healthcare Research and Quality (AHRQ) Quality Indicators (QIs) Fact Sheet: Patient Safety and Adverse Events Composite (modified version PSI 90) for ICD-9 CM/PCS, v6.0. 2016. Available at: https://www.quality-indicators.ahrq.gov/News/PSI90_Factsheet_FAQ_v1.pdf. Last accessed 7 Mar 2019.
18. Agency for Healthcare Research and Quality. CAHPS clinician and group survey. 2018. Available from: https://www.ahrq.gov/cahps/surveys-guidance/cg/index.html. Last accessed 7 Mar 2019.

Chapter 9
Patient Satisfaction Metrics

Craig Best

Introduction

Patient satisfaction has been studied and measured in earnest since the 1980s [1]. Metrics were refined over time as our understanding of patient desires has grown. Current surveys focus on the process of care rather than the outcome of the medical service and may be more appropriately referred to as surveys of patient experience. The patient experience is an important measure of medical care quality, and therefore, patient experience metrics have become as important as other measures of clinical quality such as infection rate and annual screening tests. While patient experience metrics focus on the patient's assessment of various components of care from points of access to other touch points, patients may encounter along the continuum of care, a more consumer-centric approach would consider the overall patient experience as the best endpoint. The distinction between patient satisfaction, as determined by a defined set of quantifiable metrics, and the patient experience, which includes other determinants that are sometimes outside the immediate control of the healthcare provider, is important and will be addressed in this chapter. This chapter explores the many reasons why patient experience metrics are important, reviews the most common inpatient and outpatient metrics used in the United States, and addresses some of the shortcomings associated with following and managing patient experience metrics.

C. Best (✉)
Tufts Medical Center Physician Organization, Boston, MA, USA
e-mail: cbest@tuftsmedicalcenter.org

© Springer Nature Switzerland AG 2020
D. N. Salem (ed.), *Quality Measures*, https://doi.org/10.1007/978-3-030-37145-6_9

Why Measure the Patient Experience?

To Improve the Human Condition and Relieve Suffering

First and foremost, healthcare providers should focus on patient experience to improve the human condition and to relieve suffering. While these are soft indicators of quality, as it is difficult to quantify patient suffering, it is clear that providing compassionate, empathetic care reduces the stress associated with disease and the uncertainty associated with a patient's symptoms as a diagnosis is made and treatment is considered.

It is not uncommon to see an anxious or frightened patient with symptoms that they might consider as dangerous. Patients frequently look online for information and sometimes associate their symptoms with a catastrophic disease, such as cancer. Further, they may have a family member who had a similar symptom that turned out to be life threatening. Spending time listening to patients, understanding their concerns, and addressing their concerns quickly and compassionately is an important aspect of reducing patient anxiety.

Many patients worry that their present medical condition will limit their ability to live their life as they have in the past. For example, a patient with torn ligaments in the knee may be concerned that they are not able to get back to playing tennis or get back to a competitive sport which has been important part of their life; they may worry that they can no longer provide for their family through their landscaping job. These are differently weighed concerns but important for the healthcare provider to address during the office visit for the care to be centered on the whole person.

Healthcare providers showing compassion (by understanding the individual patient's concerns and providing reassurance that the patient will get better) is important to relieve suffering. Optimism about a full recovery reduces stress and contributes to the chances of the individual getting back to their normal routine and reduces the incidence of depression [2].

Compliance with Treatment Recommendations

There is a considerable body of evidence showing that a positive experience with the healthcare provider improves compliance with treatment [3–7]. A physician, for example, who spends time with the patient explaining the importance of a medication and the consequences of not taking the medication while involving the patient in the decision is more likely to build trust with the patient and increase compliance with treatment recommendations [4].

There are a number of studies testing the hypothesis that the patient experience is associated with clinical outcomes [8–14]. The results of these studies are conflicting. One study, involving a large cohort of patients, appeared to show that higher patient satisfaction was associated with greater hospital admissions, higher overall healthcare cost, and increased mortality [14]. On the other hand, several studies show positive beneficial correlation between the patient experience and medical outcomes [8–13]. Two studies reported a lower incidence of chest pain and death after acute myocardial infarction associated with a better patient experience during hospitalization [9, 13]. Before drawing conclusions of causation between the patient experience and clinical outcomes, randomized controlled studies are needed.

The Business Case

There is a strong business case for enhancing the patient experience. The Centers for Medicare and Medicaid Services (CMS) and local health plans are asking for patient experience data and have established payment schemes based on patient experience scores. This trend is likely to continue. Direct financial incentives focused on the patient experience are embedded in the CMS value-based payment model for both hospitals and physicians.

Patients increasingly rely on social media to choose their healthcare providers. Web-based physician grading platforms such as Health Grades, Vital Signs, Yelp!, and Angie's List are directing patients to highly rated physicians. Individual physician ratings for Medicare patient satisfaction based on CG CAHPS scores are reported at the Physician Compare website (http://www.medicare.gov/physiciancompare/). For the most part, physician ratings are based on how satisfied the patient was with their doctor visit. Other factors influencing physician ratings are scheduling, access, and clinical outcomes. It is also highly likely that experiences with front office staff, medical assistants, and nursing set the stage for how the physician will be perceived by the patient. The healthcare industry has become more like other service industries such as the hospitality industry, and potential customers frequent the web before making a decision about where to seek services, including healthcare services.

Hospital ratings are posted by the federal government. Eleven HCAHPS measures are publicly reported on the government's Hospital Compare website (www.medicare.gov/hospitalcompare). Hospital Compare patient experience ratings are rolled up into a single star rating so that hospitals can be compared side by side. More than 4000 Medicare-certified hospitals participate in Hospital Compare, and consumers are encouraged to use the hospital rankings to make decisions about where they seek care. Hospital Compare, and other similar transparency efforts, encourages hospitals to emphasize the quality of care they provide through focused quality improvement efforts.

There are numerous case studies supporting the concept of customer service as a differentiator for customer decision making and, therefore, an important factor in business growth [15–17]. Medical practices and hospitals must focus on improving the patient experience to be relevant in competitive markets and to improve prospects for growth of the organization. Other factors are important for business success such as networking, marketing, and branding, but the patient experience is an extremely important determinant of business sustainability and growth, particularly in competitive markets. Consumers are looking less to what an organization says about itself and more to what other consumers are saying. Physicians making referrals to specialists and to hospitals are listening to patient feedback and making adjustments to referral patterns based on this feedback. A patient complaint to their primary care physician about substandard care received by a specialist can have a significant impact on continued referrals to that specialist. Referrals to a hospital can be impacted in a similar fashion. Positive reports about both the clinical outcome and the patient experience are necessary for continued referrals. Furthermore, patients who have a great experience are likely to refer friends and family (demonstrating customer loyalty) and could perhaps become a major institutional donor. A negative experience can have the opposite effect, leading to negative word of mouth to friends and family [18].

Healthcare organizations can mitigate poor experiences through service recovery. For example, when an office notices that physician wait times may be longer than desirable, patients should be told up front and offered an alternative to sitting in the waiting room. Some organizations offer devices that vibrate and light up when the physician is ready so that the patient can walk around and perhaps get a cup of coffee while waiting. Offering vouchers for coffee or drinks at the cafeteria is provided by some offices. If a patient or family member experiences a poor interaction during their clinical encounter, it is important for service recovery to occur quickly with an apology.

Healthcare organizations that receive high marks for the patient experience further benefit by improving staff engagement. Aurora Health, through creating a patient-centric culture, saw significant improvement in both patient and staff satisfaction [17]. Healthcare providers want to make a difference in the lives of the people they serve, and positive feedback from patients affirms that the healthcare team is making a significant impact on people's lives. Conversely, dissatisfied patients increase the number of complaints and reduce staff moral, potentially leading to higher levels of staff turnover [14] which itself can decrease office efficiency and ability to provide optimal care. High staff turnover, particularly if it involves physicians and nurses, is very costly. It has been estimated that one departing physician can cost an organization between $500,000 and $1.5 million in replacement cost when considering the cost of recruitment, sign-on bonus, and lost revenue based on the length of time to fill the vacancy [19]. Dr. Maryam Hanah of the Stanford Medicine Well MD Center estimated the cost associated with physician turnover attributable to burnout at between $250,000 and $1.0 million [20].

There are substantial benefits associated with environments that optimize the patient experience that extends to the healthcare provider. Team-based care that encourages every person on the healthcare staff to work to the top of license in a highly coordinated and collegial fashion not only provides a better, more consistent patient experience but reduces the likelihood of physician and nurse burnout [21, 22].

Malpractice risk is also reduced when patients are more highly satisfied [23–27]. The relationship between the physician and the patient as a result of excellent communication, empathy, and prioritizing the patient's needs reduces the likelihood of malpractice lawsuits even if clinical negligence is involved. A study at a large academic medical center examining the risk of malpractice claims based on physician scores on patient satisfaction surveys showed that doctors with the lowest scores of "poor" or "very poor" were twice as likely to be named in a malpractice claim compared with doctors who's lowest score was "very good" [26]. Furthermore, women who filed malpractice claims against their obstetrician-gynecologist were more likely to report interpersonal issues with the doctor. Physicians who had never been sued were more likely to be viewed by their patients as assessable, willing to communicate and concerned [23].

Focusing significant attention on the patient experience through team-based care and through nurse and physician communication is clearly the right thing to do for a healthcare organization seeking to provide the best possible care to the population it serves.

Validity of the Metrics

Establishing a set of relevant metrics requires an understanding of the various touch point patient's experience as they move through episodes of care but also requires an understanding of what matters to the patient. Factors influencing the patient experience are likely dependent on the location and unique hospital and clinic environments. However, patient experience metrics must be generalizable to allow for benchmarking with comparison groups. Therefore, standard patient experience surveys have a similar set of questions, not all of which are relevant to each clinical circumstance. Sofaer et al. criticized the HCAHPS survey for not assuring that the patient experience quality measures captured in the survey are consistent with patients' expectation of quality [28]. In order to fine-tune the factors measured, a real-time survey can be developed and tailored to the specific clinical circumstance that might involve issues like traffic to the location, parking at the location, and billing errors. Statistical analysis of the metrics using a correlation coefficient allows for comparison of individual questions or question groupings with top box patient satisfaction. This statistical analysis allows for the establishment of a hierarchy of priorities to focus on improvement efforts.

To improve the comparability and validity of results, HCAHPS surveys should not be limited to Medicare patients, they must be administered in a standardized fashion, and at least 300 surveys must be returned in a rolling four quarter period according to the HCAHPS Quality Assurance Guidelines manual found on the website www.hcahps.online.org. Individual survey questions demonstrate high reliability if at least 300 surveys are completed. All eligible hospital discharges comprise the pool from which the random sample of surveys is to be sent. Every eligible patient has an equal chance of being selected for the survey. The response rate has remained remarkably stable between 2008 and 2013 at approximately 33%. In 2013, over 4000 hospitals participated and over three million surveys were returned. Hospitals returning less than 100 surveys are publicly reported, but a footnote accompanies the result.

Patient satisfaction surveys, especially in the outpatient setting, are often criticized for low response rates. Commonly, clinicians and staff question the validity of the results when the number of returned surveys is low. Yet compared to customer satisfaction surveys in other industries, consumers of healthcare services return a higher percentage of surveys [29]. This is likely due to the importance individuals place on healthcare services. Low response rates can be addressed by looking at a

6 month rolling average or viewing individual clinician results quarterly rather than monthly.

The CMS applies a regression methodology to make a patient mix adjustment, controlling for patient variables shown to affect the measures. Demographic, health status, and other variables shown in Table 9.1 are accounted for in the results. CMS continues to partner with the Agency for Healthcare Research and Quality (AHRQ) to test and refine the HCAHPS survey.

Table 9.1 HCAHPS inpatient experience survey

Composite/item	HCAHPS survey	Response choices
Your nurse's care	*Please answer the following questions about your stay at the hospital named on the cover letter. Do not include any other hospitals in your answers.*	
	1. During your hospital stay, how were the nurse's treatment towards you with *courtesy and respect?*	○ Never ○ Sometimes ○ Usually ○ Always
	2. During your hospital stay, how often did nurses listen to you carefully?	○ Never ○ Sometimes ○ Usually ○ Always
	3. During your hospital stay, did nurses explain things in a way you can understand?	○ Never ○ Sometimes ○ Usually ○ Always
	4. After you have pressed the call button, how often did you get help as soon as you wanted it during your hospital stay?	○ Never ○ Sometimes ○ Usually ○ Always
Your doctors' care	5. How often would you say your doctors treated you with courtesy and respect during your hospital stay?	○ Never ○ Sometimes ○ Usually ○ Always
	6. How often did your doctors listen to you carefully?	○ Never ○ Sometimes ○ Usually ○ Always
	7. How often did your doctors explain things in a way you could understand during your hospital stay?	○ Never ○ Sometimes ○ Usually ○ Always
Your hospital environment	8. How often would you say your room and bathroom were kept clean?	○ Never ○ Sometimes ○ Usually ○ Always
	9. How often was the area around your room quiet at night?	○ Never ○ Sometimes ○ Usually ○ Always

Table 9.1 (continued)

Composite/item	HCAHPS survey	Response choices
Your hospital experiences	10. Did you need help from others at the hospital in getting to the bathroom or in using a bedpan?	○ Yes ○ No – [if no, go to question 12]
	11. If you got help in getting to the bathroom or in using a bedpan, how often did you get help as soon as you wanted it?	○ Never ○ Sometimes ○ Usually ○ Always
	12. Did you have any pain during your hospital stay?	○ Yes ○ No – [if no, go to questions 15]
	13. How often did the hospital staff talk with you about the amount of pain you had?	○ Never ○ Sometimes ○ Usually ○ Always
	14. How often did the hospital staff talk with you about how to treat the pain you had, during your stay?	○ Never ○ Sometimes ○ Usually ○ Always
	15. Were you given any new medications that you had not taken before, during your hospital stay?	○ Yes ○ No – [if no, go to question 18]
	16. Before hospital staff gave you new medicine, how often were you told what the medication was for?	○ Never ○ Sometimes ○ Usually ○ Always
	17. Before hospital staff gave you any new medicine, how often were you told what the possible side effects were in a way you understood them?	○ Never ○ Sometimes ○ Usually ○ Always
Leaving the hospital	18. When leaving the hospital, did you go straight to your own home, someone else's home, or to another healthcare facility?	○ Own home ○ Someone else's home ○ Another healthcare facility
	19. Did your doctors, nurses, or other hospital staff speak with you about whether you would have the help you needed when you have left the hospital?	○ Yes ○ No
	20. During your hospital stay, did you get information in writing regarding what symptoms or health issues to look out for after you leave the hospital?	○ Yes ○ No

(continued)

Table 9.1 (continued)

Composite/item	HCAHPS survey	Response choices
Overall hospital rating	*Answer the following questions regarding your stay at the hospital named on the cover letter. Do not include any other hospital stays in your answers.*	
	21. On a scale from 0 to 10, where 0 is the worst hospital possible and 10 is the best hospital possible, select a number that you would use to rate this hospital during your time of stay.	○ 0 – Worst hospital possible ○ 1 ○ 2 ○ 3 ○ 4 ○ 5 ○ 6 ○ 7 ○ 8 ○ 9 ○ 10 – Best hospital possible
	22. Is this a hospital you would recommend to your friends and family?	○ Definitely no ○ Probably no ○ Probably yes ○ Definitely yes
Understanding your care	23. Staff took my preference and those of my family or caregiver into account when deciding what my healthcare needs would be when I left during my hospital stay.	○ Strongly disagree ○ Disagree ○ Agree ○ Strongly agree
	24. After leaving the hospital, I had a good understanding of my responsibilities for managing my health.	○ Strongly disagree ○ Disagree ○ Agree ○ Strongly agree
	25. After leaving the hospital, I fully understood each purpose of my medications.	○ Strongly disagree ○ Disagree ○ Agree ○ Strongly agree ○ I was not given any medication after I left the hospital

Table 9.1 (continued)

Composite/item	HCAHPS survey	Response choices
	26. For your hospital stay, were you admitted to this hospital through the emergency room?	○ Yes ○ No
	27. How would you rate your overall health?	○ Excellent ○ Very good ○ Good ○ Fair ○ Poor
	28. How would you rate your overall mental or emotional health?	○ Excellent ○ Very good ○ Good ○ Fair ○ Poor
	29. What is the highest level or school or education you have completed?	○ Eighth grade or less ○ High school, but did not graduate ○ High school graduate or GED ○ College or 2-year degree ○ 4-year college graduate ○ More than 4-year college degree
	30. Please list if you are of Spanish, Hispanic or Latino origin or descent.	○ No, not Spanish/Hispanic or Latino ○ Yes, Puerto Rican ○ Yes, Mexican, Mexican American, Chicano ○ Yes, Cuban ○ Yes, other Spanish/Hispanic or Latino
	31. Please select the appropriate choices:	○ White ○ Black or African American ○ Asian ○ Native Hawaiian or other Pacific islander ○ American Indian or Alaska native
	32. What is the main spoken language at home?	○ English ○ Spanish ○ Chinese ○ Russian ○ Vietnamese ○ Portuguese ○ Some other language (please print below):

Survey instruments mailed out after the visit are likely to yield a different result than "real-time" surveys. Customers tend to be more generous in how they score their experience when filling out surveys at point of service. Survey results that do not account for the timing of the survey with the care delivery may introduce bias into the results.

In summary, a rigorous process was employed in the development of the most commonly used patient experience surveys, and the results of individual questions correlate well with top box patient satisfaction scores and with "would recommend" ratings. Smaller hospitals and clinicians with lower numbers of returned surveys may rightly question the validity of short-term results. These concerns can be mitigated by looking at results in a 4- or 6-month rolling average.

Inpatient Experience Metrics

Hospital Consumer Assessment of Healthcare Providers and Systems (HCAHPS) patient experience survey was developed by CMS in 2002, as a method of establishing a quality rating for the hospital inpatient experience. The survey asks recently discharged patients to answer 32 questions, including 27 questions that address multiple dimensions of the care experience. These dimensions of experience are comprised of 11 composite or single question score groupings as shown in Table 9.1. Responses to each question include never, sometimes, usually, and always. The components of the HCAHPS survey grouping are listed in the following text.

Nurse communication The relationship between nurse and patient is the most important determinant of patient satisfaction in the hospital setting [30–32]). Nurses spend considerable time with patients as they recover from the medical conditions that required hospitalization. The nurse is in constant contact with the patient, listening to their concerns, addressing their needs, executing a care plan, and serving as the intermediary between doctor and patient. It is vitally important that the nurse shows empathy, and compassion, is responsive, and communicates well with the care team. These core competencies are assessed in the HCAHPS survey.

Doctor communication The doctor-patient relationship is paramount to successful hospital treatment. Communication with the patient and key staff on the healthcare team is essential. Patients often assume their doctor is knowledgeable and skilled. Factors affecting their satisfaction with the hospital stay and ultimately their satisfaction with the doctor center around the soft communication skills or what we call "bedside manner." Did the doctor take the time to listen? Did the doctor show empathy and respect? Were things explained well and in a manner that lessened anxiety?

Staff responsiveness Was the call button answered quickly? When the patient was in need of assistance to the bathroom, was the call button answered in a manner that met the patient's expectations? Once patient expectations were communicated, was the issue addressed in a timely manner? Were staff dismissive or responsive to patient needs? When staff were busy, did they communicate a time expectation for addressing the request?

Room cleanliness   This metric addresses the patient concern about the cleanliness of the bathroom and patient's hospital room. Did housekeeping staff come daily to clean and sanitize the room?

Quietness   Hospitals are often noisy, especially in the intensive care units (ICU). Alarms go off when the intravenous line is empty or blocked, when the heart monitor detects abnormal rhythms, or when the patient presses the nurse call button. In addition, noise from telephones, televisions, and patients disrupts sleep [33–35]. Hospital staff, in constant communication, create noise in the hallways. Noise disrupts sleep, an essential component of recovery from disease and from surgery, and may add to the stress of hospitalization. Sleep improves the immune system's ability to fight off infection [36, 37] and may be beneficial for wound healing. More clinical studies are needed to establish the full clinical benefits of sleep. Therefore, a metric measuring the quietness of the hospital environment is present in the HCAHPS survey. Many units employ "quiet times" for several hours during each shift to better ensure that patients are able to rest.

Pain management   Uncontrolled pain can lead to adverse hospital outcomes [38, 39]. A postoperative patient may be unwilling to take deep breaths, thereby increasing the risk of respiratory complications. Patients experiencing pain are more likely to avoid ambulating after surgery or refuse to move limbs after joint surgery. Ambulation is critical for the prevention of deep vein thrombosis, aids in the return of bowel function after abdominal surgery, and is important for the prevention of postoperative lung complications such as atelectasis and pneumonia. Measuring how well pain was controlled during hospitalization is a HCAHPS survey measure. However, as we will discuss in the pitfalls section of this chapter, there are potential harmful consequences of placing too much focus on a pain-free hospitalization.

Medication communication   The most common reason for medication errors is poor communication. A Mayo Clinic study established that less than one third of patients knew the names of their medications and less than 40% knew the purpose of their medications. Even fewer, about 14%, knew the side effects of the medications they were taking [40]. Effective communication involves medication reconciliation (a review of the list of medications) to assure the hospital medication list corresponds to the list of medications prescribed by their doctors prior to hospitalization. If new medications are recommended and old ones removed during hospitalization, it is important that the patient and care providers post-hospitalization are on the same page. Side effects of any new medications should be carefully reviewed so patients can report unacceptable side effects. Allergies to specific medications or classes of medications should be carefully reviewed with the patient and noted in the patient chart and on wrist bands to avoid potentially dangerous medication reactions. Some hospitals have instituted bar coding of medications to assure the correct dose and correct medication are administered to all patients.

Discharge information A careful review of discharge instructions is critical for successful post-hospital recovery. Readmissions and post-hospital complications are more likely if discharge instructions are not communicated or followed. These instructions would include a careful review of discharge medications, activity limitations, and follow-up appointments or recommendations regarding follow-up appointments with specialists and with primary care doctors. Providing written instruction at discharge is important so that the patient does not need to rely on memory alone after hospital discharge.

Care transition While care transition may refer to any situation involving a change in place or person providing patient care, the HCAHPS survey has a series of three questions measuring patient perception of communication by hospital providers about the transition from hospital care to ongoing care outside the hospital – whether this care is received at a skilled nursing facility, at a rehabilitation facility, or at home. Did the provider assess the patient's ongoing need for care? Did they involve the patient in the decision about the place and type of care that would be needed? And did they provide in writing what types of things the patient should look out for after leaving the hospital? This set of questions also assesses whether medications were reviewed with the patient during the transition out of the hospital.

Hospital rating Patients are asked to give a numeric ranking of the hospital during their stay.

Willingness to recommend Patients are asked about their likelihood to recommend the hospital to friends and family. As discussed earlier in this chapter, great experiences create customer loyalty, potentially resulting in multiple referrals to the facility. The opposite is true: patients may be steered away if the patient has a bad experience.

Press Ganey has a robust set of proprietary questions to assess the hospital experience that may be used to supplement the HCAHPS survey. The primary advantage of sending a Press Ganey survey along with the HCAHPS survey is that Press Ganey provides the institution the ability to capture qualitative responses from patients in addition to the quantitative measures. The patient's written responses allow the organization the ability to make specific adjustments to improve the patient experience.

CAHPS patient satisfaction metrics have also been designed to measure the patient experience in other settings such as Nursing Homes (LTC CAHPS), Home Health (HH CAHPS), the Emergency Department (ED CAHPS), and the Operating Room (S CAHPS). Specific questions associated with each of these surveys can be found at CMS.gov.

Outpatient Experience Metrics

While there are many surveys used to measure the patient experience in the outpatient setting, two surveys, CG CAHPS and Press Ganey, are the most widely used in the United States. CG CAHPS (Clinician and Group Consumer Assessment of Healthcare Providers and Systems) survey was developed by the Agency for Healthcare Research and Quality (AHRQ) to measure the perception of the patient experience in the office setting. This survey uses 22 questions to assess the patient experience in the outpatient arena (Table 9.2). These questions fall into several cat-

Table 9.2 CGCAHPS outpatient experience survey

Composite/ item	CG CAHPS survey	Response choices
Your provider	*Please answer the following questions regarding the clinical care you have received.*	
	1. According to our records, you received care from the provider named below in the last 6 months. Is that correct? *Name of provider*	○ True ○ No
	2. Is the provider mentioned above who you usually see if you need a check-up, want advice about a health problem, or get sick or hurt?	○ Yes ○ No
	3. For how long have you been seeing this provider?	○ Less than 6 months ○ At least 6 months but less than 1 year ○ At least 1 year but less than 3 years ○ At least 3 years but less than 5 years ○ 5 years or more
Your care in the last 6 months	4. How many times did you visit this provider to get care for yourself, in the last 6 months?	○ None – If none, go to #23 ○ 1 time ○ 2 ○ 3 ○ 4 ○ 5 to 9 ○ 10 or more times
	5. Have you contacted this provider's office to get an appointment for an illness, injury, or conditions that required immediate attention?	○ Yes ○ No – If no, go to #7
	6. When you have contacted this providers' office to get an appointment for care that you needed right away, how often were you able to get an appointment as soon as you needed it?	○ Never ○ Sometimes ○ Usually ○ Always
	7. Have you made any appointments for a check-up or routine care with this provider in the last 6 months?	○ Yes ○ No, if no, go to #9

(continued)

Table 9.2 (continued)

Composite/item	CG CAHPS survey	Response choices
	8. When you have made an appointment for a check-up or routine care with this provider, how often were you able to get the appointment as soon as you needed it within the last 6 months?	○ Never ○ Sometimes ○ Usually ○ Always
	9. Have you contacted this provider's office with a medical question during regular office hours, within the past 6 months?	○ Yes ○ No – If no, go to #11
	10. When you contacted this provider's office during their regular office hours, how often were you able to get an answer to your medical question that same day?	○ Never ○ Sometimes ○ Usually ○ Always
	11. How often did your provider explain things in a way that was easy for you to understand, in the last 6 months?	○ Never ○ Sometimes ○ Usually ○ Always
	12. How often would you say your provider carefully listened to you within the last 6 months?	○ Never ○ Sometimes ○ Usually ○ Always
	13. How often did your provider seem to know the important information about your medical history, within the last 6 months?	○ Never ○ Sometimes ○ Usually ○ Always
	14. How often would you say your provider showed respect for what you had to say, in the last 6 months?	○ Never ○ Sometimes ○ Usually ○ Always
	15. How often did your provider spend enough time with you, in the last 6 months?	○ Never ○ Sometimes ○ Usually ○ Always
	16. Did your provider order a blood test, x-ray, or any other test for you, in the last 6 months?	○ Yes ○ No – If no, go to #18
	17. How often did your provider's office follow up to give you the results of any tests your provider has ordered for you, in the last 6 months?	○ Never ○ Sometimes ○ Usually ○ Always
	18. On a scale from 0 to 10, where 0 is the worst provider possible and 10 is the best provider possible, what number would you use to rate your provider?	○ 0 – Worst provider possible ○ 1 ○ 2 ○ 3 ○ 4 ○ 5 ○ 6 ○ 7 ○ 8 ○ 9 ○ 10 – Best provider possible

Table 9.2 (continued)

Composite/item	CG CAHPS survey	Response choices
	19. Have you taken any prescription medicine in the last 6 months?	○ Yes ○ No – If no, go to #21
	20. How often did you and someone from your provider's office speak about all the prescription medicines that you were taking, in the last 6 months?	○ Never ○ Sometimes ○ Usually ○ Always
Your provider's office staff	21. How often were clerks and receptionists at your provider's office as helpful as you thought they should be, in the last 6 months?	○ Never ○ Sometimes ○ Usually ○ Always
	22. How often did the clerks and receptionists at your provider's office treat you with courtesy and respect, in the last 6 months?	○ Never ○ Sometimes ○ Usually ○ Always
About yourself	23. How would you rate your overall health?	○ Excellent ○ Very good ○ Good ○ Fair ○ Poor
	24. How would you rate your overall mental or emotional health?	○ Excellent ○ Very good ○ Good ○ Fair ○ Poor
	25. Please select the age group that best fits you.	○ 18 to 24 ○ 25 to 34 ○ 35 to 44 ○ 45 to 54 ○ 55 to 64 ○ 65 to 74 ○ 75 or older
	26. Please select your gender.	○ Male ○ Female
	27. Please select what best describes your highest education level.	○ Eighth grade or less ○ High school, but did not graduate ○ High school graduate or GED ○ College or 2-year degree ○ 4-year college graduate ○ More than a 4-year college degree
	28. Please select if you are of Hispanic or Latino origin or descent.	○ Yes – Hispanic or Latino ○ No – Not Hispanic or Latino

(continued)

Table 9.2 (continued)

Composite/item	CG CAHPS survey	Response choices
	29. Please select your race. You may mark more than one answer.	○ White ○ Black or African American ○ Asian ○ Native Hawaiian or other Pacific islander ○ American Indian or Alaska native ○ Other
	30. Did you receive assistance in completing this survey?	○ Yes – If yes, go to #31 ○ No
	31. If you received help in completing this survey, how did he/she help you? You may mark more than one answer.	○ He/she read the questions to me ○ He/she wrote down the answers I gave ○ He/she answered the questions for me ○ He/she translated the questions into my language for me ○ He/she helped me in some other way

egories – access, staff experience, doctor experience, test result follow-up, overall office rating, and overall provider rating.

The Press Ganey questionnaire for assessment of the outpatient office experience draws from a large number of proprietary questions. Organizations using the Press Ganey survey can determine the length of the survey by choosing the questions they will ask of patients. Like the Press Ganey hospital survey, the outpatient survey provides the opportunity for comments, allowing for both quantitative and qualitative information about the patient experience. Patient comments offer concrete suggestions for improvement in services under the direct control of the provider office. In many cases, service improvements can be made quickly in response to patient suggestions. Positive comments are also important for building on the aspects of the patient experience the practice should continue doing. Positive comments shared with the care team impart motivation to continue working to improve the patient experience. Press Ganey, utilizing its national database, provides helpful analytics for organizations using its platform, enabling focused improvement efforts. More information about Press Ganey analytic tools and patient experience improvement programs can be found at www.pressganey.com/consulting/experience-of-care.

Additional metrics not included in HCHAPS and Press Ganey surveys should be collected and benchmarked to assess the patient experience. Phone metrics (including time to answer and dropped calls) are important access metrics. Generally, phones should be answered within 30 seconds, and dropped calls should total less than 5% of calls made. Office access metrics should also be collected. The time from request for a doctor visit to doctor appointment will vary by specialty and by the urgency of the medical problem. These metrics should be compared to appropriate clinical specialty benchmarks. Another important metric that is commonly followed in relation to the patient experience is patient complaints. Complaints may come in the form of a letter or phone call to the department manager or even the CEO of the organization. Complaints can be categorized and will often steer the organization to problem areas or system issues for focused efforts to improve the patient experience.

Patient Experience Improvement

The primary reason to assess the patient experience through metrics is to provide information to inform improvement efforts. Without metrics and patient comments, healthcare providers are relegated to guessing about the patient experience and relying on anecdotal comments. Careful data analysis of patient experience metrics provides the basis for a sound plan for improvement. However, meaningful efforts to improve patient satisfaction and achieve a great patient experience are not easy and require a sustained focus on the patient. In this section, we will provide some tips on how to approach improving the patient experience.

1. *Embrace a patient-centric culture.* Placing the patient at the center of what we do as healthcare providers is the first step to creating meaningful, actionable, and sustainable plans to improve the patient experience. Anything short of a "patient-first" culture will create obstacles to optimizing patient satisfaction as other priorities often come in conflict with doing what is best for the patient. Senior management plays a major role in establishing this culture. In both word and action, senior leadership, with board support, must clearly message to the organization that the patient comes first. Tufts Medical Center, an academic medical center in Boston, Massachusetts, has embarked on an effort to optimize the patient experience (called "Thoughtful Anticipation") by thoughtfully anticipating the needs of patients and meeting or exceeding their expectations at every encounter. By considering how we would want a family member to be treated, and then proactively delivering great service, patients are more likely to have an excellent experience. Creating a culture of service is essential for cultivating the ideal patient experience.
2. *Measure the patient experience* using both government-sponsored surveys (HCAPHS and CG CAPHS) and using additional survey tools such as Press Ganey or real-time questionnaires that allow for patient comments. Understanding the patient experience through the voice of the patient is the first step in thinking about improvement.
3. *Involve teams* of caregivers in the effort. Whether you are seeking to improve the patient experience in the hospital setting or in the office setting, all staff have an influence on patient satisfaction. This is true whether they are in direct

contact with the patient or have a back-office role as members of the healthcare team. Some of the best ideas for specific tactics to improve the patient experience will come from frontline staff or back-office staff. Make sure they are involved in the effort along with medical assistants, nurses, advance practitioners, and doctors. This inclusive approach also assists with creating the buy-in essential for achieving lasting results as well as improving staff retention.

4. *Focus on a few top drivers* of the patient experience. In most cases, it makes sense to focus on a few, high-impact areas of opportunity that are directly under the control of the team making the changes. Data analytics can assist in identifying the high-impact metrics most highly correlated with the top box patient satisfaction score or associated with "would recommend practice" score. Once these top drives have been identified, look for areas in need of improvement that are under your direct control. For instance, low scores on the ease of getting an office appointment allow the team to concentrate on phone access, schedule templates, and provider availability. Communication between the doctor or nurse and the patient is often an important driver of the patient experience during hospital stay or during an office visit. Focused efforts to improve communication may have a substantial impact on the patient experience. Specific communication strategies can be found in "Practicing Excellence: A Physician Manual to Exceptional Healthcare" by Stephen Beeson and in "The CG CAHPS Handbook" by Jeff Morris.

5. *Consider process improvement methodologies* that focus on the customer. Lean six sigma or Lean management principles focus on maintaining process steps that add customer value while eliminating wasteful steps in a process. Waste does not add value to the customer and contributes to customer dissatisfaction. For instance, long voicemail prompts followed by a request to leave a message often lead to patient dissatisfaction. Multiple phone calls often follow in an attempt to connect the patient with a nurse or secretary just so a message can be left for the doctor. More phone calls then follow to get an answer back to the patient. Mapping a process by a technique called "value stream mapping" allows the team, based on customer feedback, to eliminate steps in the process that do not add value. In most cases, streamlining processes also greatly benefits the healthcare team by reducing the time and energy to complete a task. Efficiencies created by the improved process reduce burnout and improve operational results.

6. *Hardwire a few improvements* before moving onto the next area of focus. Make sure the team is able to deliver on a few high-impact improvements every time with every patient before looking for other items to address. Management and staff leads must continually audit processes to assure they are being performed as required. Staff must be appropriately managed and new staff trained to assure compliance with patient experience standards. Physician leaders must assure all healthcare providers including doctors are meeting agreed-upon expectations. Reviewing patient experience metrics on a frequent and consistent basis along with patient comments provides an objective measure of success with a targeted improvement.

7. *Effective communication* is often a top driver of the patient experience. Do we show compassion in our words and body language? Do we listen carefully to the patient? Do we communicate empathy? Do we explain things carefully, assuring the patient understands? Do we get back to the patient quickly with results? Do we make sure to answer patient questions? Effective communication strategies are found in Steve Beeson's book "Practicing Excellence" and in "The CG CAHPS Handbook" by Jeff Morris.

8. *Manage up* your colleagues and your team. To manage up means to present your colleagues and staff in the best possible light. Comments to patients like "Isn't Dr. Salem a wonderful doctor" to describe a doctor your patient recently visited as a referral. Or "You are going to really like Dr. Yang. She is not only a great surgeon but also has a wonderful bedside manner." Statements such as these made by front office staff or referring physician about a doctor the patient is about to see for an office visit set up the visit up nicely. Doctors should also speak highly of their team members. The comment, "Donna, my nurse, is very experienced and will be able to answer any of your questions," establishes credibility for the entire team and places the patient at ease. On the contrary, nobody on the care management team benefits when negative comments are made in reference to either providers or staff. When negative comments are made to patients about facilities, processes, or team members, the person making the comment creates a negative impression for the patient about the environment in which they work.

9. *Consider adopting AIDET* or other similar communication strategy to assure patients are well informed at all times during each encounter with every individual on the healthcare team. AIDET describes a set of communication tactics that often create a positive impression during an interaction. Examples of AIDET are shown in Table 9.3.

Table 9.3 AIDET communication principles

AIDET	Keywords
A – Acknowledge	"Good morning Mrs. Kelly" (smile)
I – Introduce	"My name is Julie, I will be checking you in today." "I am Dr. Heilman. I have over 20 years of experience taking care of people who have brain tumors. Thank you for coming in today."
D – Duration	"Dr. Heilman will be with you as soon as he finishes with another patient – this should be about 15 minutes." "Let me help you get your lab tests ordered – the results should be ready about five days after the tests are completed and you will receive a phone call if the results require any follow-up or a letter will be sent about a week after results are back if they are normal" "would that be OK?"
E – Explanation	"Dr. Heilman will give you all the time you need – He is a wonderful doctor." "Would you like to get a cup of coffee at the shop downstairs and leave your number for me to call?"
T – Thank you	"Thank you for coming in today." Thank you for being on time. I heard the traffic was difficult today."

10. *Focus on staff satisfaction.* Numerous studies show that an engaged staff provide a better platform for patient engagement efforts [41–45]. A highly engaged staff appropriately aligned with the mission and vision of the organization is well positioned to focus on customer needs and concerns. Low morale among physicians and staff will interfere with efforts to focus on the patient as considerable energy will be consumed with fixing broken processes or displaying the teamwork necessary to provide a truly exceptional patient experience. Poor staff satisfaction is often associated with communication failures and lack of staff participation in decisions that affect their jobs. Because optimal communication and collegiality are essential components of both staff satisfaction and the patient experience, it is difficult to be successful in efforts to improve the patient experience without also having a highly engaged staff.

Potential Pitfalls of Patient Experience Metrics

The most significant and arguably the most legitimate concern about metrics used to determine the patient experience is that they do not assess clinical competency. Patient experience surveys are often completed after the patient has some impression of the doctor's clinical competence, yet CG CAHPS surveys do not address the question of clinical competency. Press Ganey has a question related to the patient's "confidence in the care provider," but survey metrics generally do not assess the patient's impression of the clinical competency of their providers.

The lack of focus on medical or surgical outcomes represents a substantial barrier to engaging physicians in patient experience efforts because physicians know that outcomes vary between providers and many believe that diagnostic accuracy and treatment outcomes are as important and perhaps more important than how the patient felt about their office visit or hospital stay. In one study, orthopedic surgeons felt that patient satisfaction should be almost entirely focused on surgical outcome. Yet high HCAHPS scores were not associated with surgical outcomes in a study from the University Health System of Wisconsin [46].

In addition, while patients may assume their doctor possesses superior clinical expertise when they chose a doctor, a missed diagnosis or poor surgical outcome may sour a good interpersonal interaction. At the very least, research focused on the extent to which the patient experience is influenced by clinical outcomes would be helpful and may lead to additional metrics to assess clinical competency. Considering the addition of metrics that measure the patient perception of clinical outcomes to patient experience tools could both enhance the validity of the tool and serve to engage more doctors in efforts to improve the patient experience. If clinical outcomes are a factor influencing the patient experience in the clinical setting, why not add a metric or two that measure perceived clinical competency?

In some cases, meeting patient expectations may be harmful to their health, such as overprescribing pain medications, overprescribing antibiotics, or ordering unnecessary testing. While keeping patients comfortable during their hospital stay may assist with walking and deep breathing which can reduce complications and lead to early discharge and improved pain control after surgery can even reduce the risk of opioid dependency, many experts believe some healthcare providers have focused too much attention on a pain-free hospital stay and, therefore, may have contributed to the opioid abuse crisis by prescribing too much opioid-derived pain medication. Opioids have also been shown to decrease bowel motility and respiratory effort (if given in high amounts) contributing to postoperative complications of nausea and ileus and even death from respiratory arrest [39]. These complications along with decreased mobility when opioids are overprescribed can contribute to increased length of stay. The patient should expect to have some pain after surgery or injury. While it is important to manage a patient's expectations regarding pain and to keep them safely comfortable, which has been shown to improve satisfaction, the question, "during the hospital stay, did you have any pain" may be misinterpreted by providers to suggest that hospitalized patients should be pain free. At Tufts Medical Center, the Department of Urology was able to significantly reduce length of stay by using an opioid-sparing regimen for pain control while prescribing nonsteroidal anti-inflammatory medications in a multimodal approach for postoperative patients.

Other examples of placing the patient experience ahead of sound medical judgment can occur when patients are looking for the "silver bullet" cure or the test that will explain their symptoms. A bad cold does not warrant the use of antibiotics, and their use may contribute to antibiotic resistance or allergic reaction. Yet that patient may present to the healthcare provider with the expectation that an antibiotic will be prescribed and leave dissatisfied if their expectation is not met. A patient may also present to the hospital or office with an expectation about a test they should have such as an MRI or CT scan. Sometimes, even the most carefully worded explanation for why the test should not be done will not be enough to meet the patient's expectation and result in a poor review.

While both HCCAHPS and Press Ganey are reliable well-tested standardized tools that are valuable to measure the patient experience, the combined HCAHPS and Press Ganey surveys sent to patients for completion are often too long. Both surveys are necessary if hospitals and clinics want direct patient feedback through written responses (provided only in Press Ganey). However, asking patients to fill out two surveys, containing many of the same or similar questions may impede the ability to get enough responses to make the survey meaningful. Sending one survey that asks a limited number of questions (HCAHPS or CG CAHPS) while providing the ability for written responses (Press Ganey) would be more "patient centric." Alternatively, selecting fewer questions from the Press Ganey survey may improve the survey response rate while providing additional information for a focused effort to improve the patient experience. There are a number of strategies to increase the survey response rate. The use of esurveys or text message surveys in the right population may deliver more responses. Real-time surveys performed in the office assure a higher response rate but also require some effort on the part of staff to administer the survey. Reminding patients that they will receive a survey and the office would appreciate the feedback is another tactic to improve responses.

In summary, most metrics focused on the patient experience are collected through survey tools. Many hospital and outpatient medical groups that measure the patient experience use a combination of HCCAHPS or CG CAHPS surveys with additional Press Ganey survey questions. Metrics harvested through these surveys are important measures of clinical quality and provide insights for efforts to improve the patient experience.

References

1. Kash B, McKahan M. The evolution of measuring patient satisfaction. J Primary Health Care Gen Pract. 2017;1(1):1–4.
2. Ronaldson A, Molloy GJ, Wikman A, Poole L, Kaski J, Steptoe A. Optimism and recovery after acute coronary syndromes: a clinical cohort study. Psychosom Med. 2015;77(3):311–8.
3. DiMatteo MR, Sherbourne CD, Hays RD, Ordway L, Kravitz RL, McGlynn EA, Kaplan S, Rogers WH. Physicians' characteristics influence patients' adherence to medical treatment: results from the medical outcomes study. Health Psychol. 1993;12(2):93–102.
4. Greenfield S, Kaplan S, Ware JE Jr. Expanding patient involvement in care: effects on patient outcomes. Ann Intern Med. 1985;102:520–8.
5. DiMatteo MR. Enhancing patient adherence to medical recommendations. JAMA. 1994;271(1):79–83.
6. Beck RS, Daughtridge R, Sloan PD. Physician-patient communication and health outcomes: a systemic review. J Am Board Fam Pract. 2002;15(1):25–38.
7. Safran DG, et al. Linking primary care performance to outcomes of care. J Fam Pract. 1998;47(3):213–20.
8. Stewart MA. Effective physician-patient communication and health outcomes: a review. Can Med Assoc. 1995;152(9):1423–33.
9. Fremont AM, Cleary PD, Hargreaves JL, Rowe RM, Jacobson NB, Ayanian JZ. Patient-centered process of care and long-term outcomes of myocardial infarction. J Gen Intern Med. 2001;16:800–8.
10. Sequester TD, Schneider EC, Anastario M, Odigie EG, Marshall R, Rogers WH, Safran DG. Quality monitoring of physicians: linking patients' experiences of care to clinical quality and outcomes. J Gen Intern Med. 2008;23(11):1784–90.
11. Jha AK, Orav EJ, Zheng J, Epstein AM. Patients' perception of hospital care in the United States. N Engl J Med. 2008;359:1921–31.
12. Isaac T, Zaslavsky AM, Cleary PD, Landon BE. The relationship between patients' perception of care and measures of hospital quality and safety. Health Serv Res. 2010;45(4):1024–40.
13. Meterko M, Wright S, Lin H, Lowy E, Cleary PD. Mortality amount patients with acute myocardial infarction: the influences of patient-centered care and evidence-based medicine. Health Serv Res. 2010;45(5):1188–203.
14. Fenton JJ, Jerant AF, Bertakis KD, Franks P. The cost of satisfaction. Arch Intern Med. 2012;172(5):405–11.
15. Safari DG, Montgomery HC, Murphy J, Rogers WH. Switching doctors: predictors of voluntary disenrollment from a primary physician's. Practice. Feb 2001;50(2):130–41.
16. Hill MH, Doddato T. Relationships among patient satisfaction, intent to return, and intent to recommend services provided by an academic nursing center. J Cult Divers. 2002;9(4):108.
17. Charmed PA, Frampton SB. Building the business case for patient-centered care: patient-centered care has the potential to reduce adverse events, malpractice claims, and operating costs while improving market share. Healthc Financ Manage. Mar 2008;62(3):80–5.

18. Von Wangenheim F, Bayon T. The chain from customer satisfaction via word-of-mouth referrals to new customer acquisition. J Academy Marketing Sci. 2007;35(2):233–49.
19. Shutte, L. "What you don't know can cost you: building a business case for recruitment and retention best practices." J ASPR, Summer 2002:1–7.
20. Hamidi, MS, Bohman, B, Sandburg, C, Smith-Coggins, R, de Vries, P, Albert, M, Welle, D, Murphy, M, Trockel, MT. The economic cost of physician turnover attributable to burnout. Stanford, WellMD Documents.
21. Lin Y, Huang Y. Team climate, emotional labor and burnout of physicians: a multilevel model. J Taiwan Public Health. 2014;33(3):271–89.
22. Mijakoski D, Bislimovska J, Milosevic M, Minov J. Differences in burnout, work demands and teamwork between Croatian and Macedonian hospital nurses. Cogn Brain Behav. 2015;19(3):179–200.
23. Hickson GB, Clayton EW, Entman SS. Obstetricians' prior malpractice experience and patients' satisfaction with care. JAMA (Original Contribution). 1994;272(20):1583–7.
24. Beckman HB, Markakis KM, Suchman AL, Frankel RM. The doctor-patient relationship and malpractice. Arch Intern Med. 1994;154:1365–70.
25. Levinson W, Roter DL, Mullooly JP, Dull VT, Frankel RM. The relationship with malpractice claims among primary care physicians and surgeons. Phys Pat Comm. 1997;277(7):553–9.
26. Fullam F, Garman AN, Johnson TJ, Hedberg EC. The use of patient satisfaction surveys and alternative coding procedures to predict malpractice risk. Med Care. 2009;47(5):553–9.
27. Stelfox HT, Gandhi TK, Oran EJ, Gustafson ML. The relation of patient satisfaction with complaints against physicians and malpractice lawsuits. Am J Med. 2005;118(10):1126–33.
28. Sofaer S, Crofton C, Goldstein E, Hoy E, Crabb J. What do consumers want to know about the quality of care in hospitals? Health Serv Res. 2005;40:2018–36.
29. Siegrist RB. Patient satisfaction: history, myths, and misperceptions. Virtual Mentor. 2013;15(11):982–7.
30. Schoenfelder T, Klewer J, Kugler J. Determinants of patient satisfaction: a study among 39 hospitals in an in-patient setting in Germany. Int J Qual Health Care. 2011;23(5):503–9.
31. Rafli F, Hajinezhad ME, Haghani H. Nurse caring in Iran and its relationship with patient satisfaction. Health Serv Manag Res. 2011;24(4):163–9.
32. Sweeny J, Brooks AM, Leahy A. Development of the Irish national patient perception of quality of care. Int J Qual Health Care. 2003;15(2):163–8.
33. Helton MC, Gordon SH, Nunnery SL. The correlation between sleep deprivation and the intensive care unit syndrome. Heart Lung. 1980;9(3):464–8.
34. Kahn DM, Cook TE, Carlisle CC, Nelson DL, Kramer NR, Millman RP. Identification and modification of environmental noise in an ICU setting. Chest. 1998;114(2):535–40.
35. Freedman NS, Kotzer N, Schwab RJ. Patient perception of sleep quality and etiology of sleep disruption in the intensive care unit. Am J Respir Crit Care Med. 1999;159(4):115–1162.
36. Mohren DC, Jansen NW, Kant IJ, Galama J, Van den Brandt PA, Swaen GM. Prevalence of common infections among employees in different works schedules. J Occup Environ Med. 2002;44:1003–11.
37. Patel SR, Malhotra A, Gao X, Hu FB, Neuman MI, Fawzi WW. A prospective study of sleep duration and pneumonia risk in women. Sleep. 2012;35(1):97–101.
38. Gan TJ. Poorly controlled postoperative pain: prevalence, consequences, and prevention. J Pain Res. 2010;10:2287–98.
39. Garimella V, Cellini C. Postoperative pain control. Clin Colon Rectal Surg. 2013;26(3):191–6.
40. Makaryus AN, Friedman EA. Patients' understanding of their treatments plans and diagnosis at discharge. Mayo Clin Proc. 2005;80(8):991–4.
41. Janicijevic I, Seke K, Djokovic A, Filipovic J. Healthcare workers satisfaction and patient satisfaction – where is the linkage? Hippokratia. 2013;17(2):157–62.
42. Haas JS, Cook EF, Puopolo AL, Burstin HR, Cleary PD, Brennan TA. Is the professional satisfaction of general internists associated with patient satisfaction? J Gen Intern Med. 2000;15:122–8.

43. Molyyneux J. Nurses' job satisfaction linked to patient satisfaction. AJN Am J Nurs. 2011;111:16.
44. Thornton RD, Nurse N, Snavely L, Hackett-Zahler S, Frank K, DiTomasso RA. Influences on patient satisfaction in healthcare centers: a semi-quantitative study over 5 years. BMC Health Serv Res. 2017;17:361.
45. Palese A, Gonella S, Fontanive A, Guarnier A, Barelli P, Zambiasi P, Allegrini E, Bazoli L, Casson P, Marin M. The degree of satisfaction of in-hospital medical patients with nursing care and predictors of dissatisfaction: findings from a secondary analysis. Scand J Caring Sci. 2017;31:768–78.
46. Kennedy GD, Tevis SE, Kent KC. Is there a relationship between patient satisfaction and favorable outcomes? Ann Surg. 2014;260(4):592–600.

Chapter 10
Quality Measures in Undergraduate Medical Education

David Li, Gordon Wong, and Marcia Boumil

Background and Current State of QI in Undergraduate Medical Education

The Purpose and Role of QI in UME

A traditional medical curriculum focused strictly on the diagnosis and management of disease is no longer adequate in the rapidly evolving landscape of healthcare, in which clinicians are expected to practice evidence-based medicine while minimizing patient harm and system-based errors [1]. In this context, quality improvement (QI) and patient safety (PS) have become increasingly underscored as competencies for which physician trainees should be proficient. Importantly, QI/PS has the aim of improving the process of healthcare relating to the systems issues surrounding healthcare delivery and patient outcomes while ultimately leveraging evidence-based findings to refine patient care.

The past two decades have witnessed substantial shifts in the healthcare delivery, with heightened emphasis on the integration of QI/PS initiatives toward undergraduate medical education (UME) to improve care [2]. These efforts were catalyzed in part by the Institute for Health Improvement as well as a report from the Institute of Medicine (IOM), "To Err is Human" in 2000, which concluded that most medical

D. Li
Department of Dermatology, Brigham and Women's Hospital, Boston, MA, USA
e-mail: dgli@bwh.harvard.edu

G. Wong
Department of Internal Medicine, UC Davis Medical Center, Davis, CA, USA

M. Boumil (✉)
Tufts University School of Medicine, Boston, MA, USA
e-mail: marcia.boumil@tufts.edu

© Springer Nature Switzerland AG 2020
D. N. Salem (ed.), *Quality Measures*, https://doi.org/10.1007/978-3-030-37145-6_10

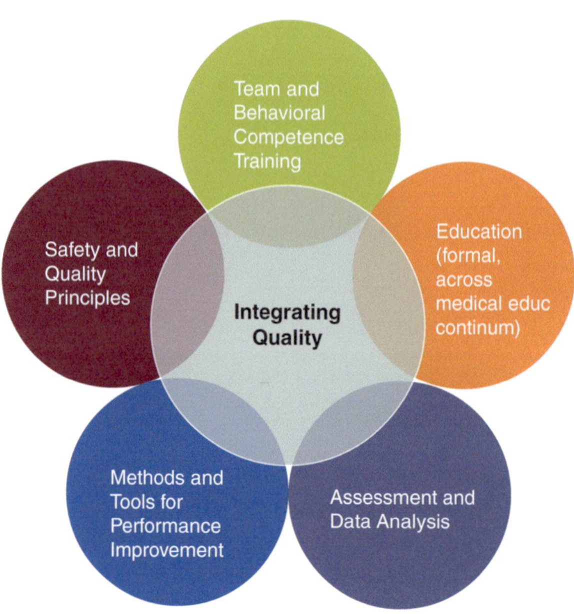

Fig. 10.1 Health care quality in Academic Medical Centers (AMCs): TEAMS model. Association of American Medical Colleges, https://www.aamc.org/initiatives/quality/52676/quality_projectmodel.html

errors are not rooted in clinician incompetency, but rather are the result of systematic processes that have failed to prevent human error [3].

Alongside these pragmatic efforts to emphasize the role of QI/PS in medicine, new regulations and accreditation requirements have spawned, resulting in changes to QI/PS education throughout US medical schools and academic medical centers [4]. These changes were in part fostered by the Association of American Medical Colleges' (AAMC) release of "Integrating Quality" (IQ), an initiative designed to guide and support medical professionals and trainees in achieving safe and high-quality healthcare [5]. The IQ initiative recommended a core model of QI/PS implementation among academic medical centers, entitled TEAMS Model, which comprises of five core factors designed to optimize healthcare quality within teaching hospitals [6]. Among these core factors is an explicit recommendation to integrate formal QI education across the UME and beyond (Fig. 10.1).

QI as a Core Competency

The purpose of QI/PS within UME is to refine processes relating to the delivery of care and optimize patient outcomes while leveraging evidence-based findings to continuously improve care in a positive feedback loop. Because the core concepts of quality in healthcare (safe, timely, efficient, effective, equitable, and patient centered) are incorporated by physicians across the spectrum of education from UME/ GME until clinical practice, it is therefore intuitive for proponents of QI to call for the engagement of learners beginning from UME [7].

In this manner, early uptake of QI/PS concepts within UME may then be more likely to be viewed by learners as a key component of practice, beyond the existing focus on diagnosis and management of disease. Likewise, early acquisition of QI knowledge during undergraduate medical training may program learners to experientially practice the optimal behaviors and conventions that may further promote a culture of quality and safety in healthcare. Thus, it is for these reasons that advocates in the healthcare arena are calling for QI/PS to be threaded throughout the entire continuum of medical education.

As of 2017, the AAMC reports that 144 of 145 (99.3%) of medical schools participating in their annual QI/PS survey acknowledged having either a required or elective course on QI/PS within the curriculum [8]. However, there is still major room for improvement and reform within UME, especially relating to specifying a clear role for QI/PS for trainees. While QI/PS is delineated as a core competency within practice-based learning and improvement, and systems-based practice within the Accreditation Council for Graduate Medical Education (ACGME) for graduate medical education (GME), the role of QI/PS as a core competency within UME is still not clearly defined (Fig. 10.2) [9, 10].

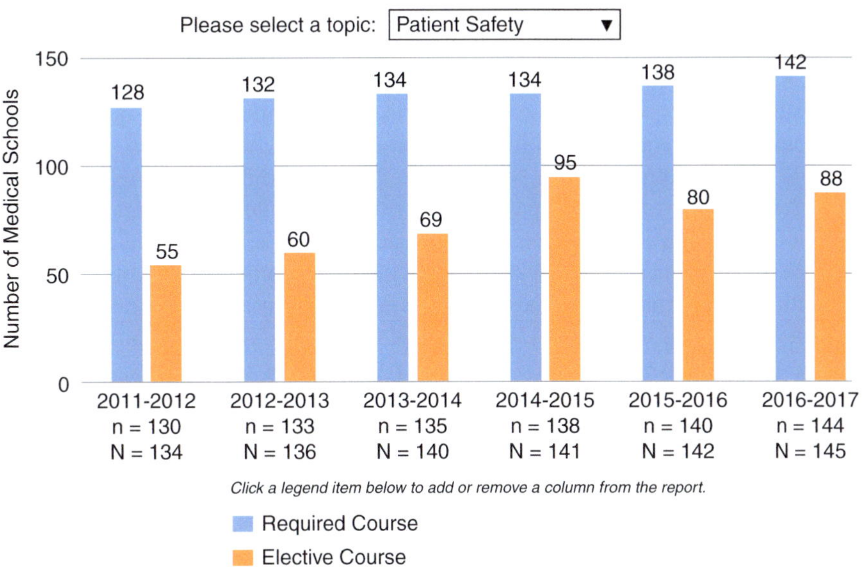

Fig. 10.2 Number of medical schools including topic in required courses and elective courses: patient safety [8]

The Role and Purpose of QI in UME (QI Data Science; Generalizability to Future Practice Settings

Effective instruction in QI as part of UME is not only important to help train physicians in quality and safety, but it is essential in general clinical practice. Understanding and applying QI principles within practice settings can create improvements in operational efficiency, patient satisfaction and safety, and health outcomes. As the landscape of healthcare reimbursement is transitioning to value-based payment methods, physician reimbursement will be tied to performance metrics and quality outcomes. Using QI processes and analytics to help physicians understand how specific performance metrics and quality outcomes are valued in value-based payment schemes will help clinicians practice more effectively. In addition, physicians will also have the option of participating in public reporting of physician quality data, such as the Physician Quality Reporting System (PQRS) which allows both individual and group practices to report information on the quality of care to Medicare and learn how often they are meeting a particular quality metric. As of 2015, PQRS began employing downward payment adjustments for individual and group practices who did not satisfactorily report quality data measures for Medicare Part B Physician Fee Schedule covered physician services in the 2013 year [29].

Implementing QI also allows practicing physicians to better participate in the federal Quality Payment Program such as the Merit-based Incentive Payment System (MIPS) or the Advanced Alternative Payment Model (AAPM), two payment tracks created under the Medicare Access and CHIP Reauthorization Act (MACRA) of 2015. Under MIPS, physician payments are adjusted based on a cumulative score based on individual performance in four categories: quality, cost, promoting interoperability, and improvement activities. Each clinician or clinician group's score is compared to a performance threshold, and final scores exceeding the threshold receive positive payment adjustments, while final scores below the threshold receive negative payment adjustments [30]. These adjustments range from +/− 5% for performance year in 2018 to +/− 9% for performance year of 2021 [30]. Exceptional performances are also eligible to receive an additional positive payment adjustment of up to 10% [30]. Under AAPM, qualifying clinicians and clinician groups are given added 5% incentive payments for high-quality, high-value care to patients and can be applied to a specific condition or patient population for reporting required quality data [31].

Finally, physician practices and healthcare institutions practicing QI have the skills to apply for accreditation programs like the American Heart Association's Center of Excellence or the Joint Commission's Certification for Primary Stroke Centers. For primary care physician groups, adopting the Patient-Centered Medical Home (PCMH) accreditation programs allows for payment incentives when patients are seen appropriately and for meeting quality and efficiency goals [32].

Recommended QI Curriculum for Medical Students

Core Recommendations for Application of QI/PS into UME

The AAMC released a report in 2013 entitled "Teaching for Quality: Report of an Expert Panel" that addresses the necessity of integrating QI/PS into the continuum of medical education, with a particular focus on promoting the development of curriculum design and competencies among faculty and students alike [4]. The vision of this report is to apply curricular assessment and educational activities across the spectrum of medication education, with the goal of amassing a sizeable force of physicians and healthcare providers who are able to engage in and lead education in QI/PS toward a reduction of unnecessary costs and avoidable medical errors. While many proponents for QI/PS are rooted in early exposure of QI/PS initiatives to students during medical school, the authors of this report recommend a more comprehensive approach which we will use as a framework to expand upon for our recommended curriculum in UME.

First, to achieve QI/PS goals for UME and eventual clinical practice, academic medical institutions (including medical schools, academic teaching hospitals, accreditation organizations) should actively work toward the integration of QI/PS concepts into clinically relevant and experiential experiences across the spectrum of physician development. This may include the development and application of QI/PS competency assessment measures across medical education while incorporating QI/PS elements into accreditation and licensing bodies for UME.

Second, while it is critical to engage learners within UME on the concepts of QI/PS, it may be even more important to require medical faculty to be at least proficient in QI/PS competencies. By utilizing a top-down, synergistic approach alongside engagement of medical student learners, UME may benefit from a body of faculty experts to serve as educators in the creation, implementation, and evaluation of training for medical students. Lastly, it is imperative that medical schools and teaching sites integrate QI/PS into foundational activities while aligning efforts to implement QI/PS concepts and engagements into UME. Collaboration between the medical school educational committee and its affiliated clinical institutions may lead to necessary infrastructure and resources for academic endeavors to study QI/PS in a real-time, problem-based fashion. The necessity of these major categories of recommendations will be expanded throughout this chapter.

Principles and Methods of QI Safety Incident Analysis: System Approaches

Several methods can be employed within healthcare for QI and safety incident analysis.

Plan-Do-Study-Act (PDSA) Cycle Widely used by the Institute for Healthcare Improvement, this model seeks to identify how changes in processes, behaviors, and capabilities affect outcomes, allowing for rapid, small changes. The PDSA cycle traditionally begins with (1) determining the nature and scope of the problem, (2) identifying what changes can be made, (3) developing a strategy for a targeted change, (4) identifying which key stakeholders need to be involved, (5) measuring and assessing the impact of the change, and (6) defining effective targeting of the strategy. As change is being implemented, data is collected, assessed, and interpreted according to predefined metrics whether implemented change yielded the intended effects. The process can be reiterated for additional improvements and changes.

Six Sigma The fundamental objective of the Six Sigma methodology looks to use measurements to refine processes and reduce variation. This is accomplished according to two submethodologies: DMAIC (define, measure, analyze, improve, control) and DMADV (define, measure, analyze, design, verify). DMAIC is an important improvement strategy that focuses on existing processes and procedures that have fallen below specified thresholds and can benefit from incremental improvement, whereas DMADV aids in the development of novel processes and products or to rework existing processes which are otherwise not amenable to smaller, stepwise changes.

Root Cause Analysis (RCA) This is a reactive process that seeks to discover the underlying cause of an error or adverse event by focusing on the multiple contributing factors and conditions. This relies not only on understanding what, when, and why the incident occurred but also on understanding what systems and processes allowed for the error to occur. Through this examination, RCA attempts to make clear which gaps and ineffective barriers exist within systems and processes that need to be addressed in order to prevent further incidents. This typically results in providing recommendations on how to address these weaknesses and how to successfully employ education, training, and system safeguards to reduce the likelihood of future errors of a similar nature.

Lean Similar to the Six Sigma philosophy, Lean (also known as "Toyota Production System") seeks to identify consumer needs and values in order to maximize helpful process elements and remove others deemed to be "no value-added." By focusing on maximizing the process functions that provide the most utility to consumers and eliminating unnecessary steps, Lean can ultimately simplify work processes, remove extraneous workarounds, clarify responsibilities, and help establish realizable goals. In order to do this, Lean usually involves all levels of personnel, from frontline to management to contribute their insight, and employs root cause analysis to identify and best track problems in real time. Proposed solutions can then be tested and measured to see results, which can uncover new insights.

Ancillary Skill Sets to Prepare Learners for QI Projects

While there are publicly available resources online (i.e., modules for QI/PS training), direct application of classroom learning through experiential projects may be most beneficial [11]. Within the reported literature, select academic programs have advocated for the use of in-classroom modules to simulate realistic problems in the hospital that may benefit from quality/safety intervention [11, 12]. These programs have found modest improvement in learner grasp and appreciation of QI/PS [13, 14]. However, the ease of integrating these modules into the medical curriculum imposing minimal interference with the traditional medical curriculum is also its notable shortcoming. While case-based scenarios may mimic reality and represent a tangible step toward integrating QI/PS within UME, the problem-based classroom learning approach may be too straightforward to elicit the creative and critical thinking needed to engage learners for unique challenges in QI/PS.

Experiential learning in the classroom should be a bridge to prepare learners to pilot individual QI/PS projects. However, other technical skill sets relating to QI practice methods are needed to help the learner navigate their projects in a rigorous and systematic manner. To this end, it is recommended that academic medical institutions integrate the core concepts of biostatistics, stakeholder engagement, medical ethics, and health services foundations into the curriculum concurrently alongside QI/PS courses. Ideally, these courses, in addition to the QI/PS curriculum, would be taught during the first 2 years of medical school. A notable example is the Dartmouth Medical School Quality Improvement and Healthcare Systems Curriculum that prepares learners for hospital-based application during core clinical rotations during the third and fourth years of medical school [15].

To facilitate experiential learning by tackling real-time problems arising in the clinical setting, learners should be paired with physician-mentors who demonstrate dedication toward QI/PS. Students should be encouraged to work with these faculty to develop and pilot their own QI/PS projects, with the aim of achieving measurable, meaningful patient outcomes that can be shared with the academic medical community. As this project will require a substantial commitment of time, medical schools should make it fulfill a capstone or another requirement such as volunteer work, clinical research, etc. By combining the in-classroom skills of QI practice methods with real-life clinical challenges aimed at improving system-based processes in the hospital, learners may then be more likely to continue such endeavors well beyond UME to foster a culture of continuous improvement within healthcare.

Assembly of All Stakeholders to Share and Use Data for QI Outcomes

Numerous stakeholders in the current healthcare arena are interested in harnessing the value of QI/PS to improve healthcare. As learners embark on real-time projects in the clinical setting, it is critical that all necessary stakeholders are engaged in a timely manner [16]. In this fashion, the learner can become at qualitative methods aimed at promoting safer patient care. To this end, the learner should also address questions that are relevant to the stakeholders who stand to benefit from data on QI outcomes.

Early engagement of key stakeholders is therefore recommended prior to the initiation of any QI/PS project. Within healthcare, Concannon et al. have defined a framework to identify key stakeholders in patient-centered outcomes research (PCOR) that can be relevant in developing a QI project: patients and the public, clinical providers in a variety of disciplines, purchasers, payers, policymakers, and product makers [17]. However, the timing of when to engage each stakeholder and how best to identify the relevant stakeholders may be a challenge; it may therefore benefit students to have a course dedicated to stakeholder engagement analysis. After all, it is imperative that learners undertake projects designed and conducted to pursue endpoints that are meaningful to the relevant stakeholders (Table 10.1).

Beyond the customization of study design and data analysis in pursuit of outcomes considered important by stakeholders, learners should also understand the importance of stakeholder engagement to identify areas of improvement within the healthcare domain under exploration. As QI/PS study initiation often requires widespread and network engagement of key stakeholders, students should be equipped with the tools to engage in qualitative data collection methods.

To this end, learners may benefit from in-classroom instruction on designing and conducting semistructured interviews, which is an interviewing technique designed to engage respondents in a formal interview utilizing an interview guide [18, 19]. This method allows the corresponding stakeholder to provide open-ended answers

Table 10.1 The 7Ps framework to identify stakeholders in PCOR and CER [17]

Category	Description
Patients and the public	Current and potential consumers of patient-centered health care and population-focused public health, their caregivers, families, and patient and consumer advocacy organizations
Providers	Individuals (e.g., nurses, physicians, mental health counselors, pharmacists, and other providers of care and support services) and organizations (e.g., hospitals, clinics, community health centers, community-based organizations, pharmacies, EMS agencies, skilled nursing facilities, schools) that provide care to patients and populations
Purchasers	Employers, the self-insured, government and other entities responsible for underwriting the costs of health care
Payers	Insurers, Medicare and Medicaid, state insurance exchanges, individuals with deductibles, and others responsible for reimbursement for interventions and episodes of care
Policy makers	The White House, Department of Health and Human Services, Congress, states, professional associations, intermediaries, and other policy-making entities
Product makers	Drug and device manufacturers
Principal investigators	Other researchers and their funders

and pseudo-tangential topics of discussion that may be unknowingly relevant to the study at hand; the interview guide allows the researcher to bring the discussion back to a preformulated trajectory should there be major digressions. Adherence to the 7Ps of stakeholder engagement may help guide learners in the employment of a rigorous study design that is geared to address outcomes meaningful to relevant stakeholders.

Communicating Learner Findings to Stakeholders

At the conclusion of a QI/PS study, researchers should engage stakeholders once more to disseminate research findings that may further promote a culture of quality improvement and safety within medicine. According to the Plan-Do-Study-Act (PDSA) cycle for implementing QI models into the clinical setting, stakeholder engagement is embedded within each of the four key steps [20, 21]. While we have discussed the importance of stakeholder engagement in the first two steps (Plan Strategy; Develop, Test Strategy), post-study surveillance and broad-scale implementation of findings are also necessary to fuel a cycle of continuous improvement, whereby researchers monitor the success of QI/PS initiative through unremitting reassessments of project success. In this way, researchers may better address the questions of "what worked, what did not work, and how to improve the process." [22]

It is therefore equally important that learner study findings and data points are communicated back to the stakeholders. As emphasis is often placed primarily on study design and testing QI/PS strategies rather than post-study surveillance, the responsibility largely lies upon the mentor to communicate key findings to relevant stakeholders. However, to fully and successfully implement a QI/PS initiative based on empiric findings, key stakeholders need to be on board (Fig. 10.3).

Implementation and Challenges

Combining Classroom Learning with Practical Projects Such as Root Cause Analysis and Safety Incident Analysis

Several challenges stand in the way of successful implementation of QI/PS concepts into real-time practice in the hospital setting. Despite these obstacles, practical projects (e.g., root cause analysis, safety incident analysis) which harness clinical research skills and in-classroom QI/PS concepts hold the promise of experiential engagements that may lead to the development of champions of QI/PS in UME and beyond. In this section, major challenges will be outlined and potential solutions presented.

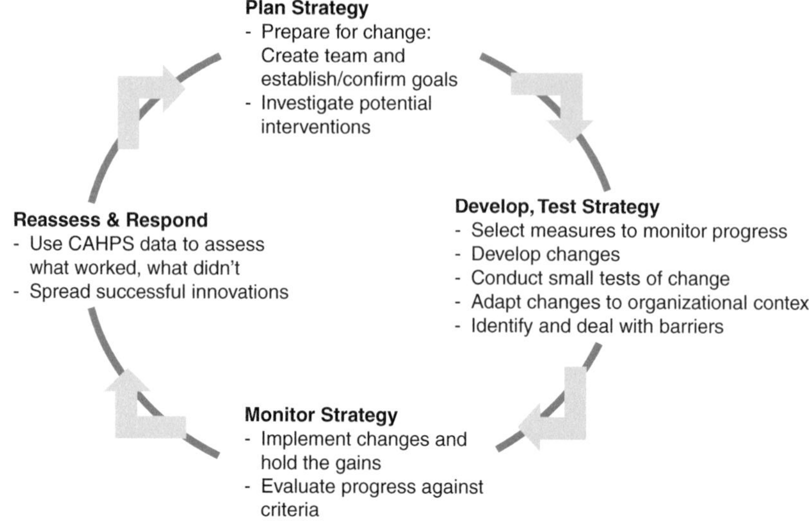

Fig. 10.3 Plan-do-study-act cycle [20]

While there have been immense efforts to bring focus toward QI/PS within healthcare, a major barrier to implementing classroom learning with practical projects in QI/PS is the diversity and level of engagement among medical education curriculum committees. To this end, obtaining support from faculty involved in clinical medicine may be challenging. The culture of medicine has been one of unwavering focus toward diagnosis and management of disease, but the concepts of QI/PS are still relatively new, and its importance may be underestimated by more traditional faculty members. Similarly, the medicine's classical commitment to individuality and professional autonomy may perceive the basis of QI/PS as threats to authority and individual practice [23]. The foundations of QI/PS lie in continuous improvement, with the unspoken assumption that the existing system is imperfect and muddled by clinical error, oftentimes human error. Faculty members who have this view of QI/PS may oppose efforts to formally incorporate practical projects into the medical curriculum.

Alongside this challenge, the existing state of QI/PS within academic medical institutions may be also marred by a lack of mentors and champions of QI/PS. Until QI/PS is formally recognized within the medical curriculum and across accreditation committees, there will likely be a shortage of faculty who are "masters" of QI/PS concepts in practice [4]. Naturally, this means a shortage of potential mentors to teach learners within UME but also a shortage of well-developed QI/PS projects for learners to participate in. As close engagement in real-world QI/PS challenges are likely to be most beneficial for students, strategizing the recruitment of key faculty members are necessary to prepare, mentor, and debrief with students is imperative.

In the short term, junior faculty involved in the disciplines of clinical research should be educated in QI/PS pursuits in order to serve as budding mentors to medical students. In the long term, early exposure of medical students and residents in the concepts of QI/PS (alongside formal competencies in QI/PS) may result in a greater number of senior faculty involved in QI/PS over time.

The logistics of integrating QI/PS training into the spectrum of UME may also pose a major challenge. It is not surprising that existing medical school curricula are time-consuming and require focused attention by learners, and the addition of further training in QI/PS may be unrealistic without corresponding shifts in existing curricula [24]. Literature has found that early quality projects without layered training did not result in the addition of quality improvement into the curriculum [25]. Similarly, hands-on projects in QI/PS may be more beneficial for learners who have acquired relevant context through classroom training in topics such as study design, root cause analysis, and safety incident analysis [26–28]. This entails the inclusion of ancillary courses early in the curriculum to prepare learners for experiential projects alongside core clinical rotations. However, to achieve this, major shifts in the curriculum of medical schools are needed to redistribute efforts involved in other educational disciplines.

Longitudinal Assessment of Learners for QI Competency

One of the difficulties in carrying out successful QI implementation in UME is that it requires hands-on projects to best allow learners to cultivate the necessary skills in a relevant context. Therefore, without the proper interval to cultivate and practice these skills, it can be difficult for assessment of QI competency. The literature suggests that the large extent of QI activities has been seen within medical residencies. Indeed, the American College of Graduate Medical Education mandates that all resident physicians undertake and complete a QI project under proper faculty supervision and evaluation [33]. QI project activities within medical residencies have traditionally been offered through dedicated elective blocks [34, 35], while some programs offer longitudinal QI curricula [35–38]. While it was found that longitudinal QI curriculum including didactics, workshops, and review sessions for residents provided the hands-on tools needed for QI knowledge and skills retention, it required balancing the different needs among learners, faculty, and the institution, along with adopting effective adult learning theory with QI/PS methodologies [39].

Current implementation of longitudinal tracks involving active QI projects within American UME is seen at the Warren Alpert School of Medicine at Brown University and Vanderbilt University School of Medicine, among others. Within the Primary Care-Population Medicine program at the Warren Alpert School, students taking part in the Longitudinal Integrated Clerkship are required to develop a quality improvement project that addresses an element of healthcare delivery at a clinical site [39]. At Vanderbilt University School of Medicine, as of January 2015, students are required to complete a cumulative 3-month-long QI course in the third or fourth year, where they develop and execute a clinically focused QI project including two PDSA cycles1 [13]. One hundred ten student QI projects were completed from January 2015 to January 2017, and 70% of Vanderbilt students rated the experience as highly clinically relevant and meaningful for their development as physicians [13].

Despite the opportunity to provide teaching and hands-on opportunities for QI, there remains to be a single method to meaningfully assess learners' knowledge and skills [14]. The most common way to assess core learning has typically involved direct faculty evaluation and feedback regarding presentation of a quality improvement project. However, how well this type of assessment properly captures learning varies by institution and evaluator. Other more standardized measures have not been reported in the literature. Ogrinc and colleagues described assessing QI knowledge in internal medicine residents using the Quality Improvement Knowledge Application Tool (QIKAT), which placed each learner in three situations with differing aims and measures requiring the learner to propose changes for improvement [28]. QIKAT was further adopted by Vinci and colleagues to assess the efficacy of a QI curriculum for internal medicine residents [40]. While QIKAT has been useful in comparing the pre-learning and post-learning QI knowledge of internal medicine in both studies, it still remains to become validated. The implementation of QI within both undergraduate and graduate medical education will involve developing more robust evaluation tools and ultimately linking QI learning to behavioral changes that improve patient-level outcomes.

References

1. Varkey P. Educating to improve patient care: integrating quality improvement into a medical school curriculum. Am J Med Qual. 2007;22:112. https://doi.org/10.1177/1062860606298338.
2. Teaching for Quality – Continuing Education and Improvement – Initiatives – AAMC. https://www.aamc.org/initiatives/cei/educatingforquality/. Accessed May 27, 2018.
3. To err is human. Washington, DC: National Academies Press; 2000. doi:https://doi.org/10.17226/9728.
4. Headrick LA, Baron RB, Pingleton SK, et al. Teaching for quality integrating quality improvement and patient safety across the continuum of medical education report of an expert panel Association of American Medical Colleges Teaching for Quality. www.aamc.org/91514/reproductions.html. Accessed May 27, 2018.
5. Integrating Quality – Initiatives – AAMC. https://www.aamc.org/initiatives/quality/. Accessed May 27, 2018.
6. TEAMS Model – Integrating Quality – Initiatives – AAMC. https://www.aamc.org/initiatives/quality/52676/quality_projectmodel.html. Accessed May 27, 2018.
7. Crossing the quality chasm: a new health system for the 21st century. 2001. http://www.nationalacademies.org/hmd/~/media/Files/ReportFiles/2001/Crossing-the-Quality-Chasm/Quality Chasm 2001 report brief.pdf. Accessed May 27, 2018.
8. Curriculum Inventory and Reports (CIR) – Initiatives – AAMC. https://www.aamc.org/initiatives/cir/406462/06a.html. Accessed May 27, 2018.
9. Wong BM, Levinson W, Shojania KG. Quality improvement in medical education: current state and future directions. Med Educ. 2012;46(1):107–19. https://doi.org/10.1111/j.1365-2923.2011.04154.x.

10. Batalden P, Leach D, Swing S, Dreyfus H, Dreyfus S. General competencies and accreditation in graduate medical education. Health Aff (Millwood). 2002;21(5):103–11. http://www.ncbi.nlm.nih.gov/pubmed/12224871. Accessed May 28, 2018
11. Institute for Healthcare Improvement: IHI Home Page. http://www.ihi.org/. Accessed May 27, 2018.
12. Institute for Healthcare improvement: embedding quality improvement in medical education: our 90-day report. http://www.ihi.org/communities/blogs/_layouts/15/ihi/community/blog/itemview.aspx?List=84e15604-08bf-4317-8323-cf46b485b7c0&ID=8. Accessed May 27, 2018.
13. Bradham TS, Sponsler KC, Watkins SC, Ehrenfeld JM. Creating a quality improvement course for undergraduate medical education. Acad Med. 2018;1:1491. https://doi.org/10.1097/ACM.0000000000002253.
14. Tartaglia KM, Walker C. Effectiveness of a quality improvement curriculum for medical students. Med Educ Online. 2015;20:27133. https://doi.org/10.3402/MEO.V20.27133.
15. Ogrinc G, Nierenberg DW, Batalden PB. Building experiential learning about quality improvement into a medical school curriculum: the Dartmouth experience. Health Aff (Millwood). 2011;30(4):716–22. https://doi.org/10.1377/hlthaff.2011.0072.
16. Roehr B. More stakeholder engagement is needed to improve quality of research, say US experts. BMJ. 2010;341:c4193. https://doi.org/10.1136/BMJ.C4193.
17. Concannon TW, Meissner P, Grunbaum JA, et al. A new taxonomy for stakeholder engagement in patient-centered outcomes research. J Gen Intern Med. 2012;27(8):985–91. https://doi.org/10.1007/s11606-012-2037-1.
18. Semi-structured interviews recording semi-structured interviews. https://www.sswm.info/sites/default/files/reference_attachments/COHEN2006SemistructuredInterview.pdf. Accessed May 28, 2018.
19. Louise Barriball K, While A. Collecting data using a semi-structured interview: a discussion paper. J Adv Nurs. 1994;19(2):328–35. https://doi.org/10.1111/j.1365-2648.1994.tb01088.x.
20. Section 4: Ways to Approach the Quality Improvement Process | Agency for Healthcare Research and Quality. https://www.ahrq.gov/cahps/quality-improvement/improvement-guide/4-approach-qi-process/index.html. Accessed May 28, 2018.
21. Pinsky L, Djuricich AM, Ciccarelli M, Swigonski NL. Forces impacting graduate medical education a continuous quality improvement curriculum for residents: addressing core competency, improving systems. https://insights.ovid.com/pubmed?pmid=15383393. Accessed May 28, 2018.
22. Batalden PB, Davidoff F. What is "quality improvement" and how can it transform healthcare? Transformation of healthcare—quality improvement. Qual Saf Health Care. 2007;16(1):2–3. https://doi.org/10.1136/qshc.2006.022046.
23. Leape LL, Berwick DM. Five years after to err is human. JAMA. 2005;293(19):2384. https://doi.org/10.1001/jama.293.19.2384.
24. Mosser G, Frisch KK, Skarda PK, Gertner E. Addressing the challenges in teaching quality improvement. Am J Med. 2009;122(5):487–91. https://doi.org/10.1016/j.amjmed.2009.01.013.
25. Parenti CM, Lederle FA, Impola CL, Peterson LR. Reduction of unnecessary intravenous catheter use. Arch Intern Med. 1994;154(16):1829. https://doi.org/10.1001/archinte.1994.00420160062008.
26. Ogrinc G, Headrick LA, Mutha S, Coleman MT, O'Donnell J, Miles PV. A framework for teaching medical students and residents about practice-based learning and improvement, synthesized from a literature review. Acad Med. 2003;78(7):748–56. https://insights.ovid.com/pubmed?pmid=12857698. Accessed May 28, 2018
27. Canal DF, Torbeck L, Djuricich AM. Practice-based learning and improvement. Arch Surg. 2007;142(5):479. https://doi.org/10.1001/archsurg.142.5.479.
28. Ogrinc G, Headrick LA, Morrison LJ, Foster T. Teaching and assessing resident competence in practice-based learning and improvement. J Gen Intern Med. 2004;19(5 Pt 2):496–500. https://doi.org/10.1111/j.1525-1497.2004.30102.x.

29. "Physician Quality Reporting Services." Centers for Medicare and Medicaid Services. Updated April 26, 2018. https://www.cms.gov/Medicare/Quality-Initiatives-Patient-Assessment-Instruments/PQRS/index.html?redirect=/pqri.
30. "MIPS Overview." Quality Payment Program. https://qpp.cms.gov/mips/overview.
31. "APMs Overview." Quality Payment Program. https://qpp.cms.gov/apms/overview.
32. "PCMH Costs, Benefits, and Incentives." American College of Physicians. https://www.acponline.org/practice-resources/business-resources/payment/models/patient-centered-medical-home/pcmh-costs-benefits-and-incentives.
33. "Common Program Requirements." American College of Graduate Medical Education. May 20, 2008. http://www.acgme.org/Portals/0/PDFs/commonguide/IVA5c_EducationalProgram_ACGMECompetencies_PBLI_Documentation.pdf.
34. Sarwar A, Eisenberg RL, Boiselle PM, Siewert B, Kruskal JB. Improving resident education in quality improvement: role for a resident quality improvement director. Acad Radiol. 2013;20(4):500–5.
35. Laiteerapong N, Keh CE, Naylor KB, Yang VL, Vinci LM, Oyler JL, Arora VM. A resident-led quality improvement initiative to improve obesity screening. Am J Med Qual. 2011;26(4):315–22.
36. Simasek M, Ballard SL, Phelps P, Pingul-Ravano R, Kolb NR, Finkelstein A, et al. Meeting resident scholarly activity requirements through a longitudinal quality improvement curriculum. J Grad Med Educ. 2015;7(1):86–90.
37. Duello K, Louh I, Greig H, Dawson N. Residents' knowledge of quality improvement: the impact of using a group project curriculum. Postgrad Med J. 2015;91(1078):431–5. https://doi.org/10.1136/postgradmedj-2014-132886.
38. Tentler A, Feurdean M, Keller S, Kothari N. Integrating a resident-driven longitudinal quality improvement curriculum within an ambulatory block schedule. J Grad Med Educ. 2016;8(3):405–9.
39. Vachani JG, Mothner B, Lye C, Savage C, Camp E, Moyer V. Impact of a longitudinal quality improvement and patient safety curriculum on pediatric residents. Pediatr Qual Saf. 2016;1(2):e005.
40. Vinci LM, Oyler J, Johnson JK, Arora VM. Effect of a quality improvement curriculum on resident knowledge and skills in improvement. BMJ Qual Saf. 2010;19(4):351–4.

Chapter 11
Resident Quality Training: More than Metrics

Mikhail Romashko and Kari E. Roberts

> The relationship between residency training and the health care delivery system is reciprocal; the fate of one affects the other. During residency, doctors acquire the habits and approaches that they carry with them throughout their careers. [3]

> Graduating residents are expected to understand how QI, PS and related concepts should be embedded into their clinical practice and how they affect health system functioning. [4]

Introduction

High-quality health care requires a physician workforce educated and engaged in patient safety and quality improvement principles and practices.

Toward the end of the twenty-first century, it became apparent that the successes of modern medicine – including tremendous advances in therapeutics and diagnostics – were tempered by an emergent crisis in health-care safety. In the late 1990s, the Institute of Medicine (IOM) commissioned a multiyear study to examine the quality of health care in the United States. This culminated in the 1999 report "To Err is Human" which revealed serious patient safety issues, marked variability in the quality of care delivered, and significant health-care disparities across the nation. In all, it was estimated that between 44,000 and 98,000 patients died each year in the United Sates as a consequence of medical error [5]. This stark message was followed by a 2001 report "Crossing the Quality Chasm" in which the IOM observed "the US health care delivery system does not provide consistent, high-quality medical care to all people," challenging the health-care community to pursue the highest quality care and outcomes for their patients and populations [2].

In response to this call to action, the Joint Commission, the Centers for Medicare and Medicaid Services, and other regulatory organizations promoted "system-based" practices and metrics to improve patient safety and quality of care. Adopting

M. Romashko · K. E. Roberts (✉)
Tufts Medical Center, Boston, MA, USA
e-mail: mromashko@tuftsmedicalcenter.org; kroberts@tuftsmedicalcenter.org

© Springer Nature Switzerland AG 2020
D. N. Salem (ed.), *Quality Measures*, https://doi.org/10.1007/978-3-030-37145-6_11

the successful practices of high-reliability industries such as aviation and nuclear power, health-care organizations created offices of Quality and Safety and tasked them with setting safety goals, identifying root causes of "close calls," and reducing variability in patient care. The ultimate goal was to create a culture of safety that was anticipatory of, not reactive to, adverse events. [6]

Valid metrics are essential as health care strives to achieve Donabedian's seven pillars of health-care quality: efficacy, effectiveness, efficiency, optimality, acceptability, legitimacy, and equity [7]. In 2019, hospitals, health-care systems, and physicians are subject to a multitude of quality metrics that are used to benchmark patient care outcomes and disease-specific processes of care, drive incentives and reimbursements, and attract consumers. Most metrics rely on easily measured, objective surrogate endpoints whose validity remains unproven. In the words of Saver and colleagues "'Quality' measures provide newer, different incentives, but may not achieve their purpose" of improving health-care quality [8]. While easily measured, these so-called "hard" metrics fail to adequately describe patient-centeredness and individual provider habits, thus excluding the influence of culture and behavior on process and outcome in clinical medicine – the so-called soft data and soft intelligence [9]. A double-edged sword, quality metrics are altruistic, driving performance improvement efforts at both the individual and organizational level, but they are also threatening, as they form the basis of performance assessments, reimbursements, and ratings. The identification of accurate and meaningful measures or metrics proves to be significantly challenging in the face of the complexity of both human disease and the system charged with the delivery of health care.

Nearly 20 years after "To Err is Human," there remains a significant gap between the provision of care at the bedside and the aspirational goals of the organization. Continued reports of horrific errors – from retained foreign bodies to medication dosing errors – remind the industry that there remains work to be done. Progress toward improvement in patient safety has been described as "frustratingly slow." [10]

For their part, physicians struggle to fully embrace the patient safety revolution on the terms defined by insurers, regulators, and social media. Many physicians acknowledge difficulty in incorporating shifting metrics into their practices, and the majority of practicing physicians have no formal education or structured experience in patient safety and quality improvement. Organizations impose a top-down implementation of quality improvement with the implicit expectation that clinicians will become effective quality champions if flooded with "hard" metric data. This approach has not only failed to effectively capture the knowledge and experience of critical stakeholders – the front-line care providers – but it has also created a situation in which they are not empowered to meaningfully engage in the reform. In academic medical centers, the compartmentalization of patient safety and quality improvement and GME perpetuates a culture in which this disconnect between providers and quality improvement is exacerbated [11]. As a result, physicians in training may not receive the mentorship and guidance that they require in order to develop competencies in this area – creating a long-term deficit in skill in this area.

It is clear that the success of the patient safety revolution requires the full engagement of physicians. We need to train physicians who adopt the critical components of quality and high reliability – including metrics and checklists – as the structured framework that facilitates efficient and appropriate delivery of patient care within the context of the individual patient-doctor relationship. Meaningful evolution of attitudes toward, and engagement in, PSQI will only be achieved if the next generation of physicians is immersed in the multidisciplinary team-based principles and practices of patient safety and quality improvement.

There is no more critical venue for this transformation than the graduate medical education (GME) system. The years spent in GME training transform medical students into independent physicians. Experience and knowledge gained during this time are foundational to the formation of professional identity and career-long practice habits.

This chapter will examine the impetus for the culture change in the American health-care system, the expectations for physicians of today and the future, and discuss the current status of GME as it relates to these evolving training goals.

Graduate Medical Education: The Foundations of Physician Culture

Graduate medical education (GME) uses an apprenticeship model to transform medical students into practicing physicians. Founded in the late 1880s, the GME system co-localized medical academia and the community, creating access to care for the medically underserved and a forum for mentored, experiential physician education. Training is rigorous, and by some accounts abusive as hospital employers control access to a prestigious, and required, extension of medical education. Institutions that sponsor GME (sponsoring institutions) have access to an affordable and captive resident workforce that multiplies the clinical capacity of the faculty and provides care to disproportionately underserved and complex patient populations. GME thus adds value to the organization with regard to capacity and reputation. There are financial benefits as well, with the federal government offset in a significant proportion of the cost of residents, in the form of both direct and indirect reimbursement to sponsoring institutions. Though conceived as a mutually beneficial relationship for trainees and organizations, a clear employer-employee relationship underlies the structure of GME.

A central tenet of physician culture is the desire to serve others competently and compassionately. Patient safety and quality care are moral imperatives, and there is the perception that anything short of error-free practice is negligence.

Physicians approach error with a combination of fear and loathing: fear of having caused harm and the potential for retribution and loathing derived from a combination of intense self- and peer-critique. Structured physician-led analysis of medical error dates to the early twentieth century when Ernest Amory Codman, a surgeon at Mass General, developed the "end result system" [12], later renamed

Morbidity and Mortality conference (M&M). Consistent with the emphasis on individual responsibility, M&Ms focused on "incidents and individuals" rather than on an analysis of root cause and system failure [3, 13], leveraging shame and fear to motivate physicians to achieve expertise [14, 15]. This tenor persists in contemporary M&Ms as demonstrated in an analysis of surgical M&M at four academic centers (2000–2001). Forty-two percent of the conferences focused on error, and individual blame was assigned in one third [16]. Though recent years have seen some softening of this "shame and blame" culture, faculty and trainees alike continue to work under the influence of this mindset that emphasizes and glorifies individual strengths and liabilities.

The years in training are characterized by a curious combination of individual pride and shame, empowerment, and dependency; the unwritten traditions, norms, and values that create the culture of medical education have been referred to as the "hidden curriculum." [17] Influential and beyond the control of the individual trainee, this curriculum emerged as the result of institutional (GME and organizational) service needs and faculty expectations [18, 19]. The GME experience shapes the professional identity of all physicians and continues to be bound by an emphasis in individual responsibility reenforced by an organizational structure characterized by a complete imbalance of power. With an emphasis on hierarchy, near exclusive reliance on individual responsibility, and intolerance for anything less than perfection, this belief system is fundamentally antithetical to the core principles of patient safety and quality improvement.

A Sentinel Event and a Call to Action

The 1984 death of a young woman named Libby Zion in a New York academic medical center, while under the care of resident physicians, fueled a very public dissection of the graduate medical education system in the United States [20].

The subsequent grand jury investigation revealed an uncomfortable reality about health-care delivery and the training of physicians in the United States: the GME workforce had simply absorbed dramatic increases in clinical acuity and patient volume over the subsequent century. There had been no concurrent growth in effective support systems (ancillary services or allied personnel) that would facilitate the provision of high-quality care by a resident physician workforce, nor were there consistent expectations regarding supervision of residents by their faculty teachers and mentors [21].

The grand jury in the Zion case convened the Bell Commission to investigate the impact of trainees' work conditions on patient care. The Commission's Report emphasized the role of sleep deprivation and physician fatigue, and as a result the primary actionable intervention was to regulate resident work hours. Thus in July 1989, New York State became the first state to regulate duty hours for GME trainees [55]. The ACGME followed suit several years later [56], and to date these restrictions remain the enduring legacy of the Zion case on physician training.

The ACGME Response: Transforming GME in the Era of the Patient Safety Revolution

> Medical education should provide trainees with the "skills, attitudes, and behaviors that will permit them to function safely and as architects of safety improvement in the future." [22]

The practice of medicine today requires that physicians possess a foundational understanding of disease pathophysiology, clinical skills, and professionalism, as well as a skillset that will enable them to navigate a complex multidisciplinary clinical landscape that is no longer in the control of the individual, but rather the organization and health-care system. Meeting the expectations of this patient safety revolution requires a significant shift in the process of educating physicians, the delivery of care to patients in all settings, and, perhaps most difficult, an evolution of physician culture.

The national debate about patient safety that emerged in the wake of the Zion case and IOM reports demonstrated that provision of high-quality, high-reliability health care required significant modifications in the way that physicians were trained. The historical model of one physician working harder, or longer, was no longer sufficient. Physicians need to work smarter and in a more multidisciplinary fashion in order to account for exponential growth of medical knowledge (beyond the scope of individual mastery) and growing appreciation for the multidisciplinary determinants of health. Physicians need to become proficient as lifelong learners in order to meet the demands of a system that expects ongoing improvements in knowledge and practice habits [23].

The ACGME responded by fundamentally overhauling graduate medical education. As part of a transition to competency-based education, the ACGME offered explicit directives aimed at the institutions that sponsored GME programs, introducing guidance, and standardization related to the education, assessment, and engagement of trainees [24, 25]. Physicians and organizations were expected to think and work as members of organizations that aspired to deliver high quality and high reliability. Educational targets (the Milestones) include multidisciplinary team work, cost-effectiveness of practice habits, participation in patient-centered care, health-care equity, quality of medical record documentation, and capacity to effectively and safely transition patient care throughout the health-care system. Though patient safety and quality improvement "learning goals" were embodied by competencies in systems-based practice (SBP) and practice-based learning and improvement (PBLI), quality concepts are embodied in 47% of all Milestones, in all specialties, emphasizing the importance of collective knowledgebase and shared appreciation for patient safety and quality improvement in post-Zion medical education [4].

In addition to mandating standard educational competencies, the ACGME introduced Clinical Learning Environment Review (CLER) site visits which offer a periodic opportunity for formative feedback in SI and GME performance in six focus areas: patient safety, health-care quality, care transitions, supervision, well-being, and professionalism [26]. The premise of this program is that the SI and their GME programs will use insights made during CLER visits to identify and act on opportunities within their local ecosystem in order to optimize the educational experience for resident and fellow physicians [27].

These three interventions – transition to competency education, incorporation of PSQI educational targets, and CLER – aspire to produce a physician workforce that possesses the skills needed today and in the future. Moving beyond sound clinical skills and medical knowledge, physicians of the future must possess the capacity to translate these aptitudes into "effective patient- and systems-level outcomes" [28] and to "advocate for system leadership and to formally engage in quality assurance and quality improvement activities." [29, 30]

Status Report 2019: Quality as a Competency: How Are we Doing?

The ACGME's CLER program offers an opportunity to assess and measure the opportunities, challenges, and successes that have been revealed during this phase of tremendous change in graduate medical education environment. In 2017, the ACGME completed the second round of CLER visits involving sponsoring institutions with more than three training programs. Similar in scope to the first round, the Executive Summary and analysis included 287 sponsoring institutions and interviews with 9292 residents, 8164 core faculty, 6043 program directors, and more than 1600 executive leaders [31]. The primary conclusion is that there is evidence of a nascent safety culture in these organizations, but there is much work yet to be done. Since the first CLER report in 2016, the authors identify growth in quality improvement knowledge; however, there remain significant opportunities in the several areas including experiential learning relevant to the patient population served by the trainees, training participation in interprofessional and interdisciplinary systems-based improvement efforts and quality improvement projects, and alignment between GME and the sponsoring institutions [32].

Most notable is the observation that despite significant investments in quality improvement at the institutional level, trainees and faculty still exhibit limited knowledge about quality improvement concepts. Exposure and engagement of trainees in organizational quality improvement efforts are "often fragmented." [31] Furthermore, there is poor alignment between trainee quality improvement efforts and CLE initiatives, thus limiting the opportunities to achieve sustained improvement in patient care.

These data demonstrate a reality that has been long recognized in graduate medical education: when the ACGME milestones mandated that resident work on quality improvement projects, organizations were not prepared to mentor or track these efforts. Quality improvement projects and patient safety initiatives are frequently the result of a top-down mandate, or a local physician-led effort that has little relationship to organizational goals. The lack of significant hands-on experience using real patient safety cases and true quality improvement data that reflect clinical practice means that its relevance is obscured; as a result, trainees underappreciate the practicality of quality improvement and forego incorporating it into their practices [6, 18]. Further, faculty continue to struggle against the tide. Instead of understanding the value of quality improvement to their patients and the community they serve, some view these efforts as "a distraction designed to satisfy ACGME requirements." [33] In the absence of sustained faculty investment in quality improvement, residents continue work in near isolation and fail to fully appreciate how this part of their education is a critical competency.

In conclusion, CLER shows us that despite improved awareness and knowledge of quality improvement, physicians (including trainees) are not demonstrating practice behaviors that target quality improvement, nor are they active participants in submitting reporting events that lead to global change. Sustained and meaningful institutional commitment in terms of resources, physician time, and alignment remains a critical missing factor. There remains much work to be done.

Challenges to Success: Relevance, Experience, and Culture

> The most fundamental change that will be needed if hospitals are to make meaningful progress in error reduction is a cultural one — Lucian Leape.

Physicians are uniquely positioned to influence the cultural changes required to support the establishment of an enduring and robust safety culture given their fundamental role in the process of health-care delivery and graduate medical education. However, as evidenced by CLER, physician engagement in quality improvement remains constrained, despite a vigorous public debate about medical error and the restructuring of physician training. A successful journey toward a just culture and high reliability will depend upon progress in three specific areas: physician attitudes, institutional-physician (faculty and trainee) alignment, and faculty development.

Physicians must acknowledge and accept that quality improvement principles are aligned with their own service-oriented value structure. As physicians embrace multidisciplinary approaches to patient care, they need to be able to trust that the systems in place are plastic enough to accommodate patient and provider needs. GME must be ground zero for this transformation as attempts to modify cultural norms once imprinted are disadvantaged. All physician faculty (not just Program Directors and educator-innovators) need to participate in these efforts and need to understand that innovation in medical education has benefit. In this era of high-throughput, high-complexity, and interprofessional care, "See one, Do one, Teach one" cannot produce competent next-generation physicians. Rather a system that integrates competency-based knowledge and clinical skills, graded autonomy, and a robust simulation experience will likely be more effective at achieving the dual goal of competency providers and high-quality reliable care [34]. Today's GME faculty learned medicine in an era that placed a premium value on individual responsibility and perfection. Institutions that sponsor GME continue to have a conflicted reliance on the affordable trainee workforce and underdeveloped ancillary structures to support clinicians. Physicians carry their training experiences as a badge of honor, and change will not be readily embraced – especially if not accompanied by investment in faculty time, development, and the systems and resources that support trainee education today.

Second, organizations must more creatively engage all physicians and recognize their contributions to the culture of safety. Efforts to leverage provider perspectives and ideas into the planning phase of quality improvement initiatives need to consider physician workflow and knowledge. For example, in many organizations, quality improvement is based at the unit level, but physician work does not share this geography; thus, physician input and perspective are not captured. Tess and colleagues observe that residents and fellows, despite being the frontline care givers in our tertiary care centers, very rarely participate in hospital or departmental quality improvement and root cause analyses [19]. Most residents continue to view quality improvement as individual provider events with an individual responsible for the solution, rather than a systems event that involves multiple team members [35]. As a result, many physician- and resident-lead quality improvement projects work in isolation from the institutional quality improvement and, as a result, are at risk of being marginalized, ignored, or redundant [11]. Top-down messaging and lack of local physician involvement means that the physician audience is disconnected from the process [36]. Physicians in training should be encouraged to work with administrators and should choose projects that align with institutional needs in order to create meaningful work that leads to sustained results [18]. Finally, SIs need to acknowledge that meaningful progress in the areas of education and integration will require time – time in schedules that have historically been dictated by patient care and distinct from (and oftentimes contrary to) the committee structures that most organizations use to guide their quality improvement efforts.

Third, there is an urgent need for faculty development in the principles and process of quality improvement. Plausible and passionate mentors for clinical care, pathophysiology, and compassionate humanism, today's medical faculty are unfamiliar and inexperienced with the terminology, techniques, and philosophy of quality improvement. Faced with their own inexperience and the limitations imposed by their training, many faculty take an oppositional position, reporting that quality improvement "distracts from actual teaching" or places a "subversive demand on educational resources." [36, 37] A downstream effect of implementing educational mandates for quality improvement, in the absence of a suitable mentorship structure, is that trainees do not see faculty engaged meaningfully in quality improvement and they in turn interpret the mandate (from their program, their institution, and the ACGME) as hypocrisy [6]. The combination of history – the rites of passage and strong emphasis on individualism – and a lack of training and experience among faculty mentors and supervisors creates a significant impediment to effective integration of physicians in these efforts [38].

Whereas GME creates providers with an overly developed sense of individual responsibility, the principles of quality improvement emphasize the importance of multidisciplinary teamwork. The interactive educational milieu characteristic of academic medical centers can facilitate and support the growth of physician knowledge and engagement, while simultaneously improving organizational sensing of risk and opportunity in quality improvement. Moving forward in the journey to create high-reliability organizations that provide high-quality care will require a fundamental shift in the culture of the academic medical center and physicians. Tess and colleagues offer a compelling model for this in their seminal article "Bridging the Gap." [19] The engagement of all stakeholders in these complex organizations must be secured in order to facilitate the cultural transformation that is required to achieve the desired benchmark of high-reliability and high-quality patient care.

One of the most promising interventions modifies an existing resource, the Morbidity and Mortality conference, in order to create a forum for physicians (faculty and residents) to learn and practice the principles of quality improvement. Restructuring the exercise to encourage a desired culture shift includes migrating the focus to systems-based issues that underlie errors, and away from the physician decision making and medical knowledge – thus the M&M becomes a Patient Safety Peer Review conference [39, 40]. Through a supervised process of error analysis, root cause identification, and action plan formulation, residents can engage in a meaningful and relevant experiential learning process. An effective M&M facilitates multidisciplinary dissection of adverse outcome and creates a forum in which nonjudgmental discussion can aid physicians in redefining the culture of blame and shame. Employing bedside providers in a constructive process that identifies system failures that contribute to suboptimal outcomes will educate and empower them, while simultaneously providing the organization with invaluable information about "soft" and individual contributions to health-care quality [41–43]. The M&M offers a setting in which the priorities of meaningful work –that which is relevant to patient care, to hospital administration, and to trainees – can be explored using actual patient encounters and data. Further repurposing an existing educational venue mitigates the conflict between patient care and valuable experiential education. The M&M reboot as a patient safety peer review conference offers stark contrast to the individualistic nature of these conferences of ages past and can facilitate the physician culture change and education required in order to fulfill Donabedian's seven pillars of health-care quality.

Measuring Success: Quality Metrics in GME

Graduate medical education is the ideal arena in which to both advance physician knowledge and experience and transform physician culture into one more receptive of the multidiscplinary model that is central to quality improvement.

As the ACGME shift to milestone and competency-based assessments has demonstrated, there is a clear expectation that outcomes of medical education and training should be measurable, discrete, and impactful – especially with regard to patient outcomes and the health of populations. Therefore, it is natural that educators would try to define quality metrics as educational outcomes.

Quality metrics must be relevant to individual providers, and they should be corrective, not punitive. Metrics should stimulate constructive improvements in both system and practice performance in order to achieve optimal patient and population outcomes. Though government- and insurer-defined metrics can motivate practice improvements and better patient outcomes, many are largely removed from the individual provider's control, knowledge, or insight. Excessive reliance on these may engender a feeling of impotence and irrelevance, especially to bedside clinicians [6, 11, 18, 19]. These "outward-facing" measures are not easily associated with true performance of individual physicians.

Ideal resident quality metrics would be meaningful and relevant, not only to the trainee but also to the patient and health system. An educationally relevant metric should "serve as an indicator that essential competencies had been acquired, integrated, and applied." [44] Unfortunately, residency training presents unique challenges to the identification of meaningful and relevant quality metrics. In specific rotation schedules, handoffs and supervisory structures mean that a single trainee has very limited impact on individual patient outcomes [28]. New approaches and metrics designed to overcome these limitations are emerging.

Surgical and procedural specialties are best suited for objective metric assessments. In addition to assessments related to discrete tasks such as endoscopy [45], educators have also designed composite measures that bundle technical skills in order to allow assessment of performance both at the bedside and in simulation-based settings [46]. Investigators at the University of Chicago extended the lessons learned through the National Surgical Quality Improvement Program (NSQIP) to their trainees. The Quality In-Training Initiative (QITI) created a model in which trainee-specific outcome reporting could be generated for senior surgical trainees for qualifying procedures [47]. Importantly, this project demonstrated an association between trainee performance and a significant reduction in resident-specific morbidity [47].

More challenging to assess are the non-technical skills such as patient education, the ability to work productively in an interprofessional team, and the effectiveness of communication across care transitions. Though these represent significant liabilities to patient outcomes and experiences, they are difficult to measure and assess from the perspective of the resident. One proposed solution takes pains to define physician-patient exemplar interactions, termed educationally sensitive patient outcomes (ESPOs). ESPOs are tasks that require a deep understanding of the relationship between the individuals (physician, patient) and the system interface; two proposed ESPOs are patient activation and clinical microsystem activation. Patient activation describes a state in which patients are informed and engaged in their own health care and has been positively associated with improved health outcomes [28, 48–50]. The clinical microsystem is the local environment – the unit-based work – in which patient care takes place [51]. Effective patient care in this setting requires that physicians work in an interdisciplinary team and understand the systems upon which patient care relies. Competent physicians must be able to activate the clinical microsystem in order to optimize patient outcomes and experience. Examples of skills critical for clinical microsystem activation are handoffs, utilization of supervision and escalation pathways, and interdisciplinary communication.

In another example, educators at Cincinnati Children's Hospital used National Quality Measures Clearinghouse (NQMC) measures as the source for quality measures that would accurately reflect the competence of residents while rotating in the emergency department. Metrics that were selected involved the most common illnesses in these setting and those that were pragmatic to resident work as markers of quality [52]. Though the quality measures have yet to be validated, a standardized approach to metric selection offers the opportunity to monitor the effectiveness of the training environment as it relates to important patient outcomes.

Two additional outstanding needs impact the development and dissemination of useful resident quality metrics. First, the electronic medical record must accurately assign individual physician performance to individual patient-level data such as patient experience surveys, providing a measure of interpersonal communication skills. Modules facilitating systematic review of documentation practices by a physician could be built into the EMR, providing opportunity for both self-study and training program oversight. Second, robust specialty- and subspecialty-specific quality metrics and practice standards must be defined using existing consensus standards [53]. In the absence of informed benchmarks for patient care and outcomes, the quality of a trainee cannot be assessed.

Conclusion

New physicians are entering a practice environment in which they will be required to understand and react to issues related to performance improvement, process improvement, and quality-based reimbursement – in other words, the fundamentals of patient safety and quality improvement. In order to prepare physicians for these changes, the ACGME restructured GME, introducing new knowledge and practice competencies related to quality improvement, a requirement for experiential learning in quality improvement, and the expectation that sponsoring institutions integrate the GME experience into the organizational safety culture.

Not surprisingly, CLER demonstrates that meeting these expectations will not be achieved solely through an educational mandate. There also needs to be a culture shift in medicine – no longer can we train individuals who will open a solo practice or expect to run a cash-only business model. Aligning quality improvement concepts and principles with patient care is fundamental to this culture shift. Quality improvement must be seen as integrated into work flow and relevant to patient care outcomes – not only in fiscal year but at the individual patient's bedside.

The years spent in GME training offer a unique and high-value opportunity for growth in physician quality improvement competence as the habits and patterns of care developed in training persist for years [54]. The natural dissemination of physicians following GME experiences offers the promise of a multiplier effect as they can carry new skills and knowledge into their practices and communities. Development of physicians as effective stewards of quality improvement will require messaging that is meaningful and relevant to patients and the members of the interprofessional health-care team, including physicians. A formal education structure for quality improvement will need to be implemented with accommodation for differences in training programs (such as procedural vs nonprocedural) and with accommodation for a diversity of career interests that could shift focus of the quality improvement to suit the trainee's interest. Time restraints inherent to the workflow of clinicians in academic medicine need to be strongly considered, as acquiring knowledge and experiential learning takes time. More thought must be given to the effective integration of GME (faculty and trainees alike) into quality improvement projects. Importantly, organizations need to consider the relative value of trainee-initiated projects that may have minimal relevance to the hospital, as opposed to system-level efforts which primarily target macroscopic, reportable measures, as there are distinct benefits and risks to both [18]. Fundamentally improved alignment between housestaff QI training and institutional priorities will enable institutions to capture the energy and service interests of these providers, harnessing them to simultaneously train themselves and improve patient care.

The mandate is clear. Training the next generation of physicians to be experts in the art and science of individual and systems-based patient care will require creativity, energy, and persistence. Culture change is never easy. Finding an optimal balance between patient- and learner-centered educational outcomes is critical. The training environment is, by reality and necessity, a microcosm of independent medical practice.

At the present time, higher education is prone to assuming that customer is the trainee. Graduate medical education might benefit from a paradigm shift: GME's customers are in fact the patients and not the trainees.

References

1. Association of American Medical Colleges. GME Track 2017; Date accessed February 24, 2018.
2. Institute of Medicine (U.S.). Committee on Quality of Health Care in America. Crossing the quality chasm : a new health system for the 21st century. Washington, DC: National Academy Press; 2001.
3. Ludmerer KM. Let me heal: the opportunity to preserve excellence in American medicine. Oxford. New York: Oxford University Press; 2015.
4. Lane-Fall MB, Davis JJ, Clapp JT, Myers JS, Riesenberg LA. What every graduating resident needs to know about quality improvement and patient safety: a content analysis of 26 sets of ACGME milestones. Acad Med. 2018;93:904–10.
5. Kohn LT, Corrigan J, Donaldson MS. To err is human: building a safer health system. Washington, DC: National Academy Press; 2000.
6. Bagian JP. The future of graduate medical education: a systems-based approach to ensure patient safety. Acad Med. 2015;90:1199–202.
7. Donabedian A. The seven pillars of quality. Arch Pathol Lab Med. 1990;114:1115–8.

8. Saver BG, Martin SA, Adler RN, et al. Care that matters: quality measurement and health care. PLoS Med. 2015;12:e1001902.
9. Martin GP, McKee L, Dixon-Woods M. Beyond metrics? Utilizing 'soft intelligence' for healthcare quality and safety. Soc Sci Med. 2015;142:19–26.
10. Leape L, Berwick D, Clancy C, et al. Transforming healthcare: a safety imperative. Qual Saf Health Care. 2009;18:424–8.
11. Blanchard RD, Pierce-Boggs K, Visintainer PF, Hinchey KT. Integrating quality improvement with graduate medical education: lessons learned from the AIAMC National Initiatives. Am J Med Qual. 2016;31:240–5.
12. Mallon B. Ernest Amory Codman: the end result of a life in medicine. Philadelphia: Saunders; 2000.
13. Leape LL. Error in medicine. JAMA. 1994;272:1851–7.
14. Orlander JD, Barber TW, Fincke BG. The morbidity and mortality conference: the delicate nature of learning from error. Acad Med. 2002;77:1001–6.
15. Harbison SP, Regehr G. Faculty and resident opinions regarding the role of morbidity and mortality conference. Am J Surg. 1999;177:136–9.
16. Pierluissi E, Fischer MA, Campbell AR, Landefeld CS. Discussion of medical errors in morbidity and mortality conferences. JAMA. 2003;290:2838–42.
17. Hafferty FW. Beyond curriculum reform: confronting medicine's hidden curriculum. Acad Med. 1998;73:403–7.
18. Liao JM, Co JP, Kachalia A. Providing educational content and context for training the next generation of physicians in quality improvement. Acad Med. 2015;90:1241–5.
19. Tess A, Vidyarthi A, Yang J, Myers JS. Bridging the gap: a framework and strategies for integrating the quality and safety mission of teaching hospitals and graduate medical education. Acad Med. 2015;90:1251–7.
20. Asch DA, Parker RM. The Libby Zion case. One step forward or two steps backward? N Engl J Med. 1988;318:771–5.
21. Court NYS. Report of the Fourth Grand Jury for the April/May Term of 1986 Concerning the care and treatment of a patient and the supervision of interns and residents at a Hospital in New York County. 1986.
22. Lucian Leape Institute at NPSF. Unmet needs: teaching physicians to provide safe patient care. Boston: National Patient Safety Foundation; 2010.
23. Miller BM, Moore DE Jr, Stead WW, Balser JR. Beyond Flexner: a new model for continuous learning in the health professions. Acad Med. 2010;85:266–72.
24. Nasca TJ, Philibert I, Brigham T, Flynn TC. The next GME accreditation system--rationale and benefits. N Engl J Med. 2012;366:1051–6.
25. Byrne LM, Miller RS, Nasca TJ. Implementing the next accreditation system: results of the 2014–2015 annual data review. J Grad Med Educ. 2016;8:118–23.
26. Wagner R, Patow C, Newton R, Casey BR, Koh NJ, Weiss KB. The overview of the CLER program: CLER national report of findings 2016. J Grad Med Educ. 2016;8:11–3.
27. Weiss KB, Bagian JP, Wagner R, Nasca TJ. Introducing the CLER pathways to excellence: a new way of viewing clinical learning environments. J Grad Med Educ. 2014;6:608–9.
28. Kalet AL, Gillespie CC, Schwartz MD, et al. New measures to establish the evidence base for medical education: identifying educationally sensitive patient outcomes. Acad Med. 2010;85:844–51.
29. Wagner R, Patow C, Newton R, et al. The overview of the CLER program: CLER national report of findings 2016. J Grad Med Educ. 2016;8:11–3.
30. The Internal Medicine Milestone Project: ABME, ACGME; 2015.
31. Co JP, Weiss KB, Koh NJ, Wagner R. CLER national report of findings 2018: executive summary. Chicago, IL: Accreditation Council for Graduate Medical Education; 2018.
32. Weiss KB, Co JPT, Bagian JP. Challenges and opportunities in the 6 focus areas: CLER national report of findings 2018. J Grad Med Educ. 2018;10:25–48.

33. Myers JS, Nash DB. Graduate medical education's new focus on resident engagement in quality and safety: will it transform the culture of teaching hospitals? Acad Med. 2014;89:1328–30.
34. Rodriguez-Paz JM, Kennedy M, Salas E, et al. Beyond "see one, do one, teach one": toward a different training paradigm. Qual Saf Health Care. 2009;18:63–8.
35. Nasca TJ, Weiss KB, Bagian JP. Improving clinical learning environments for tomorrow's physicians. N Engl J Med. 2014;370:991–3.
36. Butler JM, Anderson KA, Supiano MA, Weir CR. "It feels like a lot of extra work": resident attitudes about quality improvement and implications for an effective learning health care system. Acad Med. 2017;92:984–90.
37. Jones J, Saram DDD. Academic staff views of quality systems for teaching and learning: a Hong Kong case study. Qual Higher Educ. 2005;11:47–58.
38. Wong BM, Kuper A, Hollenberg E, Etchells EE, Levinson W, Shojania KG. Sustaining quality improvement and patient safety training in graduate medical education: lessons from social theory. Acad Med. 2013;88:1149–56.
39. Gerstein WH, Ledford J, Cooper J, et al. Interdisciplinary quality improvement conference: using a revised morbidity and mortality format to focus on systems-based patient safety issues in a VA Hospital: design and outcomes. Am J Med Qual. 2016;31:162–8.
40. Walker M, Rubio D, Horstman M, Trautner B, Stewart D. Stop the blame game: restructuring morbidity and mortality conferences to teach patient safety and quality improvement to residents. MedEdPORTAL. 2016;12:10475.
41. Deis JN, Smith KM, Warren MD, et al. Transforming the morbidity and mortality conference into an instrument for systemwide improvement. In: Henriksen K, Battles JB, Keyes MA, Grady ML, editors. Advances in patient safety: new directions and alternative approaches, Culture and redesign, vol. 2. Rockville: Agency for Healthcare Research and Quality (US); 2008.
42. Gonzalo JD, Yang JJ, Huang GC. Systems-based content in medical morbidity and mortality conferences: a decade of change. J Grad Med Educ. 2012;4:438–44.
43. Huddleston JM, Diedrich DA, Kinsey GC, Enzler MJ, Manning DM. Learning from every death. J Patient Saf. 2014;10:6–12.
44. Swing SR, Schneider S, Bizovi K, et al. Using patient care quality measures to assess educational outcomes. Acad Emerg Med. 2007;14:463–73.
45. Ortolani JB, Zhong X, Tershak DR, Ferrara JJ, Paget CJ. Quality metrics in surgery resident performance of screening colonoscopy. Am Surg. 2015;81:710–3.
46. Cox ML, Risucci DA, Gilmore BF, et al. Validation of the Omni: a novel, multimodality, and longitudinal surgical skills assessment. J Surg Educ. 2018;75:e218–e28.
47. Turrentine FE, Hanks JB, Tracci MC, Jones RS, Schirmer BD, Smith PW. Resident-specific morbidity reduced following ACS NSQIP data-driven quality program. J Surg Educ. 2018;75:1558–65.
48. Hibbard JH, Greene J, Tusler M. Improving the outcomes of disease management by tailoring care to the patient's level of activation. Am J Manag Care. 2009;15:353–60.
49. Hibbard JH, Stockard J, Mahoney ER, Tusler M. Development of the Patient Activation Measure (PAM): conceptualizing and measuring activation in patients and consumers. Health Serv Res. 2004;39:1005–26.
50. Mosen DM, Schmittdiel J, Hibbard J, Sobel D, Remmers C, Bellows J. Is patient activation associated with outcomes of care for adults with chronic conditions? J Ambul Care Manage. 2007;30:21–9.
51. Nelson EC, Batalden PB, Huber TP, et al. Microsystems in health care: Part 1. Learning from high-performing front-line clinical units. Jt Comm J Qual Improv. 2002;28:472–93.
52. Schumacher DJ, Holmboe ES, van der Vleuten C, Busari JO, Carraccio C. Developing resident-sensitive quality measures: a model from pediatric emergency medicine. Acad Med. 2018;93:1071–8.
53. Haan CK, Edwards FH, Poole B, Godley M, Genuardi FJ, Zenni EA. A model to begin to use clinical outcomes in medical education. Acad Med. 2008;83:574–80.

54. Asch DA, Nicholson S, Srinivas S, Herrin J, Epstein AJ. Evaluating obstetrical residency programs using patient outcomes. JAMA. 2009;302:1277–83.
55. https://govt.westlaw.com/nycrr/Document/I4fe39657cd1711dda432a117e6e0f345?viewType=FullText&originationContext=documenttoc&transitionType=CategoryPageItem&contextData=(sc.Default)&bhcp=1).
56. Accreditation Council for Graduate Medical Education, ACGME highlights its standards on residents duty hours. May 2001.; Available at: https://www.acgme.org.

Chapter 12
The Role of the Hospital Board of Trustees in Ensuring Quality Care

Stanley Goldstein and Jeffrey Weinstein

Getting Beyond Average: The Hospital Board of Trustees Role

In February 2007, the Institute for Healthcare Improvement launched the Boards on Board program, which sought to engage board leadership in clinical quality.[1] Subsequently, the National Quality Forum and others have called on hospital boards to focus on quality.[2]

This chapter will address the call to action to board of directors and trustees of hospitals and hospital systems to become leaders in ongoing efforts to improve patient safety and overall healthcare. We explore the foundation of the board's fiduciary duties to become involved in safety and quality and provide examples of efforts across the world to employ board-led initiatives and finally to provide concrete examples of how focused attention to quality and safety initiatives by the board of trustees and quality of care committee of the board at Tufts Medical Center in Boston, Massachusetts, measurably improved safety, quality, and patients experience at this tertiary/quaternary teaching hospital.

The role of hospital board members is best expressed by the fiduciary duties that are owed by such governors to the institutions they serve. The Governance Institute

---

[1] Institute for Healthcare Improvement. Getting boards on board [Internet]. Cambridge, MA: IHI; [cited 18 Sep 2008]. Available from: http://www.ihi.org/IHI/Programs/Campaign/BoardsonBoard.htm. Google Scholar.

[2] National Quality Forum. Hospital governing boards and quality of care: a call to responsibility. Washington, DC: NQF; 2 Dec 2004. Google Scholar.

S. Goldstein (✉) · J. Weinstein
Tufts Medical Center, Boston, MA, USA
e-mail: jweinstein@tuftsmedicalcenter.org

© Springer Nature Switzerland AG 2020

D. N. Salem (ed.), *Quality Measures*, https://doi.org/10.1007/978-3-030-37145-6_12

serves as the leading, independent source of governance information and education for healthcare organizations across the USA. In their article entitled "A Framework for Effective Governance" by Roger W. Witalis, FACHE, WITALIS & Company, Inc. published by the Governance Institute in April of 2013, those fiduciary duties of board members to the running of the hospital are detailed. Those duties are as follows:

1. *The Duty of Care*: The duty of care requires board members to have knowledge of all reasonably available and pertinent information before taking action. Directors must act in good faith, with the care of an ordinarily prudent person in similar circumstances, and in a manner he or she reasonably believes is in the best interest of the organization.
2. *The Duty of Loyalty*: The duty of loyalty requires board members to discharge their duties unselfishly in a manner designed to benefit only the corporate enterprise and not board members personally. It incorporates the duty to disclose situations that may present a potential for conflict with the corporation's mission, as well as protection of confidential information.
3. *The Duty of Obedience* (for those institutions that operate as a not-for-profit organizations): The duty of obedience requires board members to ensure that the organization's decisions and activities adhere to its fundamental corporate purpose and charitable mission as stated in its articles of incorporation and bylaws and other binding corporate documents. These duties cannot be assessed or applied in isolation. Rather, all three are interrelated and collectively inform what is appropriate governance practice for any given board. Of particular relevance to not-for-profit, multihospital systems is the duty of obedience. This is because multihospital systems have both local and/or regional and system/corporate-level governance structures. In order for the different levels of governance to operate effectively, and not to work at cross-purposes, board members at each level must understand and adhere to the duties and responsibilities delegated to their level by the system's governing articles, bylaws, and other documents. In other words, the duty of obedience informs the scope of the duty of care and the duty of loyalty. While all board members have a duty of care and a duty of loyalty to the particular organization they serve, in fulfilling those duties they must act in accordance with their duty of obedience to the organization's specific purposes, bylaws, and binding commitments and the purposes and structure of the overall system of which the organization is a part. For system-level officers and directors, this means acting in accordance with the system's articles and bylaws, and in the system's best interests, as defined and informed by those articles and bylaws.

Adhering to the fiduciary duties, concepts, and precepts, the board provides oversight in important areas of operations including financial oversight, strategy development and implementation, philanthropy, and overall direction to and review of management performance.

"But first among the Board's core responsibilities is Quality Oversight." Mr. Watalis enunciates that "Boards have a legal, ethical, and moral obligation to keep patients safe and to ensure they receive the highest quality of care." While there is significance and importance to the board's other oversight responsibilities, the responsibility for quality and safety is foremost. The Governance Institute's governance framework also seeks to draw clear lines between governance and management. The Governance Institute defines the "role of governance" as the process of exercising accountability by setting policy, making decisions, and overseeing implementation:

- Setting policy: Approving statements of intent to guide and constrain subsequent decision making and limit choices. Policy statements may include definitions of core duties and responsibilities, statements of intended direction, or statements of expectation. They can be prescriptive or prohibitive.
- Decision making: Making ultimate choices and reaching agreements within the context of approved policy. The board may retain full decision-making authority or delegate authority, with limits, for the preparation of recommendations to the board.
- Overseeing implementation: Oversight the process of ensuring that tasks and authority are being executed in ways that meet board expectations as expressed in its policies and decisions. Oversight provides monitoring, assessment, and feedback and provides the context for corrective action.

The "role of management," on the other hand, is to deliver results by implementing policy and decisions as set forth by the governing board, managing operations, and reporting on performance. Boards need to be continually reminded of the distinction between governance and management to avoid the tendency to micromanage and "meddle" in operations.

The role of Hospital Boards of Trustees is to ensure that management executes its day-to-day operations in accordance with strategic initiatives formulated by the board. These strategies are in part intended to assure the hospital achieves its mission and at its most fundamental core has the resources and determination to provide for its patients in a safe, effective, and high-quality manner. Every hospital in America touts its attention to quality care and patient safety. Ask any hospital executive and she will quote those quality measures that put the hospital's operations in the best light. This is the best way to ensure average performance.

It is up to the board to demand that the management sets quality goals that are aspirational and, in fact, audacious. Highly engaged executive leadership teams working with highly engaged boards in a trusting partnership can be the source of will for the entire organization. In the context of business operations, it is always best for each participant to have a boss. With respect to quality and safety, the board has to act like the demanding boss of the executive management to drive to zero countenance for failings in patient safety and in the delivery of quality patient care.

As hospitals try to drive rapid improvement, boards have an opportunity and a responsibility to make better quality of care the organization's top priority. The board's responsibility for ensuring and improving care cannot be delegated to the medical staff and executive leadership; ensuring safe and harm-free care to patients is the board's job, at the very core of each member's fiduciary responsibility. With respect to safety and quality, an activated board, in partnership with executive leadership, can set system-level expectations and accountability for high performance and elimination of harm. Properly conducted this tandem leadership work can dramatically and continually improve the quality and safety of care. In fact, hospital quality improvement has been a topic of conversation for over a century: "I am Called Eccentric for Saying in Public that Hospitals, if They Wish to be Sure of Improvement: …" Must find out what their results are. Must analyze their results to find their strong and weak points. Must compare their results with those of other hospitals. Must care for what cases they can care for well, and avoid attempting to care for cases which they are not qualified to care for well. Must welcome publicity not only for their successes, but for their errors, so that the public may give them their help when it is needed. Must promote members of the medical staff on the basis which gives due consideration to what they can and do accomplish for their patients. Such opinions will not be eccentric for a few years hence (E.A. Codman, M.D. A Study in hospital efficiency, 1916). Much more has been written over the past decade of the need to make hospitals safer and to provide all patients the highest levels of care. How dangerous is it to be hospitalized? Well recent articles identified the following: Hospitals are typically thought of as places where lives are saved, but statistics show they are actually one of the most *dangerous* places you could possibly frequent.[3,4] Each day, more than 40,000 harmful and/or lethal medical errors occur, placing the patient in a worse situation than what they came in with.[5] According to a 2013 study,[6,7] preventable medical errors kill around 440,000 patients each year – that is more than 10 times the number of deaths caused by motor vehicle crashes! Hospitals have become particularly notorious for spreading lethal infections. According to 2014 statistics[8,9] by the US Centers for Disease Control and Prevention (CDC), 1 in 25 patients end up with a *hospital-acquired infection*. In 2011 alone, 75,000 people died as a result.[8] Medicare patients may be at even greater risk. According to the 2011 Healthgrades Hospital Quality in America Study,[10] 1 in 9 Medicare patients developed a hospital-acquired infection. So, what is the role of the board in quality and safety?

---

[3] The Crux, SHOCKING: This is one of the most dangerous places in America.

[4] New York Times January 26, 2016.

[5] HealthGrades 2011 Healthcare Consumerism and Hospital Quality in America Report.

[6] Journal of Patient Safety 2013 Sep;9(3):122–8.

[7] NPR September 24, 2013.

[8] CDC.gov Health Care Associated Infections.

[9] New England Journal of Medicine 2014;370:1198–208.

[10] Consumer Reports, America's Antibiotic Crisis.

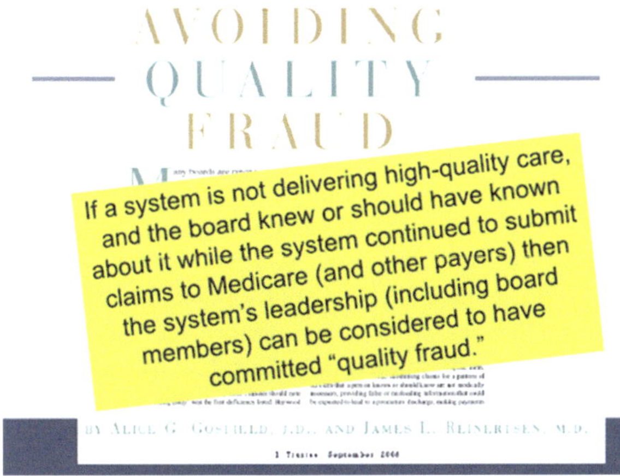

We have determined that the most important pursuit and oversight of a hospital board is in ensuring the provision of safe and high quality of patient care. The obvious next question is how?

Do No Harm

The Board Must Set Clear, Concise, and Measurable Goals

The Children's Hospitals' Solutions for Patient Safety Network (SPS Network) is a good example of how to affect patient safety and quality of care, in this instance for pediatric care. This is an organization of 130 children's hospitals working together to help each individual hospital make progress "on a journey to zero harm: so that every child receives safe care every time they enter our hospitals."

With this audacious goal, the board set out clear, concise, and measurable goals. They were defined as follows: *40% reduction in hospital-acquired conditions (HACs), 20% reduction in 7-day readmissions, 50% reduction in serious safety events (SSEs), and 25% reduction in DART – days away, restricted, or transferred.* These goals are the measuring rods for the overall objective of providing safe and quality healthcare, with no exceptions. In order to continually improve, this organization has stated that:

> "We must act with urgency and discipline, focusing on outcomes through a combination of high reliability concepts and quality improvement science methods. We learn through testing and partnering with families and frontline staff."

Every hospital, clinic, and physician office claims to strive to provide high quality and safe care. But how many make it an urgent tenant of everything they do? Healthcare providers work in highly regulated environments that are financially challenged by fiscal realities. Costs and expenses of operating a healthcare organization go up inexorably each year, especially the costs of technologies, equipment, and pharmaceuticals. At the same time, that costs and expenses are going up, while commercial and government payer reimbursements are going down. This unbalance leads to a juggling act that may compromise the ultimate objective. "No margin, no mission" is an oft-repeated reason proffered for decisions that may have an impact on the achievement of the goal of providing care without harm at the highest levels of quality. But note, in its mission statement, SPS Network recognizes the need to act with "urgency." Healthcare institutions should act with the same sense of urgency it provides to the generation of profit to the performance of safe and quality care. Likewise, the effort must be disciplined. All effort should be made to be laser focused on outcomes data. Nothing is more powerful in this quest than the accumulation of data. Raw data, transparent data, and data that is not subjected to spin or interpretation lead to bending the rule of achieving zero harm to patients while delivering high quality and in most cases complex healthcare. Then with the unvarnished truth of data, the application of quality improvements in a scientific manner is required. The board delegates some of its quality- and safety-related work to a committee of the board, often referred to as the quality of care and safety committee. In an effort to the achievement of minimum levels of safety and quality of care, state legislatures impose certain regulatory compliance requirements of hospitals. As an example in Massachusetts, the Board of Registration in Medicine has the Quality and Patient Safety Division (QPSD) that uses a unique approach to help healthcare facilities maintain the highest levels of healthcare quality. QPSD operates under the basic premise that the people who deliver excellent patient care every day – doctors, nurses, pharmacists, and other professionals – know what needs to be done to ensure that Massachusetts continues to have the highest healthcare quality in the world. Utilizing collaboration and data analysis, the QPSD brings vital tools and information to healthcare facilities to help them meet their patient safety and quality goals. The QPSD oversees institutional systems of quality assurance, risk management, peer review, and credentialing. These activities are known collectively as the institution's "Patient Care Assessment (PCA) Program." The systems comprising a facility's PCA program must be overseen by both physician and corporate leadership and must actively involve all healthcare providers as well as other employees at the institution. In Massachusetts, the PCA and other regulations of the Department of Health and the Board of Registration in Medicine are the "table stakes" of healthcare delivery in the Commonwealth. But in reality, we are striving for much more than table stakes, much more than satisfying the minimum requirements to ensure licensure. The goal is perfection: no harm and best outcomes every time, no matter what. The Board of Registration in Medicine says this about the PCA process, "The QPSD function is unique among the nation's state licensing boards, as the legislature placed oversight of institutional quality assurance in an agency that licenses physicians, but not healthcare facilities". This rationale is compelling: institutional quality assurance will not succeed without meaningful physician leadership and participation.

In order to ensure that the institution sees safety and quality as urgent matters of attention, every board meeting must begin with the honest state of quality and safety at the institution. Reports from the chief medical officer and the head of the medical staff should inform the Board of Registration for every unexpected negative outcome. Through Massachusetts General Law, chapter 305 of the Acts of 2008, hospitals and ambulatory surgery centers are required to report serious reportable events (SREs) to the Massachusetts Department of Public Health (DPH). As defined, SREs are (i) adverse events that are of concern to both the public and healthcare professionals and providers, (ii) clearly identifiable and measurable and thus feasible to include in a reporting system, and (iii) of a nature such that the risk of occurrence is significantly influenced by the policies and procedures of the healthcare facility.

The law prohibits hospitals from charging for these events or seeking reimbursement for SRE-related services. Through regulation, the Department has defined SREs to meet the National Quality Forum's definitions of 28 such events. See Appendix A for the 28 such events. The board and the quality of care and safety committee must insist on complete transparency because without the cold light of day being shown on these incidents, meaningful improvements cannot be achieved. The board must review recognized quality and safety data measures; it must seek to understand what is presented and track the aims of the program and the performance trajectory. In this effort, the board should insist on the development of a comprehensive dashboard of quality and safety measures. All of the aims of the dashboard must be clearly defined and measurable. The board must hold management accountable for any harm to patients while at the same time supporting positive changes to improve safety and quality. The board should demand to understand the trends, trajectories, and strategic imperatives to accomplish the achievement of zero harm and best outcomes. As the boss, administrative and medical staff leadership must be held accountable for results, behaviors, and implementation of changes to improve outcomes. Establishment of a culture of safety and quality fosters transparency, honest self-reflection, and ameliorative behavior. Improvements and successes must be rewarded and celebrated. A review of the medical literature highlights the fact that the board's involvement in safety and quality is not unique to healthcare in the USA. It is a worldwide topic of interest.

A report from Health Service Executive Quality Improvement Division, 11 September 2017 ISBN 978-1-78602-056-7 Quality Improvement Division Health Service Executive Dr. Stevens' Hospital Dublin D08 W2A8 Ireland outlines a framework developed with reference to international leading practices which have included a review of relevant publications and material from the UK (including Ireland), the USA, Australia, Canada, and New Zealand. Additionally, this scholarly review included a summary of board leading practices in improving quality and safety from an international perspective. Many of the concepts discussed above make up recommended oversight by boards of healthcare institutions.

- From England:

   Place the quality of patient care, especially patient safety, above all other aims. Engage, empower, and hear patients and caregivers at all times. Foster whole-heartedly the growth and development of all staff, including their ability and support to improve the processes in which they work. Embrace transparency unequivocally and everywhere, in the service of accountability, trust, and the growth of knowledge. (Extract from the National Advisory Group on the Safety of Patients in England, A Promise to Learn, a Commitment to Act, 2013).

- From Canada: Practices for Improving Quality and Safety

The capability of boards and board quality committees to function effectively and to move appropriately between fiduciary and strategic modes relies on boards and senior leadership capacity to develop trust and a strong collaborative relationship, while not undermining the board's duty to ask challenging questions.

- From Scotland: Measurement for Improving Quality and Safety

Improvement focused oversight is better serviced by measurement processes (Statistical Process Control and Run Charts) that encourage action when the data signals concerns or success – rather than requiring effort of actions responding to inherent variation in the data being considered.

- From the USA, the Netherlands, and Taiwan

In the article "Assessing patient safety culture in hospitals across countries" C. Wagner M. Smits J. Sorra C.C. Huang from the International Journal for Quality in Health Care, Volume 25, Issue 3, 1 July 2013, Pages 213–221, https://doi.org/10.1093/intqhc/mzt024. Published: 09 April 2013, the authors compared and contrasted healthcare organizations in the USA, the Netherlands, and Taiwan with respect to patient safety culture. "In this article, we have compared the patient safety culture in a sample of hospitals of the Netherlands, Taiwan and the USA. Based on the 12 culture dimensions of the Hospital SOPS, the results showed that Teamwork within units is a strong area in the participating hospitals in all three countries. A weak area in all three countries is the culture dimension handoffs and transitions."

The worldwide effort to improve safety and quality in hospital settings is a universal undertaking. The goals associated with these efforts will all be improved with attention from the highest levels of the organization. Tufts Medical Center is a leading academic medical center in Boston, Massachusetts, the primary teaching hospital for Tufts University School of Medicine and the primary tertiary care facility for the Wellforce Inc. system. At Tufts Medical Center, the board of trustees has taken a very proactive approach to quality and safety. Quality of care and safety has become the single most important priority of the board. Historically, the board was focused on the financial performance of the institution; after all, "no margin, no mission." However, beginning in 2004, the board began to elevate its understanding of the importance of quality and safety as part of its governance role. A major shift occurred with the introduction of many more physicians to the board. With this added complement of knowledgeable caregivers came a comfort level with medicine that allowed for increased scrutiny and the advancement of the science and practice of medicine.

The quality of care committee had been a long-standing committee of the board. But in the newly constituted board, the workings of the committee were expanded beyond those needed to meet regulatory requirements. The committee is chaired by a non-physician, independent, or "outside" member of the board of trustees. The committee is led by the Chief Medical Officer of the Medical Center and includes among others the President of the medical staff, the Medical Center President and CEO, the Chief Nursing Officer, the Vice President of Risk Management, and the Director of Quality of Care as well as numerous other clinical leaders from across the adult and pediatric medical community. Additionally, others that are part of the quality of care committee are members of the patient family advisory council and local community leaders. The committee meets monthly, and the efforts of the committee are reviewed in detail at every meeting of the board of trustees. The quality of care committee develops annual plans for quality and safety. The plans are intended to provide the committee and the board with a measurable method of overseeing quality and safety initiatives. The metrics are process, outcomes, and patient experience related and are established and monitored by national and regional organizations such as the US Department of Health and Human Services, Agency for Healthcare Research and Quality, National Committee for Quality Assurance, Centers for Medicare and Medicaid Services (CMS), Hospital Compare website, Leapfrog Hospital Survey, and Vizient Quality and Accountability Study of the leading academic medical centers in the USA. Other organizations' healthcare outcomes, safety, and quality metrics are also monitored for specialties and subspecialties. Included in this grouping are health insurance companies and the Association of American Medical Colleges and its subdivisions.

Specific initiatives to improve performance against these benchmarks are presented to the committee and board and form the basis for regular review. The Medical Center's monthly performance in safety and quality is compared to national and regional benchmarks as published by each organization. Performance is meticulously charted. Trends, trajectories, improvements, and worsening performance are noted in dashboards. Board leadership is a key component to creating a culture of quality and safety throughout the organization. The attention paid to these efforts on a daily basis permeates the organization, from the Chairman of the Board to the housekeeping and security staffs. The annual quality and safety plan which is approved by the board is driven by its commitment to quality and safety and to the goal of zero harm and high-quality patient care.

As stated in the plan: "Governance, leadership, frontline staff and the organized medical staff work together to promote a culture of safety and reliability. The goal is to have a culture characterized by teamwork with open discussion about quality and safety with a particular focus on systems and processes, supported by robust data and benchmarking. Also key to the achievement of the organization's goals is the active engagement and participation by patients and families through the Patient Family Advisory Council and as active members of the Quality of Care Committee." The board has articulated its intentions with the following statements in the plan which detail the Mission, Values, and Guiding Principles central to the workings of the quality of care committee. Taken together they imbue the culture of safety and quality of care in the organization:

The Mission of Tufts Medical Center
"We strive to heal, to comfort, to teach, to learn, and to seek the knowledge to promote health and prevent disease. Our patients and their families are at the center of

everything we do. We dedicate ourselves to furthering our rich tradition of health-care innovation, leadership, charity and the highest standard of care and service to all in our community".

The Values of Tufts Medical Center
- *Respect for Every individual*: We will treat each person we work with and care for with respect.
- *Honesty and Fairness*: We will be truthful, equitable, and open in all our relationships
- *Delivery of the Highest Quality Service*: We will always strive to deliver the highest quality service and care to our patients, their families, and our colleagues.
- *Constant Pursuit of Excellence*: We will continuously strive to meet or exceed our patients' and colleagues' expectations.
- *Guiding Principles*: We focus on the patient in everything we do. We practice open communication in order to improve our processes and build trust. We expect the management to lead by example and remove the barriers to meet our goals. We are a learning organization that respects and encourages innovation, creativity, and risk-taking. We succeed with employee involvement, which is continuously encouraged, recognized, and rewarded. We collaborate to achieve our goals. We embrace cultural diversity.
- *Creating a Culture of Safety*: A patient safety culture can be defined as the shared values, beliefs, norms, and procedures related to patient safety among members of an organization, unit, or team. Patient safety is an organization-wide, inte-grated, and coordinated approach designed to avoid injuries to patients from the care that is intended to help them. Safety is a priority and a property of systems and processes. Tufts Medical Center is committed to the ongoing assessment of the culture of safety within the medical center using evidence-based surveys to evaluate the culture and the effectiveness of interventions to strengthen the cul-ture of safety over time. Priorities are identified and categorized based on the Institute of Medicine's (IOM's) six aims of healthcare:

    - *Safe* (e.g., supporting the just culture model as a framework for event investi-gation and response to events)
    - *Timely* (e.g., reducing wait times and delays, timely test results)
    - *Effective* (e.g., reducing preventable mortality, sepsis management, stroke care) *Efficient* (e.g., timely data analytics, clinical documentation improvement)
    - *Equitable* (e.g., reducing variation in our care, cultural diversity strategy)
    - *Patient centered* (e.g., patient rights and values guide all clinical decisions)

- Guiding all of our efforts to drive quality and safety are the following four pil-lars: (a) creating a culture of safety, (b) improving high-risk processes, (c) ensur-ing excellent patient experiences, and (d) effectively managing care transitions.

The annual quality and safety plan prioritizes activities in each of these domains each year. Goals are set and metrics are developed to measure progress. At each meeting of the committee, progress is reviewed and corrective action recommended as appropriate. Highlights are reviewed with the full board at each board meeting. The following is a sample of some of the tools used to guide our efforts. These are examples of slides that are reviewed at every board of trustees meeting held at Tufts Medical Center. Founded on principles of transparency and honesty, these inform the board of the challenges and successes of the never-ending quest to perfect healthcare.

▶ Credentials

  ▪ Approval recommended
    VOTE

▶ Critical events (PCAC)

▶ Initiatives

  ▪ Team training

  ▪ QI education for house staff

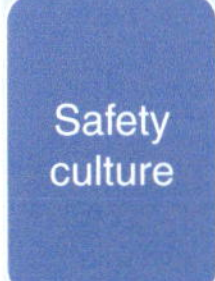
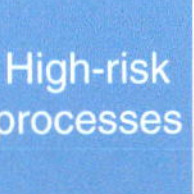
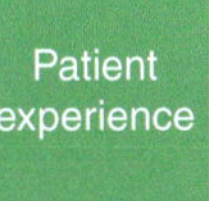
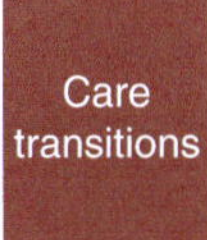

Inpatient teams
- Improving call button response time (North 4)
- Neuroscience improved discharge time (Proger 5N)
- Improving discharge satisfaction (MIU-OB)

Ambulatory Teams
- Reducing no-shows in general pediatrics
- Improving valet parking services
- Text-based appointment reminders in adult primary care

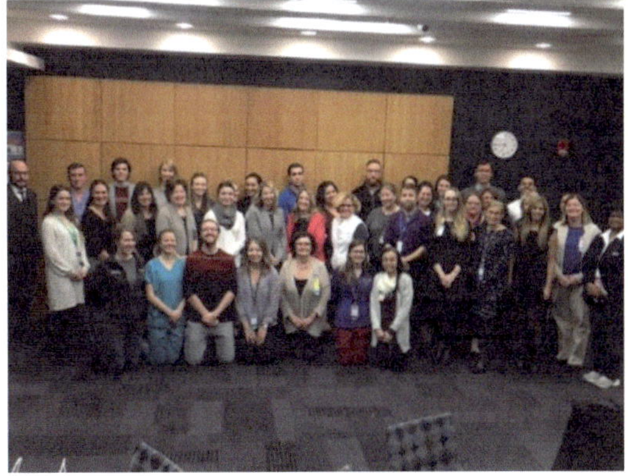

Best volume   **Best outcomes**

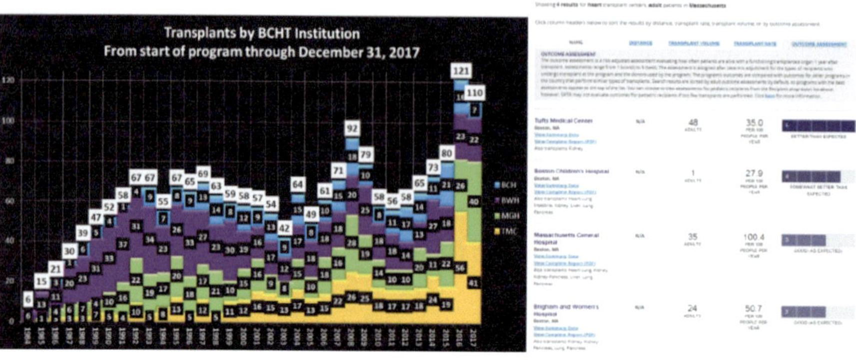

Tufts Medical Center — HARM BUBBLE QUARTERLY VIEW - September 2019

Metric	Q3 2019	Prior Quarter	Change Q/Q	Goal	3 Year Rolling Quarterly Trend
Falls with Injury Rate/1000 patient days	0.61	0.46	0.15	≤ 0.30	
CLABSI rate/1000 line days (all inpt units)	0.30	0.34	−0.03	≤ 0.51	
CAUTI Adult Med Surg rate/1000 catheter days	1.33	1.33	0.00	≤ 2.4	
Serious Med Errors per 1000 pt days	0.25	0.15	0.10	≤ 1.0	
Pressure Injuries Med/Surg	0.36	0.86	−0.49	≤ 1.0	
Pressure Injuries ICU	6.48	7.83	−1.34	≤ 4.0	

Tufts Medical Center

INTEGRATED QUALITY DASHBOARD - September 2019

SAFE	Oct	Nov	Dec	Jan	Feb	Mar	Apr	May	Jun	Jul	Aug	Sep	Trends	FY19	FY18	FY17
Serious Safety Events	0	1	0	2	3	0	3	0	1	2	1	1		14	25	
Serious Safety Events Rate/10,000 patient days	1.2	1.2	1.1	1.0	1.1	1.0	1.0	0.7	0.7	0.7	0.7	0.6		2.6		
Preventable Harm Rollup	21	20	22	14	13	11	12	10	18	10	17	11		15	17	
Workplace Injury Events	5	8	4	3	4	4	5	5	4	5	3	3		4.4	5.3	5.3
Days lost due to Workplace Injuries	36	41	26	8	16	8	11	17	56	37	15	108		31.6	36.9	71.5
Workplace assaults	5	16	18	10	13	12	16	5	9	5	12	14		11.3	9.2	6.8
Falls # Total / With Injury (excl NICU)	15 / 3	21 / 5	20 / 3	17 / 3	17 / 3	15 / 1	14 / 3	15 / 2	21 / 5	16 / 3	25 / 6	12 / 5		208/42	197/43	193/31
Falls Rate/1000 patient days	1.9	2.8	2.5	2.1	2.3	1.9	1.9	2.0	3.0	2.1	3.2	1.6		2.3	2.2	2.1
Falls with Injury Rate/1000 patient days	0.38	0.67	0.38	0.37	0.40	0.13	0.41	0.27	0.71	0.40	0.77	0.65		0.46	0.48	0.34
Serious medication errors reaching the patient #	4	2	3	2	3	1	2	1	1	1	5	1		2.2	3.3	2.8
Rate/1000 patient days	0.44	0.23	0.33	0.22	0.35	0.11	0.23	0.11	0.12	0.11	0.53	0.11		0.39	0.38	0.32
Central line-associated bloodstream infections (CLABSIs) #	1	0	3	3	0	3	1	0	1	0	2	0		1.2	1.3	1.5
Overall rate/1000 line days (all inpt units)	0.4	0.0	1.4	1.5	0.0	1.5	0.5	0.0	0.5	0.0	0.9	0.0		0.6	0.6	0.7
Pediatric rate/1000 line days (includes all pedi units)	3.7	0.0	2.7	3.1	0.0	0.0	2.3	0.0	0.0	0.0	0.0	0.0		1.0	0.9	0.8
Catheter-associated urinary tract infections (CAUTIs) #	6	3	5	2	2.0	1.0	1.0	1.0	2.0	1.0	1.0	2.0		2.3	3.0	2.9
ICU rate/1000 line days (excl NICU)	5.5	4.5	5.4	2.8	1.5	1.6	0.0	1.3	3.3	0.0	1.4	1.5		2.5	2.2	1.7
Adult Med Surg Units rate/1000 line days (incl NSIMC)	4.3	0.0	2.5	0.0	2.1	0.0	2.4	0.0	0.0	2.1	0.0	2.4		1.3	3.1	3.3
Pediatric Units rate/1000 line days (excl NICU)	0.0	0.0	0.0	0.0	0.0	0.0	0.0	0.0	0.0	0.0	0.0	0.0		0.0	1.7	0.0
Pressure Injuries (quarterly prevalence study) *	18	16	16	15	14	15	14	16	19	11	8	17		179	185	152
Pressure Injuries (avoidable)	2	2	4	1	1	1	0	1	0	0	0	0		12	9	
Adult ICU	6.18	6.86	8.51	3.87	7.40	7.56	7.33	8.72	7.48	7.29	3.90	8.26		6.92	6.50	5.98
Adult Med/Surg	1.43	1.36	0.74	1.60	0.58	0.37	0.38	0.20	1.99	0.00	0.35	0.74		0.81	1.10	0.81
Pediatrics	1.49	0.64	0.73	0.73	1.60	2.76	2.48	2.41	0.00	1.45	0.71	2.28		1.47	1.53	0.94
Serious reportable events (SREs) #	1	6	6	3	5	6	6	6	7	5	4	2		4.8	3.3	3.3
AHRQ PSI-90 Composite (observed/expected)	1	1	1	1	1	1	1	1	1	1	1	1		0.9	1.0	0.9
AHRQ PSI-90 Composite (# of cases)	9	10	4	5	4	5	8	6	4	6	8	6		6.3	6.9	6.5
Hand hygiene performance, Goal: ≥ 95%	95%	92%	93%	91%	95%	93%	94%	94%	93%	93%	91%	93%		93%	92%	92%

TIMELY	Oct	Nov	Dec	Jan	Feb	Mar	Apr	May	Jun	Jul	Aug	Sep	Trends	FY19	FY18	FY17
Emergency Dept wait time in minutes, from arrival to provider	28	28	39	41	38	43	47	44	42	42	42	41		40	28	33
Emergency Dept wait time in minutes, from disposition to floor	174	139	186	194	227	164	143	142	142	143	207	173		170	141	157
Lag time in days for new patients to obtain appointment	29.1	28.9	29.6	27.9	28.0	27.8	28.4	29.5	32.1	32.7	31.4	33.4		30.1	28.7	31.0
Percentage of ambulatory patients scheduled within 14 days	56.2	56.2	54.7	51.7	54.4	55.4	54.2	55.8	62.2	53.4	57.8	53.1		53.0	55.3	55.8
Call center abandonment rate*** (Adult Call Center)	15%	13%	11%	11%	10%	12%	12%	14%	10%	10%	10%	13%		12%	18%	21%
Call center abandonment rate (Adult - Non CC)	15%	9%	4%	5%	3%	3%	2%	3%	3%	8%	6%	3%		5%	9%	10%
Call center abandonment rate (Pediatric Call Center)	14%	15%	13%	15%	12%	12%	13%	13%	15%	13%	14%	12%		14%	19%	16%

GENERAL	Oct	Nov	Dec	Jan	Feb	Mar	Apr	May	Jun	Jul	Aug	Sep	Trends	FY19	FY18	FY17
Discharges	1,494	1,209	1,460	1,305	1,418	1,564	1,452	1,515	1,396	1,527	1,481	1,437		1,438	1,446	1,542
Clinic Volume	38,769	37,016	33,308	37,105	33,091	36,256	35,194	35,688	32,039	33,356	33,172	36,983		35,165	33,247	31,210
Medicare Case Mix Index (CMI)	2.11	2.54	2.83	2.46	2.54	2.45	2.43	2.39	2.23	2.39	2.58	2.53		2.51	2.49	2.42
Total Case Mix Index (CMI)	2.21	2.12	2.09	2.00	2.03	2.12	1.99	2.00	2.03	2.02	2.19	2.20		2.09	2.12	2.08

Notes:
*Pressure injury data is from our quarterly prevalence study, with calendar year totals displayed in the fiscal year columns
**UHC (University HealthSystem Consortium) methodology is used to track and standardize these metrics
***Abandonment Rate = the percent of callers that hang up before an agent answers.

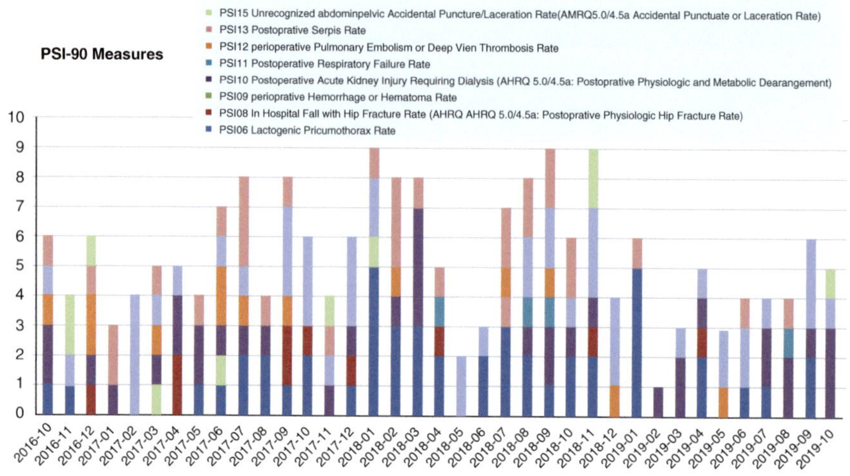

AHRQ Version 2019 used

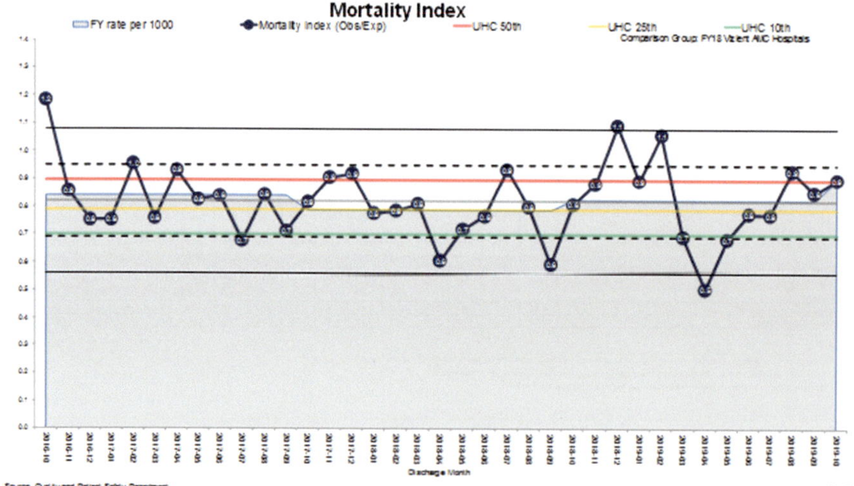

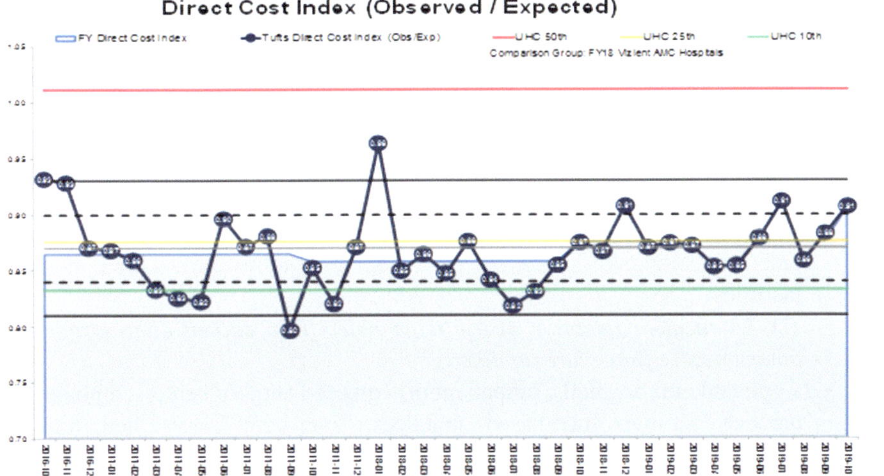

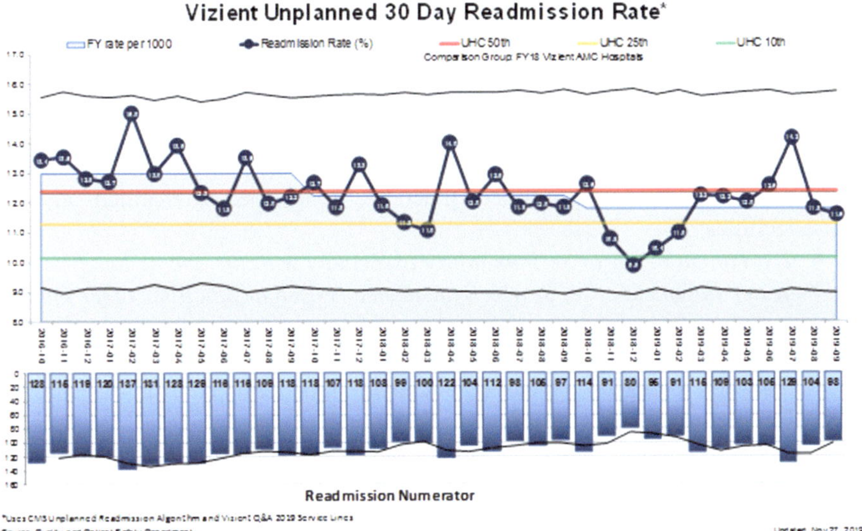

Appendix A

Serious Reportable Events

1. Surgical or Invasive Procedure Events
    - 1A. *Surgery or other invasive procedure performed on the wrong site (updated)*
    - Applicable in: hospitals, outpatient/office-based surgery centers, ambulatory practice settings/office-based practices, long-term care/skilled nursing facilities

- 1B. *Surgery or other invasive procedure performed on the wrong patient (updated)*
- Applicable in: hospitals, outpatient/office-based surgery centers, ambulatory practice settings/office-based practices, long-term care/skilled nursing facilities
- 1C. *Wrong surgical or other invasive procedure performed on a patient (updated)*
- Applicable in: hospitals, outpatient/office-based surgery centers, ambulatory practice settings/office-based practices, long-term care/skilled nursing facilities
- 1D. *Unintended retention of a foreign object in a patient after surgery or other invasive procedure (updated)*
- Applicable in: hospitals, outpatient/office-based surgery centers, ambulatory practice settings/office-based practices, long-term care/skilled nursing facilities
- 1E. *Intraoperative or immediately postoperative/postprocedure death in an ASA Class 1 patient (updated)*
- Applicable in: hospitals, outpatient/office-based surgery centers, ambulatory practice settings/office-based practices

2. Product or Device Events
   - 2A. *Patient death or serious injury associated with the use of contaminated drugs, devices, or biologics provided by the healthcare setting (updated)*
   - Applicable in: hospitals, outpatient/office-based surgery centers, ambulatory practice settings/office-based practices, long-term care/skilled nursing facilities
   - 2B. *Patient death or serious injury associated with the use or function of a device in patient care, in which the device is used or functions other than as intended (updated)*
   - Applicable in: hospitals, outpatient/office-based surgery centers, ambulatory practice settings/office-based practices, long-term care/skilled nursing facilities
   - 2C. *Patient death or serious injury associated with intravascular air embolism that occurs while being cared for in a healthcare setting (updated)*
   - Applicable in: hospitals, outpatient/office-based surgery centers, long-term care/skilled nursing facilities

3. Patient Protection Events
   - 3A. *Discharge or release of a patient/resident of any age, who is unable to make decisions, to other than an authorized person (updated)*
   - Applicable in: hospitals, outpatient/office-based surgery centers, ambulatory practice settings/office-based practices, long-term care/skilled nursing facilities
   - 3B. *Patient death or serious injury associated with patient elopement (disappearance) (updated)*

- Applicable in: hospitals, outpatient/office-based surgery centers, ambulatory practice settings/office-based practices, long-term care/skilled nursing facilities
- 3C. *Patient suicide, attempted suicide, or self-harm that results in serious injury, while being cared for in a healthcare setting (updated)*
- Applicable in: hospitals, outpatient/office-based surgery centers, ambulatory practice settings/office-based practices, long-term care/skilled nursing facilities

4. Care Management Events
   - 4A. *Patient death or serious injury associated with a medication error (e.g., errors involving the wrong drug, wrong dose, wrong patient, wrong time, wrong rate, wrong preparation, or wrong route of administration) (updated)*
   - Applicable in: hospitals, outpatient/office-based surgery centers, ambulatory practice settings/office-based practices, long-term care/skilled nursing facilities
   - 4B. *Patient death or serious injury associated with unsafe administration of blood products (updated)*
   - Applicable in: hospitals, outpatient/office-based surgery centers, ambulatory practice settings/office-based practices, long-term care/skilled nursing facilities
   - 4C. *Maternal death or serious injury associated with labor or delivery in a low-risk pregnancy while being cared for in a healthcare setting (updated)*
   - Applicable in: hospitals, outpatient/office-based surgery centers
   - 4D. *Death or serious injury of a neonate associated with labor or delivery in a low-risk pregnancy (new)*
   - Applicable in: hospitals, outpatient/office-based surgery centers
   - 4E. *Patient death or serious injury associated with a fall while being cared for in a healthcare setting (updated)*
   - Applicable in: hospitals, outpatient/office-based surgery centers, ambulatory practice settings/office-based practices, long-term care/skilled nursing facilities
   - 4F. *Any Stage 3, Stage 4, and unstageable pressure ulcers acquired after admission/presentation to a healthcare setting (updated)*
   - Applicable in: hospitals, outpatient/office-based surgery centers, long-term care/skilled nursing facilities
   - 4G. *Artificial insemination with the wrong donor sperm or wrong egg (updated)*
   - Applicable in: hospitals, outpatient/office-based surgery centers, ambulatory practice settings/office-based practices
   - 4H. *Patient death or serious injury resulting from the irretrievable loss of an irreplaceable biological specimen (new)*
   - Applicable in: hospitals, outpatient/office-based surgery centers, ambulatory practice settings/office-based practices, long-term care/skilled nursing facilities

- 4I. *Patient death or serious injury resulting from failure to follow up or communicate laboratory, pathology, or radiology test results (new)*
- Applicable in: hospitals, outpatient/office-based surgery centers, ambulatory practice settings/office-based practices, long-term care/skilled nursing facilities

5. Environmental Events
   - 5A. *Patient or staff death or serious injury associated with an electric shock in the course of a patient care process in a healthcare setting (updated)*
   - Applicable in: hospitals, outpatient/office-based surgery centers, ambulatory practice settings/office-based practices, long-term care/skilled nursing facilities
   - 5B. *Any incident in which systems designated for oxygen or other gas to be delivered to a patient contains no gas, the wrong gas, or are contaminated by toxic substances (updated)*
   - Applicable in: hospitals, outpatient/office-based surgery centers, ambulatory practice settings/office-based practices, long-term care/skilled nursing facilities
   - 5C. *Patient or staff death or serious injury associated with a burn incurred from any source in the course of a patient care process in a healthcare setting (updated)*
   - Applicable in: hospitals, outpatient/office-based surgery centers, ambulatory practice settings/office-based practices, long-term care/skilled nursing facilities
   - 5D. *Patient death or serious injury associated with the use of physical restraints or bedrails while being cared for in a healthcare setting (updated)*
   - Applicable in: hospitals, outpatient/office-based surgery centers, ambulatory practice settings/office-based practices, long-term care/skilled nursing facilities

6. Radiologic Events
   - 6A. *Death or serious injury of a patient or staff associated with the introduction of a metallic object into the MRI area (new)*
   - Applicable in: hospitals, outpatient/office-based surgery centers, ambulatory practice settings/office-based practices

7. Potential Criminal Events
   - 7A. *Any instance of care ordered by or provided by someone impersonating a physician, nurse, pharmacist, or other licensed healthcare provider (updated)*
   - Applicable in: hospitals, outpatient/office-based surgery centers, ambulatory practice settings/office-based practices, long-term care/skilled nursing facilities
   - 7B. *Abduction of a patient/resident of any age (updated)*

- Applicable in: hospitals, outpatient/office-based surgery centers, ambulatory practice settings/office-based practices, long-term care/skilled nursing facilities
- 7C. *Sexual abuse/assault on a patient or staff member within or on the grounds of a healthcare setting (updated)*
- Applicable in: hospitals, outpatient/office-based surgery centers, ambulatory practice settings/office-based practices, long-term care/skilled nursing facilities
- 7D. *Death or serious injury of a patient or staff member resulting from a physical assault (i.e., battery) that occurs within or on the grounds of a healthcare setting (updated)*
- Applicable in: hospitals, outpatient/office-based surgery centers, ambulatory practice settings/office-based practices, long-term care/skilled nursing facilities

Chapter 13
Quality Improvement and Population Management in Adult Primary Care

Julie Tishler, Kristin T. Huang, and Deborah Blazey-Martin

Ambulatory Quality Measures: A History

Over the past 10 years, with the implementation of an increasing number of quality measures and a heightened awareness of the need for population health management, we have experienced a revolution in the way we care for patients in the ambulatory setting. In 2008, the Institute for Healthcare Improvement coined the Triple Aim, which holds that health systems must be designed with three foundational goals: improving the health of populations, enhancing the individual experience of care, and reducing the per capita costs of healthcare. The premise was simple; if primary care providers, those responsible for all care in their panels of patients, managed diabetes, hypertension, and other chronic diseases through a population-based approach, their patients would remain healthier and avoid expensive downstream emergency department visits and hospitalizations. In addition, if primary care practices could increase rates of cancer screening and primary preventive care, they would have the opportunity to prevent, diagnose, and address health conditions at earlier stages, before they became more difficult and expensive to treat. The expectation was that patients would have a better experience, health would improve, and costs would go down.

The challenge for most ambulatory practices was that they had neither the technology nor the skills required to manage patients from a population perspective. In 2008, most practices were still using paper records, which could not practically be used to collect population-level data. A 2004 random sample of US healthcare facilities found that only 13% of respondents had implemented an electronic health record (EHR); 10% did not have or did not plan to have an EHR system [1]. In 2008, only 22% of US hospitals had adopted EHR technology. It quickly became apparent

J. Tishler · K. T. Huang · D. Blazey-Martin (✉)
Internal Medicine and Adult Primary Care, Tufts Medical Center, Boston, MA, USA
e-mail: dblazey-martin@tuftsmedicalcenter.org

© Springer Nature Switzerland AG 2020

D. N. Salem (ed.), *Quality Measures*, https://doi.org/10.1007/978-3-030-37145-6_13

that without significant financial incentives, hospitals and practices could not afford to implement the expensive EHR systems required to practice the kind of quality-based population health believed indispensable to decreasing healthcare costs and achieving the Triple Aim.

From this necessity, the 2009 Health Information Technology for Clinical and Economic Health (HITECH) Act was created to incentivize physicians and hospitals to implement qualified EHR technology. Not all EHRs would qualify for the incentives; the EHR must be designed for "Meaningful Use" to make population management possible. Vendors had strict rules for certification of their EHRs; in a three-stage process, they created IT infrastructure for standardized data capture, clinical decision support, and improvement of patient outcomes. The financial incentives to practices were sufficient to aid in purchasing certified technology, and the penalties for those practices that chose to ignore the HITECH Act were great enough that most took notice. By 2015, 88.3% of nonfederal acute care hospitals in the USA had adopted a certified EHR [2].

With the ability to measure population performance, insurers developed quality contracts as an innovative new risk-sharing arrangement that paid primary care practices an additional per member per month dollar amount for achieving pre-defined prevention and disease management process and outcome targets on their primary care panels. Over time, more practices have implemented EHRs capable of building reports and providing data to physicians identifying which patients needed outreach to improve care for their population.

However, while hospitals and practices worked to adopt Meaningful Use technology, the skills needed for population management were not yet available in most primary care practices. The "patient-centered medical home" (PCMH) created a primary care practice model focused on population management. States and private accrediting bodies, such as the National Committee for Quality Assurance (NCQA), supported programs that trained and certified practices in the PCMH model. The concept was built upon team-based care, in which responsibility for patient care would be shared across a team with every member working to the top of their license. The certification process involved building population reporting capacity, radically changing the primary care staffing model to include pre-work to ensure metric-driven care during the office visit, and population-based outreach to patients between visits. Operations were reworked so that patient data were now entered into structured data fields that could be compiled into reports for population health management. The anticipated return on this investment was to come from improved quality performance in risk-bearing contracts, better patient satisfaction, and the decreased cost of higher quality care.

With new EHRs and an awareness of the importance of population management in primary care, insurers saw an encouraging decrease in costs of care for patients in their risk contracts [3]. As practices improved the quality of care, insurers raised the bar for their measures. Merely educating physicians and their staffs and providing data to primary care practices were no longer sufficient to continue improving performance. Quality improvement required a change in the model of care beyond the early PCMH, with additional support to providers in managing the patient registry reports and many other support functions, including data entry and outreach. Additional staff support to primary care practices was needed for improving outcomes and decreasing cost, both at the time of visit and in between. A team of nurse care managers to outreach to complex patients, social workers to aid with behavioral health management, and pharmacists to review medication lists and improve transitions of care became the new standard [4, 5]. This robust team approach to population management in primary care is embodied in the Chronic Care Model and operationalized in National Committee for Quality Assurance certification as a Patient-centered medical home (PCMH). This model has been shown to improve patient outcomes in a number of chronic diseases including diabetes and hypertension and to reduce emergency room utilization in a variety of clinical care settings, including academic health centers, community health centers, veteran administration practices, and community primary care [5–8].

Each year, more insurers have jumped on the bandwagon with their own preferred risk arrangements, quality measures, and new models of care. The Centers for Medicare and Medicaid Services (CMS) introduced their Medicare Accountable Care Organization (ACO) models in 2011 through the Affordable Care Act (ACA). In the ACO model, primary care practices were given an annual member cost per year target and took responsibility for total medical expense. Meeting minimum quality measures and patient experience standards became a gate for sharing in cost savings. However, the CMS quality measures did not perfectly align with any of the measures supported by the multitude of private insurers touting pay-for-performance (P4P) plans, adding to the chaos and confusion at the practice level. In 2018, MassHealth, the Medicaid insurance for the state of Massachusetts, also established an ACO model of care with its own distinct quality measures, including screening for social needs.

Primary care providers are now held accountable not only for preventive care, chronic disease management, and behavioral health but also for utilization, including emergency department visits, total medical expenses, and hospital readmissions. The burden placed on primary care practices over the past 10 years in the name of the Triple Aim has come at a cost. In 2018, Merritt Hawkins surveyed physicians and found that 78% experience symptoms of burnout at least some of the time [9]. A work-time study performed by the American Medical Association found that for every hour spent seeing patients in the office, nearly 2 additional hours are spent on EHR documentation and other paper work [10]. Many are now shifting from the Triple Aim to the Quadruple Aim, which adds "improving the work life of healthcare providers, including clinicians and staff" [11]. The team approach to addressing care with self-management support coaching, integrated behavioral healthcare, and management of referrals should take pressure off of the physician, but there are mixed reports in the literature on the impact of the patient-centered medical home model on physician burnout [12, 13]. We are still early in the ambulatory quality and population health revolution, and as our operations, skills, and tools continue to improve, hopefully the well-being of physicians and other caregivers will follow.

Implementation of Quality Improvement in an Academic Primary Care Setting

We present here our approach to population management and quality improvement in a large academic primary care practice affiliated with a tertiary care hospital in downtown Boston. We care for over 40,000 patients with a diverse payor mix and high case mix index, with over 35 attending physicians and 75 resident physicians. We serve the Chinatown and South Boston neighborhoods, as well as patients from many outlying communities. One of our five teams is especially equipped to care for our significant Asian population. As of 2019, our primary care practice participates in multiple commercial risk agreements, a CMS Next-Generation ACO, and a Medicaid ACO. We are currently responsible for over 35 different quality measures encompassing as many as six domains with different targets and ranges for success, including preventive care, chronic disease management, utilization, behavioral health, total medical expenses, and hospital readmissions.

Guiding Principles

As primary care physicians have become responsible for an overwhelming number of differing quality measures from multiple insurers, our practice has established guiding principles regarding how to choose quality measures to target for improvement. In order to make substantive improvements, we have worked hard to create a culture of continuous improvement in our practice, approaching data with curiosity and embracing change. We have also found it necessary to focus on only a few measures at a time, enabling us to make systems-level changes to effect long-lasting improvements. This has necessitated prioritizing the measures on which we work.

Foundational to our prioritization has been the Triple Aim, focusing on the health of populations, the patient experience of care (including quality and satisfaction), and reductions in healthcare costs. We therefore prioritize initiatives that will improve population health and have real impact in the lives of our patients, either immediately or downstream as supported by evidence-based literature. For example, correct medication reconciliation after a transition of care has an immediate effect on the health of many individual patients, especially after a hospitalization where inappropriate medications could well lead to a readmission [14, 15]. In contrast, an individual patient may not appreciate the benefits of well-controlled blood pressure immediately, yet blood pressure control has been shown to have clear downstream benefits [16, 17]. We focus on a handful of process and outcome measures that we believe will have an important impact on our patients' lives, health, engagement, and satisfaction with care. Our initiatives seek to be cost-neutral.

We have also embraced a fourth component that has commonly become known as the Quadruple Aim: staff experience or joy in work. It is our belief that higher levels of employee satisfaction lead to increased patient satisfaction and improved safety [13]. Staff burnout has impacted our practice as it has nationwide [9, 12]. Unreliable and inefficient systems contribute to patient and staff dissatisfaction as well as to poor quality and gaps in care. We believe quality improvement has the power to combat burnout and increase provider satisfaction with work by addressing these problems from a systems-level perspective, empowering our staff to participate in our progress. Thus, some of our quality initiatives are focused on improving clinic operations and reducing inefficiencies.

A fifth principle that guides our approach to quality measures is health equity. While various payors and insurers have different quality measures and pay-for-performance incentives, we believe it is important to be payor-blind when managing the health of a patient population. We set our practice's quality standards for all patients using evidence-based medicine and best practices. The current Massachusetts Medicaid ACO recognizes the issue of health equity in providing care to low-income and traditionally underserved populations by explicitly providing additional resources including community healthcare workers to provide additional support to achieve quality goals in care [18–20].

Implementation

Empanelment is central to identifying patients and their designated primary care provider within our practice in order to manage their care and their health. We define our patients as those who have had a visit to our practice within the past 1200 days. We regularly update our empanelment by running reports on patients who have been seen in the practice but whose provider field has been left blank.

Data transparency and reporting is another cornerstone of how we approach our quality improvement work. We have created a Physician Quality Dashboard (Table 13.1) that tracks a select group of quality metrics for each physician in the practice. The report lists individual physician rates, goal rates where appropriate, the practice average, and rates in attending patients vs. resident patients.

It is important that the reports we provide to our clinicians are actionable. Each quarter, we choose one to two measures (such as hypertension control or pneumococcal immunization) and provide hard copy lists to our providers of their patients who are not meeting those measures. For example, we might send a provider's overall rate of pneumococcal 13-valent immunization as well as a detailed list of all patients over 65 who do not have a documented pneumococcal 13-valent immunization in our EHR. Clinicians are also able to manipulate the electronic report within Excel to find their lists of patients who are out of compliance for any specific measure. These lists can be used for targeted, team-based outreach. In this way, our report includes both treetop and ground-level detailed views of the data.

In order to design and implement our systems-based quality improvement initiatives, we have a *dedicated quality improvement team* that we call "Change Team"

Table 13.1 Ambulatory physician quality dashboard

Health condition	Measure	Metric	Goal
Diabetes	Diabetes is well-controlled	HbA1c < 7.5%	
	Diabetes is uncontrolled	HbA1c > 9.0%) [21]	
	Two A1c process measurements	% of patients with two or more A1Cs in 1 year	80%
	No A1C in 1 year	% of patients with 0 A1Cs in 1 year	<2% year
Hypertension [22]	Blood pressure control	SBP < 140 and DBP < 90	60%
	Blood pressure process	BP is rechecked if triage blood pressure is high	75%
Cancer screening [23]	Colorectal cancer screening	Rate for appropriate patients	71%
	Breast cancer screening	Rate for appropriate patients	82%
	Cervical cancer screening	Rate for appropriate patients	93%
Infectious disease	Hepatitis C screening	Rate for appropriate patients	
	Pneumococcal 13-valent immunization	Rate for patients ages 65 and older	70%

that meets weekly. This multidisciplinary team is comprised of physicians, nurses, administrators (both front line and managerial), and a data/technology expert. We use the Model for Improvement to run PDSA (Plan/Do/Study/Act) cycles and execute small tests of change that we then study, iterate, and adapt as needed until ready for widespread implementation [24]. The weekly iterative process is crucial to driving improvements forward. In addition, there is a larger quality improvement committee that meets once every 2 months for a wider audience of ideas as it relates to the Change Team's work. We have focused on two to three improvement areas per year where systems-based improvements are tested, designed, and implemented in Change Team. We align these measures with the annual practice-wide physician quality incentive bonus goals and with our data reporting.

Quality Improvement in Practice: Practical Examples in the Primary Care Setting

Automating Point-of-Care Hemoglobin A1c Testing

An example that highlights the Change Team's use of PDSA cycles to accelerate and refine a clinical improvement is our implementation of automated point-of-care (POC) hemoglobin A1c (HbA1c) testing. Point-of-care A1c testing has been shown to improve glycemic control [25, 26], patient and provider satisfaction [27], and operational practice efficiency [28]. However, despite acquiring POC HbA1c machines for each of our five clinic teams, the machines were not well-utilized. Individual clinicians could request that a medical assistant perform the test, but this was done inconsistently. There was then a 7-minute lag time while waiting for the machine to process the sample, resulting in a delay of care for the patient. Since the machines required weekly use of costly controls to ensure accuracy, the lack of utilization also meant that they were not financially efficient for the practice.

The Change Team began a process to increase POC HbA1c testing on appropriate patients and decrease the delay. Initially, automated lists of each clinician's patients for the day were printed and left on the clinician's door. The list included relevant information about each patient, including their last HbA1c value and the date this lab was drawn. The clinician then circled any patient who would need the POC HbA1c and gave the list to one of the MAs on the team. Subsequently, the medical assistant started the POC HbA1c testing process during triage, such that the result would be available by the time the clinician was ready to see the patient or shortly thereafter.

However, since our practice does not have a 1:1 medical assistant-to-clinician ratio and since there was only one hard copy of each list, patients were often missed if a different medical assistant triaged the patient. Also, not every clinician made use of the list, bringing us back to the original problem of underutilization.

The Change Team sought to automate the process further. Our IT specialist modified our electronic health record (EHR) such that a red alert appears on the MA's computer screen during triage if a patient is due for an HbA1c test. We set up a simple algorithm to determine which patients would qualify as "due" for a HbA1c test: if the last HbA1c on file was more than 6 months ago for any diabetic patient, or if the last HbA1c on file was $\geq$3 months ago for those patients whose last HbA1c was $\geq$7.5%. If the medical assistant sees the red alert in the patient's electronic chart, they perform the POC HbA1c test for that patient during the initial triage. The result is immediately entered in the EHR and a hard copy printout is also given to the clinician clipped to the patient's encounter form.

Medical assistants were trained in this workflow by the supervising nurse practitioner. We piloted this first on one team to ensure all challenges were addressed before disseminating throughout our entire practice. We created buy-in from clinicians for automating the process by highlighting the value of reduced delays in obtaining the results of the POC HbA1c test and having accurate HbA1c data on every appropriate patient at the time of clinical interaction.

We generated a weekly report on the rate at which each medical assistant was performing the test when appropriate. Medical assistants struggling with the new workflow were given individual retraining. High-functioning medical assistant teams were celebrated.

Our baseline rate of POC HbA1c testing when due by our protocol was less than 20% in August 2016. This rose to 75–85% and has been maintained over the past 3 years despite significant turnover in medical assistant staff (Fig. 13.1). Our baseline rate of appropriate HbA1c testing overall (at least two HbA1c on all diabetic

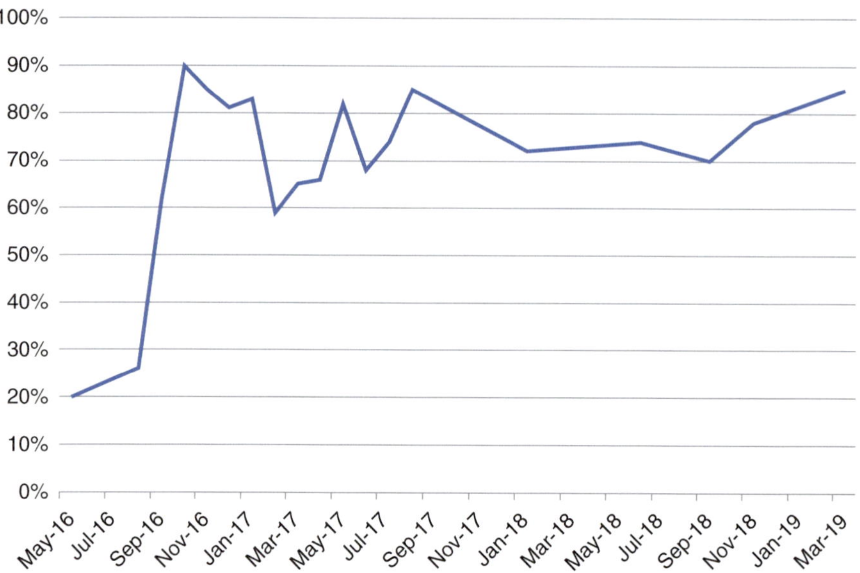

Fig. 13.1 POC A1c rates from March 2016 to May 2019. May 2016: Automated POC A1c process piloted on one of our practice's five teams. August 2016: Automated POC A1c process disseminated to entire practice

patients per year) was 66% in May 2016, and this rose to 79% in April 2019. Our overall rate of diabetes control (defined as HbA1c < 7.5%) has remained unchanged at 44%, demonstrating the challenge of improving outcomes even with improvements in related process measures.

Hypertension Control

Appropriate blood pressure control is essential to prevent cardiovascular morbidity and mortality [16]. Hypertension control is also a key metric for many insurance quality contracts. The following example illustrates how we approached improving this quality measure on a population health level using several key components.

First, we created a hypertension registry of each patient who carried a diagnosis of hypertension on their problem list. The registry includes key characteristics, such as comorbidities, last blood pressure reading and date, next appointment, and number of antihypertensive medications prescribed. From this registry, we generate quarterly reports to our physicians of all their patients with uncontrolled hypertension (we defined this as patients whose last blood pressure measurement included a systolic blood pressure ≥ 140 or diastolic blood pressure ≥ 90). Providers and their frontline team could then use these reports for individual outreach.

Second, we perform bimonthly practice-based automated outreach phone calls to patients with uncontrolled hypertension without an upcoming appointment. The automated message reminds them that they are due for an appointment and to please call us to schedule one.

Third, we harnessed our EHR to create visual prompts for medical assistants and clinicians, alerting them when a patient's blood pressure is high. When the medical assistant inputs a patient's triage blood pressure that is ≥ 140/90, a button appears to prompt the medical assistant to print a patient education handout regarding behavioral modification to improve blood pressure control. The handout is then given to the clinician, which serves as a reminder that the patient's triage blood pressure is elevated and should be rechecked. A second visual alert in the EHR – a red "Hi" next to the blood pressure field of the clinician's note, which is pre-populated with the patient's triage blood pressure – serves as another signal to the clinician. At the end of the visit, after manually repeating the patient's blood pressure, the clinician decides whether the patient should receive the handout.

Lastly, we aim for transparency with data by sending out regular, practice-wide emails including the percentage of each provider's patients with hypertension who are well-controlled, as well as the percentage of time that clinicians are re-measuring a patient's blood pressure if the triage blood pressure is high.

Collectively, these efforts have helped us improve our rates of blood pressure re-measurement when initial blood pressure is elevated from 43% in March 2017 to 72% in March 2019 and have improved our practice rate of hypertension control from 72% in August 2016 to 78% in April 2019 (Fig. 13.2).

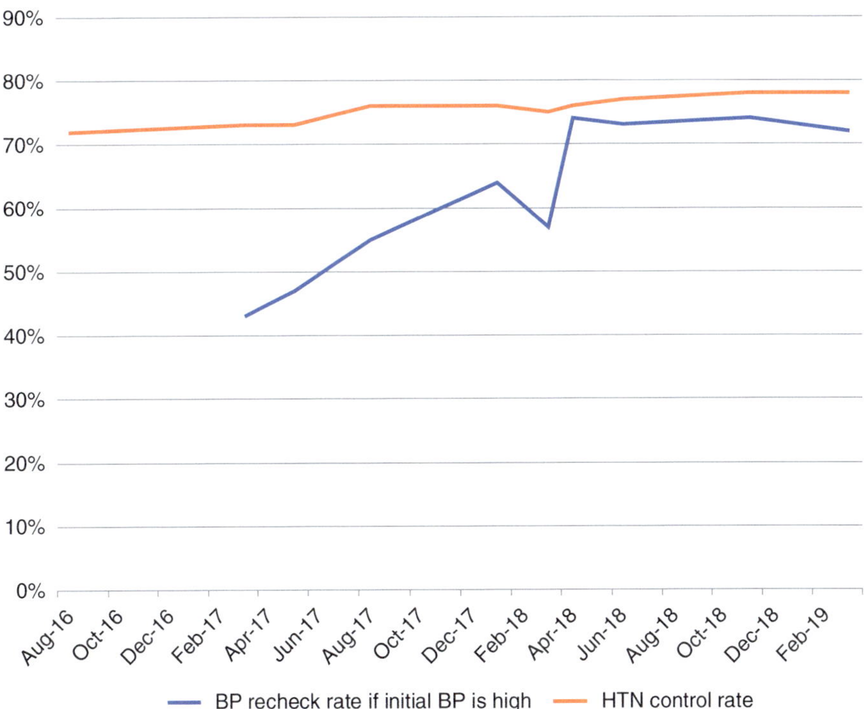

Fig. 13.2 Rates of BP recheck if initial BP is high and rates of HTN control in our practice, August 2016 to March 2019

Improving Adherence to Guidelines for Prescribing and Monitoring Opioids

While insurers and ACOs do not currently assess our practice based on how we care for our patients on chronic opioid therapy, given the growing epidemic of opioid-related morbidity and mortality in the USA [29, 30], we made it a priority to ensure that these patients receive the highest quality care possible. The Centers for Disease Control and several pain societies have published guidelines for appropriate management of chronic opioid therapy that are underutilized by primary care physicians [31, 32]. Standardizing prescribing and monitoring of chronic opioid medications also serves to address the fourth aim of provider satisfaction, by developing a team-based approach and practice standards to support providers in the care of challenging patients with chronic opioid requirements.

To address this, we developed a multicomponent, team-based opioid management system with EHR support. Our strategy included the following:

1. *Creating a patient registry*: Identification of the target population was necessary to track metrics and enable population health management efforts. A registry of patients was created based on the presence of the diagnosis code for "chronic pain, opioid requiring (ICD-10 F11.20)." Monthly reports are generated for providers listing their patients who are regularly prescribed opioids as well as any overdue monitoring measures for each patient, such as an annual patient-provider agreement, a biannual urine drug screen, or a regular review of the state prescription monitoring program.
2. *Standardization of chronic opioid prescribing policies*: Standardization of prescribing patterns includes 28-day prescriptions to avoid the need for weekend prescriptions, a regular review of the state prescription monitoring program by the prescriber or physician assistant team member, and a minimum requirement of biannual urine drug screen. Policy expectations were communicated to patients via explicit annual agreements signed by both prescribers and patients and recorded in our EHR.
3. *Development of a risk-assessment algorithm*: An algorithm to assess risk of opioid misuse was designed using validated screening tools (including the Opioid Risk Tool [33] and the Current Opioid Misuse Measure [34]) to evaluate patients at the time of opioid initiation or for patients new to our practice (Fig. 13.3). Using these tools, we can assign a risk category to each patient and institute the recommended different monitoring strategies. Lastly, we defined patient behaviors that were grounds for termination from opioid therapy.
4. *Team-based case management*: Two physician assistants were hired with 0.5 FTE dedicated to serving as population health specialists and case managers for a panel of 430 patients who are chronically prescribed opioids. The physician assistants regularly review patient panels, appropriateness of opioid prescriptions, and timeliness of urine drug screen monitoring and then discuss any situations requiring attention with the provider.

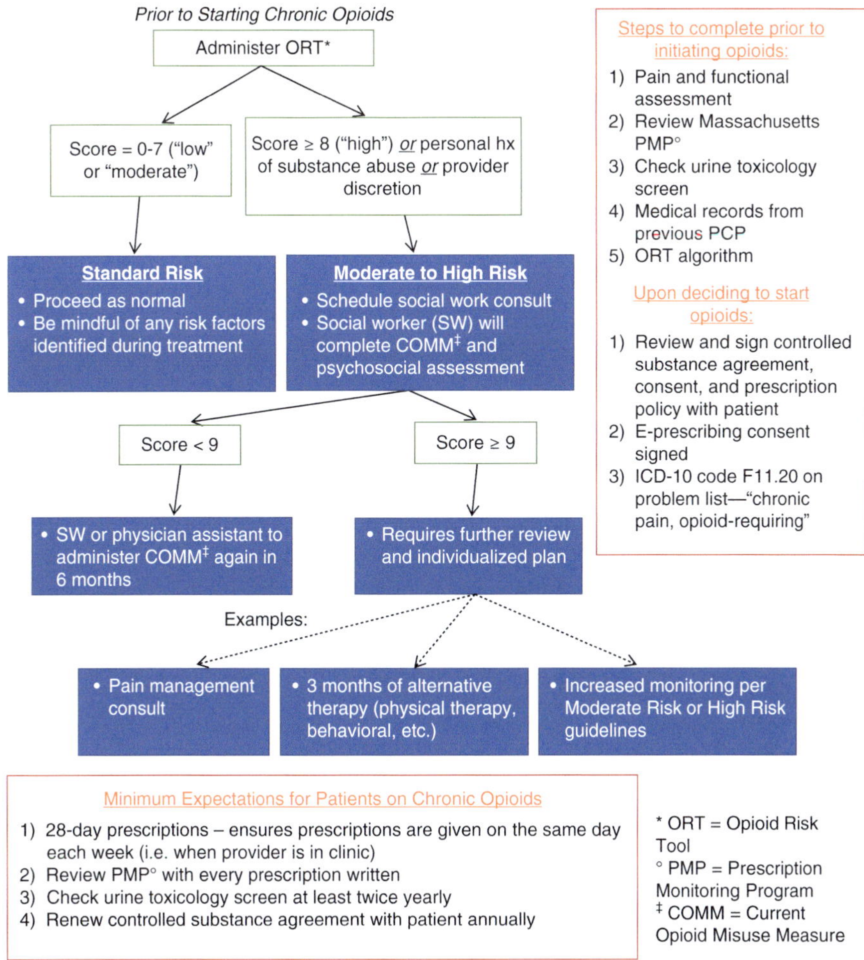

Fig. 13.3 Algorithm for initiation of chronic opioid therapy or for patients new to the practice

5. *EHR support module*: A tool, or "component," in our EHR was designed to centralize all activities related to chronic opioid prescribing. First, this component serves as a prescription management tool for controlled substances. Second, it facilitates communication among clinicians with a designated area to document aberrant patient behavior. Third, the component helps providers adhere to monitoring guidelines by streamlining access to all recommended practices, including one-click access to the state prescription monitoring program, ordering a urine drug screen, printing the patient-provider controlled substance agreement, and documenting when these procedures were last done. Lastly, it serves as a repository for opioid management resources and patient resources.

Between September 2015 and September 2016, the percentage of patients on chronic opioid therapy with a signed controlled substance agreement within the preceding year increased from 46% to 76% ($p < 0.0001$), while the percentage of patients with a urine drug screen done within the past 6 months rose from 23% to 79% ($p < 0.0001$). The percentage of patients whose state prescription monitoring program profile had been checked by a primary care team member in the past year rose from 45% to 97% ($p < 0.0001$). These results have been maintained as of April 2019.

Conclusion

The revolution in quality and population health management has required dramatic and rapid changes in ambulatory medicine. Primary care practices successfully adapting to this new environment require an EHR capable of generating reports on selected measures and a staff able to interpret these reports and engage patients in their care. As our practice has matured in population management and grappled with the multitude of payors setting expectations for us, we have found that guiding principles based on the Quadruple Aim and health equity have served us well in choosing metrics on which to focus. Using our Change Team to pilot and implement quality improvement initiatives not only allows us to improve performance in our risk contracts and ACOs but also makes a lasting impact on the health of all of our patients and of our practice.

References

1. Watzlaf VJ, Zeng X, Jarymowycz C, Firouzan PA. Standards for the content of the electronic health record. Perspect Health Inf Manag. 2004;1:1.
2. Henry J, Pylypchuk Y, Searcy T, Patel V. Adoption of electronic health record systems among US non-federal acute care hospitals: 2008–2015. ONC Data Brief. 2016;35:1–9.
3. Song ZR, Rose S, Safran DG, Landon BE, Day MP, Chernew ME. Changes in health care spending and quality 4 years into global payment. N Engl J Med. 2014;371(18):1704–14.
4. Patel MS, Arron MJ, Sinsky TA, Green EH, Baker DW, Bowen JL, et al. Estimating the staffing infrastructure for a patient-centered medical home. Am J Manag Care. 2013;19(6):509–16.
5. Coleman K, Austin BT, Brach C, Wagner EH. Evidence on the chronic care model in the new millennium. Health Aff. 2009;28(1):75–85.
6. van den Berk-Clark C, Doucette E, Rottnek F, Manard W, Prada MA, Hughes R, et al. Do patient-centered medical homes improve health behaviors, outcomes, and experiences of low-income patients? A systematic review and meta-analysis. Health Serv Res. 2018;53(3):1777–98.
7. Pourat N, Chen X, Lee C, Zhou W, Daniel M, Hoang H, et al. Assessing the impact of patient-centered medical home principles on hypertension outcomes among patients of HRSA-funded health centers. Am J Hypertens. 2018;32(4):418–25.
8. Woodard LD, Adepoju OE, Amspoker AB, Virani SS, Ramsey DJ, Petersen LA, et al. Impact of patient-centered medical home implementation on diabetes control in the veterans health administration. J Gen Intern Med. 2018;33(8):1276–82.

9. Jha A, Iliff A, Chaoui A, Defossez S, Bombaugh M, Miller Y. A crisis in health care: a call to action on physician burnout. Partnership with the Massachusetts Medical Society, Massachusetts Health and Hospital Association, Harvard T.H. Chan School of Public Health, and Harvard Global Health Institute; 2018.
10. Sinsky C, Colligan L, Li L, Prgomet M, Reynolds S, Goeders L, et al. Allocation of physician time in ambulatory practice: a time and motion study in 4 specialties. Ann Intern Med. 2016;165(11):753.
11. Bodenheimer T, Sinsky C. From triple to quadruple aim: care of the patient requires care of the provider. Ann Fam Med. 2014;12(6):573–6.
12. Wagner EH, LeRoy L, Schaefer J, Bailit M, Coleman K, Zhan CL, et al. How do innovative primary care practices achieve the quadruple aim? J Ambul Care Manag. 2018;41(4):288–97.
13. Rathert C, Williams ES, Linhart H. Evidence for the quadruple aim: a systematic review of the literature on physician burnout and patient outcomes. Med Care. 2018;56(12):976–84.
14. Heaton PC, Frede S, Kordahi A, Lowery L, Moorhead B, Kirby J, et al. Improving care transitions through medication therapy management: a community partnership to reduce readmissions in multiple health-systems. J Am Pharm Assoc. 2019;59(3):319–28.
15. Liu VC, Mohammad I, Deol BB, Balarezo A, Deng L, Garwood CL. Post-discharge medication reconciliation: reduction in readmissions in a geriatric primary care clinic. J Aging Health. 2018;31(10):1790–805. https://doi.org/10.1177/0898264318795571.
16. Staessen JA, Li Y, Thijs L, Wang JG. Blood pressure reduction and cardiovascular prevention: an update including the 2003–2004 secondary prevention trials. Hypertens Res. 2005;28(5):385–407.
17. Reboussin DM, Allen NB, Griswold ME, Guallar E, Hong Y, Lackland DT, et al. Systematic review for the 2017 ACC/AHA/AAPA/ABC/ACPM/AGS/APhA/ASH/ASPC/NMA/PCNA guideline for the prevention, detection, evaluation, and management of high blood pressure in adults: a report of the American College of Cardiology/American Heart Association Task Force on Clinical Practice Guidelines. J Am Coll Cardiol. 2018;71(19):2176–98.
18. Chisolm DJ, Brook DL, Applegate MS, Kelleher KJ. Social determinants of health priorities of state Medicaid programs. BMC Health Serv Res. 2019;19:7.
19. Machledt D. Addressing the social determinants of health through medicaid managed care. Issue Brief (Commonw Fund). 2017;2017:1–9.
20. Gottlieb L, Ackerman S, Wing H, Manchanda R. Understanding medicaid managed care investments in members' social determinants of health. Popul Health Manag. 2017;20(4):302–8.
21. 2020 Topics & Objectives: D-5.1 Reduce the proportion of persons with diabetes with an A1c value greater than 9 percent Healthy People 2020: Office of Disease Prevention and Health Promotion; 2017. Available from: https://www.healthypeople.gov/2020/topics-objectives/topic/diabetes/objectives.
22. 2020 Topics & Objectives: S-12 Increase the proportion of adults with hypertension whose blood pressure is under control Healthy People 2020: Office of Disease Prevention and Health Promotion 2017. Available from: https://www.healthypeople.gov/2020/topics-objectives/topic/heart-disease-and-stroke/objectives.
23. Cancer Objectives Health People 2020: Office of Disease Prevention and Health Promotion; 2017. Available from: https://www.healthypeople.gov/2020/topics-objectives/topic/cancer/objectives.
24. Langley G, Nolan K, Nolan T, Norman C, Provost L. The improvement guide: a practical approach to enhancing organizational performance. Danvers: Jossey-Bass Inc. Google Scholar; 1996.
25. Cagliero E, Levina EV, Nathan DM. Immediate feedback of HbA(1c) levels improves glycemic control in type I and insulin-treated type 2 diabetic patients. Diabetes Care. 1999;22(11):1785–9.
26. Miller CD, Barnes CS, Phillips LS, Ziemer DC, Gallina D, Cook CB, et al. Rapid A1c availability improves clinical decision-making in an urban primary care clinic. Diabetes Care. 2003;26(4):1158–63.

27. Laurence CO, Gialamas A, Bubner T, Yelland L, Willson K, Ryan P, et al. Patient satisfaction with point-of-care testing in general practice. Br J Gen Pract. 2010;60(572):e98–e104.
28. Lewandrowski EL, Yeh S, Baron J, Crocker JB, Lewandrowski K. Implementation of point-of-care testing in a general internal medicine practice: a confirmation study. Clin Chim Acta. 2017;473:71–4.
29. Paulozzi LJ, Jones CM, Mack KA, et al. Vital signs: overdoses of prescription opioid pain relievers–United States, 1999–2008. MMWR Morb Mortal Wkly Rep. 2011;60(43):1487.
30. Overdose death rates: National Institute of Drug Abuse; updated 2018. Available from: https://www.drugabuse.gov/related-topics/trends-statistics/overdose-death-rates.
31. Dowell D, Haegerich TM, Choou R. CDC guideline for prescribing opioids for chronic pain—United States, 2016. Morb Mortal Wkly Rep. 2016;65(1):1–49.
32. Chou R, Fanciullo GJ, Fine PG, Adler JA, Ballantyne JC, Davies P, et al. Clinical guidelines for the use of chronic opioid therapy in chronic noncancer pain. J Pain. 2009;10(2):113–30. e22.
33. Webster LR, Webster RM. Predicting aberrant behaviors in opioid-treated patients: preliminary validation of the opioid risk tool. Pain Med. 2005;6(6):432–42.
34. Butler SF, Budman SH, Fernandez KC, Houle B, Benoit C, Katz N, et al. Development and validation of the current opioid misuse measure. Pain. 2007;130(1–2):144–56.

Chapter 14
Quality of Quality Measures

Yazan Daaboul, Saahil Jumkhawala, and Deeb N. Salem

Introduction

Medical errors are a major cause of morbidity and mortality among both hospitalized and ambulatory patients. It has been estimated that preventable medical errors may be attributable to up to 98,000 deaths annually in the United States [1]. Over the past decade, there have been substantial efforts to reduce the rate of medical errors and improve the overall quality of healthcare. Nonetheless, despite improvements in access to healthcare, higher utilization of healthcare services, and rising costs, there has been inconsistent improvements in patient outcomes (Table 14.1). The ongoing mismatch between the amount of services and the quality of healthcare has subsequently turned patient safety into a national priority and mandated the development of programs that aim to identify gaps in quality of care and develop reliable and cost-effective quality metrics that predictably improve patient outcomes.

In 2010, the Affordable Care Act (ACA) developed the pay-for-performance (P4P) program, which was designed to link financial incentives or penalty to provider performance. The objective of the P4P program was to encourage healthcare organizations to simultaneously optimize quality of care and reduce unnecessary costs in multiple settings, including in-patient hospitalizations as well as outpatient ambulatory visits [2]. The Center for Medicare and Medicaid Services (CMS) played a key role in developing various P4P models to address hospital reimbursements, including the Hospital Value-Based Purchasing Program (VBP), the Hospital Readmissions Reduction Program (HRRP), and the Hospital-Acquired Condition

Y. Daaboul · S. Jumkhawala · D. N. Salem (✉)
Department of Medicine, Tufts Medical Center, Tufts University School of Medicine, Boston, MA, USA
e-mail: dsalem@tuftsmedicalcenter.org

© Springer Nature Switzerland AG 2020

D. N. Salem (ed.), *Quality Measures*, https://doi.org/10.1007/978-3-030-37145-6_14

Table 14.1 Report card: blue cross blue shield AQC metrics [108]

Quality metric	Care that matter analysis
Quality indicator[a]: Good	
1. Diabetes and eye exams Adults 18–75 years with diabetes had at least one eye exam within the last 2 years	Evidence supports reduced eye damage in diabetes with screening eye exams
2. Early testing: Cervical cancer Women 21–64 years received a PAP smear in the past 3 years, or ages 30–64 years had PAP and HPV testing in the last 5 years	Conclusive evidence that cervical cancer screening reduces mortality in the population specified, and the benefit outweighs the anxiety and hassle of testing
3. Early testing: Colorectal cancer Adults 51–75 years are tested for early colorectal cancer, with colonoscopy in the last 10 years, sigmoidoscopy in the last 5 years, or stool test in the last year	Early testing by these methods reduces the amount of colon cancer and death from colon cancer
4. Strep throat and testing Children ages 2–18 years receiving antibiotics for strep throat have a strep test within 3 days	Good evidence supports verifying strep throat before antibiotic treatment due to similarity with viral causes that are not affected by antibiotics
Quality indicator: suggested modification	
5. Diabetes and blood pressure Adults 18–75 years with diabetes had blood pressure checked this year, and most recent result is less than 140/90 mmHg	Good evidence supports reducing blood pressure below 140/90 mmHg which reduces heart attacks, strokes, and death in type II diabetes. Such evidence is not available for type I diabetes, and so these patients should not be included
6. Diabetes and kidney disease Adults 18–75 years with diabetes were tested for evidence of early-onset kidney disease in the past year	Patients with early-stage kidney disease do benefit from early detection and treatment. Established type I diabetes guidelines suggest initiating testing 5 years after diagnosis. Testing should not apply to those with life expectancy shorter than the potential gain from preventing kidney damage
7. Early testing: Chlamydia in teens Sexually active women 16–20 years were tested for chlamydia last year	Evidence supports testing for chlamydia in the absence of symptoms. An annual schedule is arbitrarily chosen and may be too frequent
8. Early testing: Chlamydia in adults Sexually active women 21–24 years were tested for chlamydia last year	As above, this is supported with evidence but annually is arbitrary and may be too frequent
9. Antibiotics for bronchitis Adults 18–64 years diagnosed with acute bronchitis are not prescribed antibiotics within 3 days	Patients with chronic lung conditions should be excluded since early treatment of respiratory symptoms may be helpful
10. Antibiotics for upper respiratory tract infection Children diagnosed with upper respiratory tract infections do not receive antibiotics	Good evidence indicates that antibiotics for simple upper respiratory tract infections are more harmful than helpful. However, antibiotics for prolonged moist cough may be beneficial
Quality indicator: poor	
11. Depression: Short term For a 16-week period, adults with depression who have started an antidepressant missed less than 30 days of treatment, determined by whether or not they filled their prescriptions at the drug store	Although there is good evidence that antidepressants work only for severe depression, this metric incorrectly includes mild–moderate depression as well. The time periods chosen are arbitrary and do not reflect studied cutoffs. The metric denies patient choice to stop treatment due to side effects or switch to other effective or potentially preferable therapies

Table 14.1 (continued)

Quality metric	Care that matter analysis
12. Depression: Long term For a 6-month period, all adults with depression who were started on an antidepressant missed less than 51 days	As above, this metric inappropriately includes mild–moderate depression. The time periods are again arbitrary. Patient choice for effective alternative treatments and side effect avoidance is denied
13. Diabetes and testing blood sugar Adults 18–75 years with diabetes had long-term blood sugar (A1C) tested in the last year	No evidence suggests that the simple act of testing long-term blood sugar itself leads to reduced harm from diabetes
14. Diabetes and blood sugar goals Adults 18–75 years with diabetes had long-term blood sugar (A1C) less than 9% when last tested this year	No A1C goal has been established as optimal. The benefits of intensive A1C lowering (slight reductions in heart attack, eye damage, and amputation) are less well established than the harms (dangerously low blood sugar, weight gain, emotional distress, and cost). An A1C goal of 9% has not been studied and is therefore arbitrary
15. Checkups for infants Children less than 15 months receiving regular checkups	Good evidence suggests there is no benefit for a particular number of checkups, with three visits being no worse than six visits in the first year of life
16. Checkups for children Children ages 3–6 years who receive at least one checkup annually	Although widely considered good practice, there is no evidence that annual checkups for children are beneficial
17. Checkups for adolescents Adolescents received at least one checkup with primary care or OB-GYN doctor annually	There is no evidence that annual checkups for adolescents are beneficial
18. Blood pressure goals Adults aged 18–85 have last blood pressure measured at less than 140/90 mmHg in the last year	Treating very high blood pressure is important, but major review committees do not agree on specific goals. They recommend higher goals for ages above 60 years. Good evidence suggests treating pressures only slightly above 140/90 mmHg is not beneficial for patients without cardiovascular risks
19. Early testing: Breast cancer Women 50–74 received at least 1 mammogram within the last year	Although mammograms slightly reduce the chance of dying from breast cancer itself, they do not reduce the overall chance of dying. This may pressure clinicians and women to choose a test that does not suit their preferences

Adapted from the "Report Card: Blue Cross Blue Shield AQC Metrics". v1.0. Available at www.carethatmatters.org

1. Convincing evidence that action changes clinical outcomes
2. Desirable consequences outweigh undesirable consequences (including consideration of consequences of quality measure implementation)
3. Population adequately specified for appropriately targeted quality measure implementation
4. Intervention adequately specified for appropriately performed implementation
   - If all four criteria are met, measure will be designated as "Meets criteria"
   - If criteria one and/or two not met, measure will be designated as "Does not meet criteria"
   - If criteria three and/or four not met, measure will be designated "Meets criteria with suggested modification"

[a]Dynamed criteria for appropriateness for clinical implementation:

(HAC) reduction program. Generally, these P4P models prespecified quality metrics as benchmarking methods to compare structure, process, outcomes, efficiency, as well as quality-related reporting of data, and then they provided reimbursements or penalties based on the compliance of individual healthcare providers with these metrics [3–5]. These new P4P models were a considerable paradigm shift from the preexisting fee-for-service programs, which at the time had similarly focused on providing access to healthcare but at the expense of generating excessive healthcare costs with no improvement in the quality of provided care [6].

Simultaneously, a public reporting strategy has been developed to address healthcare quality. Public reporting provided healthcare providers, patients, and third-party payers with information regarding the performance of these providers and payers, the ability to compare quality of care and costs, and the degree of patient satisfaction [7–9]. Public reporting was thought to offer the advantage of helping patients make informed decisions about their health, including the decision to choose their providers, the location and cost of their care, and insurance plans. Agencies that sponsor public reporting have been made available either at a federal level, such as the Agency for Healthcare Research and Quality (AHRQ) and Centers for Medicare and Medicaid Services, state level, or through private nonprofit or employer-based organizations. While they were initially implemented in the 1980s, public reporting strategies advanced substantially in the pay-for-performance era in an effort to accurately reflect true quality of care [8, 9].

The combination of all these quality metrics that link payment to quality of outcomes was hypothesized to be an appealing strategy to address the limitations of the traditional fee-for-service approach that reimbursed healthcare providers solely based on the volume of services. Despite their importance, these metrics have insofar proven to be flawed and are also yet to demonstrate a clear association with actual hard patient outcomes [1, 10–15]. This lack of association between quality metrics and outcomes has historically been related, at least in part, to the lack of robust evidence in demonstrating improvement in either process-of-care outcomes or patient outcomes (Table 14.2), as well as to underestimating key nuances and losing important data when translating these objective quality metrics into the real-world setting [14, 15].

Deficiency in the Validity of Quality Metrics

Intensive Insulin Therapy Among Critically Ill Patients

Hyperglycemia is common among critically ill diabetic and non-diabetic patients, in part due to physiologic and adaptive stress responses in critical illness, namely, inhibition of insulin by inflammatory cytokines and stress hormones, as well as due to side effects of medications commonly administered in the critical care setting [16, 17]. Aggressive pharmacologic reduction of hyperglycemia has historically

Table 14.2 Complications reported from studies evaluating quality measures in clinical practice [15]

Quality measures/indicator examined	Reported complication
Perioperative beta-blockers [50]	Increased mortality, risk of stroke and hypotension, decreased risk of non-fatal myocardial infarction
Intensive insulin therapy in critically ill patients [26, 109]	Increased hypoglycemic episodes, increased mortality
Preemptive antibiotics for suspected community-acquired pneumonia [110]	No association between early antibiotics and outcomes
Blood pressure control in chronic kidney disease [43]	Increased mortality rates with lower diastolic pressures
Patient satisfaction in surgical care [74, 111, 112]	No association between hospital compliance with surgical quality measures
Prophylactic antibiotics for major surgical procedures [113]	No correlation with surgical site infection rates
Heart failure performance measures [114]	No correlation with rehospitalization or 60–90-day post-discharge mortality
Length of hospital stay [115]	Increased rates of mortality with short length of stay
30-day readmissions [116, 117]	Multiple factors that lead to readmission, < 20% deemed preventable
Venous thromboembolism [36]	Limited utility from surveillance bias
Hospital-acquired pressure ulcers [118]	Difference in administrative vs. surveillance incidence
Patient safety indicators [77, 119–122]	Inability to assess preventable events, low positive predictive value

Adapted from Esposito et al. [15]

received little attention, but real-world observational studies have since demonstrated an association between hyperglycemia and mortality, increased rate of infections postoperatively, and increased length of stay. These findings raised the hypothesis of reducing hyperglycemia among critically ill patients to improve patient outcomes [18, 19]. In 2001, the first randomized trial for intensive insulin therapy was conducted exclusively among surgical critically ill patients ($n = 1,548$). Intensive glycemia control at or below 110 mg/dL significantly reduced mortality and morbidity, as compared with conventional therapy (4.6% vs. 8.0%, $p < 0.04$). Notably, the benefit of intensive insulin therapy in the trial was first observed as early as a few days during the hospitalization period and remained unchanged through 1 year [20]. A trial of similar design in the nonsurgical medical intensive care unit demonstrated a reduction in morbidity, but not mortality, with intensive insulin therapy. Based on these studies, the American Association of Clinical Endocrinologists in 2007 and the American Diabetes Association in 2008 recommended strict glucose control in critically ill patients, but nonetheless made a clear distinction between the mortality benefits observed in surgical patients vs. the absence of mortality benefit in nonsurgical medical patients [21, 22]. Despite the clear discrepancy in the guidelines, quality metrics were enthusiastically adopted in both surgical and nonsurgical patients. Indices of quality measures, including mean blood glucose levels, number of patients with extreme hyperglycemia and hypoglycemia, glucose variability, and time in target glucose range, were subsequently developed to quantify glucose control and to measure hospital compliance to this quality metric [23–25].

Since then, the larger NICE-SUGAR trial, a pragmatic study that enrolled both medical and surgical patients, randomized patients to either intensive glucose control (target glycemia range 81–108 mg/dL) vs. conventional control (target glycemia of 180 mg/dL) ($n = 6,104$) [26]. In contrast to earlier studies, intensive glucose control was associated with increased mortality among critically ill patients (27.5% vs. 24.9%, OR = 1.14, 95% CI (1.02–1.28), $p = 0.02$), with no difference in treatment effect in the subgroups of surgical and medical patients when analyzed individually. NICE-SUGAR highlighted the risk of tight glycemic control and suggested a potential deleterious and harmful effect of insulin among critically ill patients. Accordingly, the enthusiasm surrounding intensive glucose monitoring and control that had been generated prior to NICE-SUGAR lapsed, and the determination of the effect of glucose control and outcomes among non-surgical critically ill patients remains an unmet need.

Rate of Postoperative Venous Thromboembolism

Venous thromboembolism (VTE) is a common, preventable complication and a major cause of morbidity and mortality in the postoperative setting. The cumulative incidence of postoperative VTE is estimated to be approximately 5% to 10% in the short-term postoperative period [27, 28]. In clinical trials, VTE prophylaxis postoperatively has been demonstrated to be a cost-effective measure associated with significant reduction in VTE events and improved outcomes [29–33]. In 2001, the AHRQ's "Making Healthcare Safer" report recommended the use of mechanical and pharmacologic VTE prophylaxis. Based on the compelling evidence from both clinical trials and observational data, VTE prophylaxis was considered in the top 10 list of strongly encouraged patient safety practices [34]. To ensure compliance, the agency also developed its Patient Safety Indicator 12, a risk-adjusted postoperative VTE rate measure. This safety indicator was then endorsed by the National Quality Forum in 2008 and has since been included in quality improvement and pay-for-performance programs, as well as public reporting data, namely, the Medicare and Medicaid Services 2015 Value-Based Purchasing Program (Centers for Medicare and Medicaid Services Hospital Value-Based Purchasing).

As VTE prophylaxis gained attention and was used as a hospital quality metric, studies demonstrated a surprisingly positive correlation between higher VTE prophylaxis adherence rates and higher VTE event rates, which was contradictory to the data from the existing literature [35, 36]. Upon further investigation, however, this observation was eventually determined to be confounded by surveillance bias due to increased hospital staff vigilance and availability of imaging modalities to detect VTE events within hospitals of higher structural quality, as compared with hospitals of lower structural quality. Despite the evidence in support of VTE prophylaxis, the measurement method of VTE events as a quality metric in the Patient Safety Indicator 12 was inherently flawed due to confounding of surveillance and detection bias and paradoxically masked true quality of care [35, 36].

Intensive Blood Pressure Control Among Patients with Chronic Kidney Disease

Chronic kidney disease (CKD) is associated with an increased risk of cardiovascular morbidity and death [37–39]. Elevated blood pressure in patients with CKD is considered the most important reversible risk factor for disease progression to renal failure and end-stage renal disease [40]. In a meta-analysis of 18 randomized controlled trials for patients with CKD ($n = 15,924$), intensive systolic blood pressure reduction has been associated with a significant 14% reduction in the likelihood of all-cause death, as compared with less-intensive systolic blood pressure reduction.

Based on these findings, the 2004 National Kidney Foundation Kidney Disease Outcome Quality Initiative (NKF K/DOQI) recommended a blood pressure goal of less than 130/80 mmHg for all individuals with CKD [41]. Then in the 2012 Kidney Disease: Improving Global Outcomes report, the guidelines recommended a similar blood pressure goal of 130/80 mmHg in CKD patients with albuminuria and 140/90 mmHg in CKD patients without albuminuria [42]. Notably, these targets emphasized an intensive reduction of blood pressure to achieve a systolic goal but paid little attention to the potential detrimental effects of lowering the diastolic blood pressure with this intensive blood pressure reduction approach.

In 2013, an observational study among 651,749 US veterans with CKD demonstrated that the highest mortality risk was among patients in both extremes of blood pressures, and blood pressure mortality in fact followed a U-shaped curve. While systolic blood pressure was an important determinant of risk in CKD, diastolic blood pressure was of similar importance. A diastolic blood pressure of less than 70 mmHg was associated with a significantly increased risk of mortality, and the outcome benefits observed with achieving an intensive reduction in systolic blood pressure were offset by very low levels of diastolic blood pressure [43], and intensive blood pressure was therefore proven to be of no net clinic benefit. Interestingly, as quality measures incorporating indicators for CKD and blood pressure control were being processed in the USA, the emergence of this data precluded their final release, and to date there remains no updated quality indicators for the management of CKD.

Use of Perioperative Beta-Blockers in Noncardiac Surgery

Worldwide, approximately 100 million adults undergo noncardiac surgery each year, of whom 10 to 40 million sustain a major adverse cardiac event. Early studies hypothesized that catecholamine surge during the perioperative period may result in hemodynamic alterations and lead to an increased rate of myocardial ischemia. Accordingly, it has been suggested that the use of beta-blockers in the perioperative period may reduce myocardial contractility and may, in turn, reduce myocardial oxygen demand and the risk of myocardial ischemia. Early on, modest-sized randomized trials confirmed this hypothesis and demonstrated a reduction in the risk of myocardial infarction with beta-blockers when evaluated through 2 years among patients who undergo noncardiac surgery [44, 45].

These promising findings led to the development of the landmark DECREASE I trial (Dutch Echocardiographic Cardiac Risk Evaluation Applying Stress Echo). In DECREASE I, patients were enriched for high-risk features, i.e., the presence of both clinical risk factors and positive stress test on dobutamine echocardiography, and were then randomized – in a non-blinded fashion – to receive either bisoprolol or placebo perioperatively at least 7 days before noncardiac surgery ($n = 112$). Bisoprolol was associated with a tenfold reduction in the primary endpoint of the composite of cardiovascular (CV) death or non-fatal myocardial infarction (MI) through 30 days (3.4% vs. 34.0%, $p < 0.001$), as well as the incidence of individual outcomes, i.e., CV death alone (3.4% vs. 17.0%, $p = 0.02$) and non-fatal MI alone (0% vs. 17.0%, $p < 0.001$). Interestingly, DECREASE I was in fact terminated prematurely following the first interim analysis due to the overwhelming efficacy observed in the bisoprolol group.

Given the overwhelming benefit, the results from the DECREASE I trial led to the class I recommendation in the 2002 American Heart Association (AHA)/American College of Cardiology (ACC) joint guidelines for the use of perioperative beta-blockers among high-risk patients with known ischemia and undergoing vascular surgery [46]. Following this recommendation, the National Quality Forum also recommended the use of perioperative beta-blockers and further included this recommendation in the list of "30 safe practices for better healthcare." Also, the AHRQ endorsed the use of perioperative beta-blocker as an important quality metric and identified it as one of the "clear opportunities for safety improvement" in healthcare [47, 48]. Subsequently, the results of five additional trials (DECREASE II–VI trials) demonstrated findings consistent with that of DECREASE I when various patient populations were evaluated, and the recommendation for the use of perioperative beta-blockers was further incorporated into the 2009 US and European guidelines [49].

In 2011, however, the validity of the methodology of the DECREASE family of trials was brought into questioning. Following a series of extensive investigations, the results were largely discredited due to misconduct and fabrication of results, as well as absence of source data, absence of consent forms, fictitious events that did not match the source documentation, and falsified methods and outcome data. As it was determined that the DECREASE results were actually falsified, the hypothesis of perioperative beta-blockers and the reduction in mortality had to be readdressed. Accordingly, the large, multicenter POISE randomized trial re-evaluated the efficacy and safety of perioperative use of beta-blockers. Patients were randomly assigned to receive either metoprolol or placebo on the day of surgery ($n = 8,351$). Although metoprolol reduced the risk of perioperative MI (5.8% vs. 6.9%), this reduction was offset by a significant increase in all-cause mortality (3.1% vs. 2.3%) and stroke (1.0% vs. 0.5%) through 30 day [50]. A subsequent meta-analysis of nine randomized trials for perioperative beta-blockers in noncardiac surgery ($n = 10{,}529$), excluding the DECREASE trials, eventually demonstrated no efficacy with beta-blockers in the perioperative setting [51], and society guidelines eventually deemed there was lack of sufficient data to strongly recommend the use of perioperative beta-blockers in noncardiac surgery.

Of importance, however, the changing guidelines, along with the misconduct of the DECREASE trial investigators, highlighted the risk of using nationwide metrics for quality assessment prematurely. In fact, this overt promotion favoring the use of beta-blockers perioperatively may have driven an excessive unnecessary use of beta-blockers among patients undergoing noncardiac surgery and increased the risk of mortality in this patient population. Numerically, this risk is substantial, where based on the results of the POISE trial, for every 1000 patients who undergo non-cardiac surgery, the use of perioperative beta-blocker has been associated with an excess of 13 deaths and 6 stroke events [50].

Flawed Technologies that Quantify Outcomes

Flawed Methodology and Statistical Designs

Despite the increasing implementation of the pay-for-performance (P4P) program in quantifying quality of care, its efficacy and success have been limited due to flaws related to the program's methodology and statistical design. Overall, it has been difficult to determine sound methods that accurately and cost-effectively measure quality of care. While the failure of the P4P program has been attributed, at least in part, to the lack of robust evidence, and conversely the abundance of unreliable data, this failure has also been a consequence of inherent principle flaws in the program design itself [52–55]. First, these programs have historically been criticized for either oversimplifying measures or extremely complicating them. Further, the P4P models have been thought to overcompartmentalize important patient factors and are subsequently impractical in quantifying clinically relevant patient risk and comorbidities. For instance, a P4P program that focuses on hypertension may only assess clinicians on antihypertensive management and will neglect other aspects of patient preventative care, such as diabetes, obesity, and smoking. This often results in the unintended consequence of prioritization of care to meet the predefined success criterion for the P4P program at the expense of other similar and equally substantial elements in patient care [52–55]. Alternatively, an extensive P4P program is also problematic because it may be confusing and unrealistic. Clinicians may be demotivated early and are more likely to abandon the program altogether or approach the program with an emphasis to address the measured metrics rather than overall quality [56].

Second, the P4P program has historically failed to accurately adjust for patient risk. While patient outcomes are directly associated with the overall profile of comorbidity and risk, this is often not reflected in P4P programs [14, 53, 57]. When risk is not accounted for, P4P programs may unjustly penalize hospitals that provide excellent quality of care and, conversely, reward those that do not. While Medicare adjusts for age and level of education, it has no protocols to adjust for comorbidities or diagnoses. Accordingly, hospitals that accept higher proportion of patients with dual Medicare and Medicaid eligibility are often penalized for poor patient outcomes that are often related to unpreventable patient factors rather than the quality of provided care. For instance, in 2015, the Rush University Medical Center – a tertiary care center in Chicago – received the lowest patient safety score in the US News and World Report Best Hospital Rankings, but paradoxically had high scores for patient safety measures based on both the Leapfrog Group measures and the University Healthcare Consortium [58]. This discordance in safety reports led to investigations, which eventually determined that the US News and World Report Best Hospital Rankings had falsely included patients who were transferred from peripheral sites to the medical center and who were often medically complex with significant comorbidities and at high risk of death during the hospitalization. The inclusion of these transferred patients, or even the lack of risk adjustment, was a fundamental statistical flaw in the calculation of complication rates and had no actual correlation with the quality of care provided at the medical center.

Finally, it has previously been demonstrated that despite their use and their powerful influence on physician reimbursement rates, the methodologies in these programs are not necessarily verified and may actually be inaccurate. For instance, the Medicare Physician Fee Schedule program that determines physician payments has been shown to be significantly inaccurate when comparing data related to time estimates for common surgical procedures from the database of the Relative Value Scale Update Committee (RUC) of the American Medical Association vs. database from the Surgeons National Surgical Quality Improvement Program (NSQIP) [59]. In fact, the discrepancy between the two databases resulted in a substantial impact on the variation of surgeons' incomes over the course of several years. The differences between the databases were not systematic (i.e., both negative and positive differences were present) and ranged substantially from 30 to 160 million dollars. This led to excessive reimbursement rates for specific surgical specialties, such as orthopedics and urology, and significantly lower payments to other specialties, such as cardiothoracic, vascular, and neurosurgery [59]. Interestingly, when these variations in methodologies were re-evaluated, approximately half of these inaccuracies were actually reduced, suggesting that these methodological flaws are reversible in nature and may be improved if monitoring and optimization of these data sources are prioritized [59].

The Metric of Patient Satisfaction

Public reporting is a quality metric strategy that utilizes patient satisfaction to infer quality of care [60]. To achieve this, regulatory agencies, such as the Joint Commission on Accreditation of Healthcare Organizations and the National

Committee on Quality Assurance, required that healthcare providers include patient satisfaction in their development process of their quality indicators and also demanded that health plans publicly report patient satisfaction data [61]. To date, available satisfaction assessment tools encompass all aspects of patient encounters, including evaluation of pain management, patient education, parental needs in pediatric care, discharge teaching, provision of information, as well as nonclinical measures, such as parking and food services [62–65].

Despite their honorable purpose, patient satisfaction surveys provide a subjective perspective and may not necessarily reflect accurate delivery or quality of care. First, patient satisfaction assessment tools, which are typically in survey form, are often methodologically flawed and have historically suffered suboptimal degrees of reliability and validity [66–70]. More importantly, correlating reimbursement, quality of care, and patient satisfaction may pressure providers to comply with patient needs, even when these needs are medically futile, potentially harmful, or unnecessary [71–73]. In a prospective, nationwide survey for patient satisfaction, healthcare utilization, and outcomes ($n = 36,428$), patients in the highest satisfaction quartile had paradoxically higher likelihood of inpatient admissions (adjusted odds ratio [OR] 1.12, 95% CI 1.02–1.23), an increase in total expenditures (adjusted OR 8.8, 95% CI 1.6–16.6), and a 26% increased odds of all-cause death (adjusted OR = 1.26, 95% CI (1.05–1.53), as compared with patients in the lowest satisfaction quartile [74].

While an assessment of the overall patient experience and satisfaction may be important, the overemphasis on the association between satisfaction and patient outcomes and the degree of reimbursement that depends on this satisfaction may be problematic and potentially counterproductive. Accordingly, patient satisfaction data should perhaps be utilized more judiciously in the appropriate context and cautiously interpreted to prevent the pitfall of unintended consequences, namely, patient rehospitalization and death.

Patient Safety Indicators

The AHRQ developed patient safety indicators (PSIs) as screening tools to monitor for the development of preventable complications and adverse events, as well as to target opportunities for improvement. PSIs use prespecified flags based on hospital billing data, length of stay, and other discharge data to extrapolate information regarding patient safety at an epidemiological level [75, 76]. PSIs have been thought to be particularly appealing because they are often readily available at the time of patient discharge and are easily measurable.

Despite their use, however, PSIs have not been well-validated, and the evidence for their association with patient outcomes and other quality metrics remains controversial and inconsistent [77, 78]. First, the methodological technique to obtain PSIs, which is usually based on billing data and International Classification of Diseases (ICD) codes, has been debatable. In a meta-analysis evaluating the predictive value of ICD codes against the standard of clinician review to detect 5 PSIs, including development of iatrogenic pneumothorax, central line-associated bloodstream infection, postoperative hemorrhage or hematoma, postoperative deep venous thromboembolic event, or accidental puncture or laceration, the validity of ICD codes was significantly lacking or was moderate at best. The mean predictive value of using ICD codes ranged from as low as 49.0% to up to 80.9% [79].

Also, frequently used PSIs, such as the development of decubitus ulcer or infection due to medical care, were not only not associated with other measures of healthcare quality, but the relationship was paradoxically inverse when evaluated among Medicare enrollees across 4,504 acute-care hospitals [77]. Also, it has previously been demonstrated that there is no association between the accreditation scores granted by the Joint Commission on Accreditation of Healthcare Organizations (JCAHO) and the performance status as evaluated by the AHRQ based on the PSI assessment [80]. Despite the lack of scientific evidence to support their use, PSIs unfortunately remain to be increasingly used by public reporting organizations and payers as a metric for quality of care, and for this reason, its utility should perhaps be re-evaluated in the light of the available evidence [77].

Unanticipated Outcomes of Quality Measures

Readmission Rates and Mortality Outcomes

Over the past decade, the US Centers for Medicare and Medicaid Services (CMS) has aimed to incentivize hospitals to reduce their 30-day readmission rates among Medicare patients. This initiative has been largely based on CMS's assumption that high readmission rates are modifiable factors that may potentially be reduced with improved adherence to its quality metrics. Subsequently, in 2010, the Patient Protection and Affordable Care Act developed the Hospital Readmissions Reduction Program (HRRP) to publicly report hospitals' 30-day readmission rates and to penalize those with a higher than expected rate of readmissions. Since the program's implementation, however, concerns have been raised with regard to the lack of reliability and validity of the proposed quality metrics, the use of substandard statistical modeling with suboptimal discrimination capacity, as well as the unfairness of the program's penalty system [81–85]. Despite risk adjustments, the program could not account for differences in patient disease severity across various hospital types, i.e., community hospitals vs. academic hospitals vs. safety-net hospitals [86–88]. As patient acuity in academic and safety-net hospitals is usually higher than in community hospitals, the rate of 30-day readmissions was naturally more frequent in these hospitals, as compared with the rate in community hospitals. This has resulted in unjustly penalizing these hospitals by the HRRP and reducing reimbursements to hospitals that actually require the most amount of resources to care for the high acuity patients they host.

Although the HRRP has been effective in reducing the rate of 30-day readmissions, there has been no reduction in overall mortality following the implementation of the program. When longitudinal data before and after the implementation of the HRRP for heart failure were evaluated, there was an inverse association between the change in the 30-day rate of readmission over time and the respective mortality rate. Specifically, despite a reduction of 2.1% in the rate of readmission from 2008 to 2014, there was a paradoxical increase by 1.3% in the rate of mortality [89]. Ironically, this program has inadvertently favored out-of-hospital deaths that occurred shortly after discharge, as the HRRP penalty system has accounted only for readmissions but not account for deaths outside the hospital. It remains unclear as to why the heart failure mortality rate increased following the implementation of the HRRP program, but it is plausible to hypothesize that with the incentive to reduce readmission rates, there is the unintended consequence of forcing clinicians and hospitals to inappropriately delay heart failure hospitalizations beyond 30 days to comply with the HRRP's quality metrics but at the expense of potential harm, access to care, and patient safety [89, 90].

In a large analysis using Medicare data of pre- and post-implementation of HRRP for readmissions for heart failure ($n = 4$ million hospitalizations), acute myocardial infarction ($n = 1.7$ million hospitalizations), and pneumonia ($n = 3.5$ million hospitalizations), there was overall no significant change in the in-hospital or 30-day post-discharge mortality following the HRRP implementation for any of the diagnoses despite a significant reduction in the rate of readmissions [91]. Also in 2014, chronic obstructive pulmonary disease (COPD) was also affected by HRRP, and hospitals have since been penalized for high COPD readmission rates [92, 93]. Despite the implementation of this measure, there remains limited data to support that adherence to quality metrics truly reduces COPD readmissions. More importantly, readmission for COPD did not correlate with mortality and was demonstrated to be a measure that is significantly confounded by readmissions for other diseases (e.g., pneumonia, acute myocardial infarction, stroke, and heart failure) as opposed to being an isolated factor for readmission. Similar concerns regarding stroke readmission rates have also been raised, namely, the absence of association between stroke quality metrics with mortality outcomes and the poor discrimination capacity of these metrics, knowing that they do not adjust for stroke severity or hospital case mix index [94].

Traditional and Novel Approaches for Quality Measurement

With ongoing developments in healthcare delivery, approaches to measuring quality have continued to be reimagined for appropriateness and relevance. As such, exploration of novel methods has been imperative to ensure high standards of care in an ever-changing healthcare landscape. A fundamental question at the base of this debate has been related to the degree to which these quality metrics should be evaluated, namely, whether an expanded measurement approach vs. a scaling back approach is more appropriate [95, 96].

Expanded Measurement Approach

A first approach to measuring quality is that of expanded measurement, in which a growing number of measures are used to finely gauge quality. Such a method has been employed by the Medicare's merit-based incentive payment system (MIPS), a payment track created under the Medicare Access and CHIP Reauthorization Act of 2015 (MACRA) [95]. In this system, healthcare providers are evaluated based on performance in the categories of quality, cost, promoting interoperability, and improvement activities. Each of these four categories is further divided into subcategories that are aggregately a score. Performance in these categories is weighted and subsequently scored in order to determine payment adjustments on a sliding scale.

The nature of the expanded measurement approach allows for comprehensive evaluation of physician performance on myriad-specific standardized metrics. These metrics can be further expanded to encompass more granulated levels of information, providing flexibility in the long-term application of such approaches. Well-delineated quality metrics also allow for providers to have more clarity regarding the benchmarks and standards to which they are held.

However, this approach comes with its fair share of limitations, in the forms of expense, limited evidence, and physician dissatisfaction. Physician practices nationwide have been estimated to spend upward of $15 billion annually in the collecting and reporting of their healthcare metrics [95]. Further, within the long list of measurements exist some with limited evidence supporting improved health outcomes through their use [95, 97, 98]. Clinician dissatisfaction has been another concern with such a far-reaching set of metrics, as requiring clinicians to work within a large set of parameters has the possibility of being overly prescriptive in practice. This burden, in combination with the additional hours and labor associated with reporting numerous outcomes, is likely to contribute to increasing rates in physician burnout and dissatisfaction.

Scaling Back Approach

Conversely, quality may be measured by a more judiciously chosen subset of metrics, an example being those intended by the Centers for Medicare and Medicaid Services (CMS) Meaningful Measures initiative [95]. Through this method, quality of care is measured through a less prescriptive framework that seeks to highlight only the areas of utmost priority for quality measurement. By reducing the number of metrics by which clinician performance is measured, the scaling back approach theoretically allows for more autonomy in practice. Similarly, the costs associated with reporting a large set of metrics is reduced, thereby allowing for reallocation of funds and time to other patient-care objectives. This "less is better" approach seeks to reduce the burden on clinicians and allow providers to adapt to the environment of their practices, in which specific quality measurement standards may not always be appropriate.

Importantly, the global decrease in the measurement of quality is not necessarily singly beneficial. Implementing overarching goals, rather than specific metrics, prevents the overseeing organization from standardizing aspects of quality measurement. While core measurements do often provide more flexibility for patient care organizations in terms of management and practice, data available to the regulatory organization or insurer is limited and may preclude any meaningful chance for development or improvement.

Novel Targeted Supplemental Data Collection Approach

Neither the expanded measurement nor the scaling back approach is without its own sets of particular drawbacks [96]. Given that the goal remains to improve quality while recognizing specific areas of weakness in care, the challenge lies in choosing sets of quality measures that adequately gauge for quality while still allowing for variation in delivery within different circumstances of care. One proposed method of quality measurement that could fulfill these needs is that of targeted supplemental data collection [95]. This method seeks to exclude low-performing providers and focus alternative payment models on the remaining population. In this way, extra supplemental information would only be collected from providers whose preliminary measures fall below certain predetermined standards.

The potential benefit of a targeted supplemental data approach would be in decreasing the costs associated with data collection, while still retaining the collection of data necessary for quality assessment. By recognizing performers who systematically perform toward the lower end of the quality spectrum on certain measures, this approach could theoretically serve to improve quality delivery without the potential wasted burden associated with the generalized application of single measures. Further, resources could be more effectively utilized to determine whether low performers remain so in subsequent testing, providing additionally specific measurement of quality performance when implemented properly.

This approach identifies an "initial pass" set of core measures for which the value of collecting is warranted in almost all cases, due in combination to the importance of the metrics and to the relatively low labor of their collection [95]. Some examples include patient death, patient access to care, and patient experience. Using these metrics is also particularly worthwhile because of the relative difficulty of rigging their measurements. Scores on these measures can be looked upon as indicative of whether additional data collection would be appropriate to more accurately measure performance to identify low performers. Recognizably, even this novel approach would not necessarily be fitting for all situations. The challenge of many discordant metric systems is still existent and requires additional research to provide effective solutions geared toward striking the right balance.

Improving the Quality of Quality Measures

With the goal of evaluating quality and performance, selecting metrics with evidence of association with improved health is of foremost importance. Many currently used metrics are chosen with regard to convenience, ease of collection, or associations based on flawed observational studies, rather than due to their proven cause-effect relationship with improved health outcomes as a modifiable and preventable risk [99, 100]. Notably also, accountability measures are geared such that the primary endpoints of assessment are health outcomes, such as readmissions, nosocomial infections, and death [95]. However, payment programs that incorporate such metrics are less primed to evaluate for the underlying processes that result in the outcomes, thereby overlooking the frameworks and circumstances within which these outcomes occur. Therefore, there should be novel guidelines to create efficient, cost-effective, and reliable strategies to select for high yield quality metrics pertaining to important health outcomes.

Utilizing Metrics with Reliable Evidence of Efficacy and Safety and Improving Quality Measures Research to the Level of Clinical Research

In 2018, the editors of the Journal of the American Medical Association (JAMA) recognized the substandard evidence behind quality measures and issued a letter calling for quality improvement for quality improvement studies, namely, improvement in statistical and design methodology. Overall, this included emphasis on generalizability, use of hard outcomes rather than processes as endpoints, and simultaneous examination of benefits as well as adverse outcomes of measures [101].

Similar to clinical research for efficacy and safety for drugs or devices, quality metrics as an endpoint should be considered at the same level of accountability and should also demonstrate utility in modifying outcomes effectively and safely [101]. To date, the majority of quality metrics are unfortunately chosen based on flawed observational data that demonstrate a potentially confounded association between risk exposure and outcomes, and inferences are then made to assume causality. Over time, these inferences have become at the core of daily healthcare practice with no evidence of their true efficacy. To prove efficacy, however, methods of quality improvement must have evidence of benefit with regard to health outcomes and relative cost-effectiveness and be determined a priori as prespecified endpoints in adequately powered clinical trials, when feasible, to substantiate their true non-confounded effect, as well as their practicality and safety in implementation [97].

Responsiveness to Patient Preference

In addition to being evidence based, favorable quality metrics should relate to patient-centered outcomes, rather than disease-oriented outcomes or intermediate endpoints. In addition to patient satisfaction, quality care should be aligned with outcomes prioritized by the patients being served. The US National Institutes of Health PROMIS program and International Consortium for Health Outcomes Measurement (ICHOM) serve as two authorities that compile lists of such outcomes, such as effective addiction care and reduction of food insecurity [97]. Given that patient satisfaction scores still remain a large factor in the majority of algorithms on which healthcare providers are ranked or reimbursed, this serves as additional incentive for organizations to prioritize those outcomes that are most valued by patients.

Balanced Trade-Off Between Outcomes and Relative Costs

Given the limitations of the fee-for-service landscape in healthcare, cost-consciousness is another important consideration. Although quality benchmarks can serve as a new approach to improve the health of populations on a large scale, it does not necessarily incentivize providers to contemplate appropriateness and judicious use of diagnostic tests and interventions [102]. Quality measurements should therefore serve as a vehicle to incorporate such themes, incentivizing the provision of value care in all aspects. To the same end, focus on metrics that result in greater value in terms of health improvement within available resource constraints should be prioritized [103]. Similarly, quality interventions should be evaluated on the effects that they can have on downstream foregone interventions and procedures, resulting in perpetuated savings of cost and disease in the future. Recognizing and addressing social determinants of health is a crucial practice in this regard.

Generalizability of Measures Across Specialties

Although there are not always quality measures that are appropriate in all environments, efforts should be made to select and implement quality metrics that are sufficiently generalizable to result in the benefit for the majority of clinical settings. Having streamlined quality objectives that can universally be demonstrated to improve care can help align incentives along multiple providers in the healthcare system in a purpose similar to that of cost-effectiveness [104]. While professional societies and specialty groups continue to highlight individualized metrics fitting for their selected missions, quality metrics can serve as valuable tools to incentivize multidisciplinary collaboration and discussion even among previously discordant clinical entities [105]. Non-specialized medical entities such as the US Preventative Services Task Force (USPSTF) and American Medical Association (AMA) may potentially play integral roles in the formal establishment of such objectives.

Reduced Reliance on Claims Data

At present, claims data remain an essential tool by which organizations like the CMS are able to assess performance on quality benchmarks. For the field of quality improvement to continue evolving more toward improving health outcomes, reliance on such data must be reduced [106, 107]. One reason for this is the lack of transparency inherent in the use of such data, often resulting in frustration among providers about the methods used for their evaluation [106, 107]. Similarly, errors in coding and temporal lags in reporting of such data also contribute to the distrust in their use. While these data will remain useful in quality measurement given their relative prevalence and ease of access, efforts to explore additional data as reference can serve as opportunities for more targeted and transparent performance measurement.

Conclusions

In conclusion, the development of a pay-for-performance model based on quality metrics to determine reimbursements and ranking of providers is perhaps an appealing alternative to the traditional fee for services, but still struggles with substantial flaws and is yet to demonstrate a clear association with actual patient outcomes. Despite the importance of these metrics and their increasing implementation in quantifying quality of care, optimizing their efficacy and success remains an unmet need due to flaws related to their validity, inconsistent methodology, and lack of robust and reliable data to support their utility. This excessive noise surrounding quality metrics has dramatically affected their use over time, raising arguments questioning the quality of these quality metrics. As such, the longevity of a quality metrics system as a strategy in healthcare cannot sustain without having strong and robust evidence to back them up, and guidelines should be developed to create effective, safe, cost-conscious, and reliable strategies that select for high-yield quality metrics pertaining solely to important, measurable, and modifiable health outcomes.

References

1. James JT. A new, evidence-based estimate of patient harms associated with hospital care. J Patient Saf. 2013;9(3):122–8.
2. Epstein AM, Lee TH, Hamel MB. Paying physicians for high-quality care. N Engl J Med. 2004;350(4):406–10.
3. Goodman DC. Benchmarking the US physician workforce. An alternative to needs-based or demand-based planning. JAMA. 1996;276(22):1811–7.
4. Rosenthal GE, Harper DL. Cleveland health quality choice: a model for collaborative community-based outcomes assessment. Jt Comm J Qual Improv. 1994;20(8):425–42.
5. Rosenberg AL, Hofer TP, Strachan C, Watts CM, Hayward RA. Accepting critically ill transfer patients: adverse effect on a referral center's outcome and benchmark measures. Ann Intern Med. 2003;138(11):882–90.
6. Wolfe A. Institute of medicine report: crossing the quality chasm: a new health care system for the 21st century. Policy Polit Nurs Pract. 2001;2(3):233–5.
7. Lindenauer PK, Remus D, Roman S, Rothberg MB, Benjamin EM, Ma A, et al. Public reporting and pay for performance in hospital quality improvement. N Engl J Med. 2007;356(5):486–96.
8. Hibbard JH, Stockard J, Tusler M. Hospital performance reports: impact on quality, market share, and reputation. Health Aff (Millwood). 2005;24(4):1150–60.
9. Marshall MN, Shekelle PG, Leatherman S, Brook RH. The public release of performance data: what do we expect to gain? A review of the evidence. JAMA. 2000;283(14):1866–74.
10. Scott A, Peter S, Ait Ouakrim D, Willenberg L, Naccerella L, Furler J, et al. The effect of financial incentives on the quality of health care provided by primary care physicians. Cochrane Database Syst Rev (John Wiley & Sons, Ltd). 2010;9:CD008451.
11. Eijkenaar F, Emmert M, Scheppach M, Schöffski O. Effects of pay for performance in health care: a systematic review of systematic reviews. Health Policy. 2013;110(2–3):115–30.
12. Houle SKD, McAlister FA, Jackevicius CA, Chuck AW, Tsuyuki RT. Does performance-based remuneration for individual health care practitioners affect patient care? Ann Intern Med. 2012;157(12):889.
13. Gillam SJ, Siriwardena AN, Steel N. Pay-for-performance in the United Kingdom: impact of the quality and outcomes framework–a systematic review. Ann Family Med. 2012;10(5):461–8.
14. Mendelson A, Kondo K, Damberg C, Low A, Motúapuaka M, Freeman M, et al. The effects of pay-for-performance programs on health, health care use, and processes of care. Ann Intern Med. 2017;166(5):341.
15. Esposito ML, Selker HP, Salem DN. Quantity over quality: how the rise in quality measures is not producing quality results. J Gen Intern Med. 2015;30(8):1204–7.
16. Kavanagh BP, McCowen KC. Clinical practice. Glycemic control in the ICU. N Engl J Med. 2010;363(26):2540–6.
17. Lena D, Kalfon P, Preiser JC, Ichai C. Glycemic control in the intensive care unit and during the postoperative period. Anesthesiology. 2011;114(2):438–44.
18. Falciglia M, Freyberg RW, Almenoff PL, D'Alessio DA, Render ML. Hyperglycemia-related mortality in critically ill patients varies with admission diagnosis. Crit Care Med. 2009;37(12):3001–9.
19. Krinsley JS. Association between hyperglycemia and increased hospital mortality in a heterogeneous population of critically ill patients. Mayo Clin Proc. 2003;78(12):1471–8.
20. van den Berghe G, Wouters P, Weekers F, Verwaest C, Bruyninckx F, Schetz M, et al. Intensive insulin therapy in critically ill patients. N Engl J Med. 2001;345(19):1359–67.
21. American Diabetes A. Standards of medical care in diabetes–2008. Diabetes Care. 2008;31(Suppl 1):S12–54.

22. Rodbard HW, Blonde L, Braithwaite SS, Brett EM, Cobin RH, Handelsman Y, et al. American Association of Clinical Endocrinologists medical guidelines for clinical practice for the management of diabetes mellitus. Endocr Pract. 2007;13(Suppl 1):1–68.
23. Preiser JC, Chase JG, Hovorka R, Joseph JI, Krinsley JS, De Block C, et al. Glucose control in the ICU: a continuing story. J Diabetes Sci Technol. 2016;10(6):1372–81.
24. Rafael Machado T, Jean-Charles P. Reporting on glucose control metrics in the intensive care unit. Eur Endocrinol. 2015;11(2):75–8.
25. Fahy BG, Sheehy AM, Coursin DB. Perioperative glucose control: what is enough? Anesthesiology. 2009;110(2):204–6.
26. Investigators N-SS, Finfer S, Chittock DR, Su SY, Blair D, Foster D, et al. Intensive versus conventional glucose control in critically ill patients. N Engl J Med. 2009;360(13):1283–97.
27. Grosse SD, Nelson RE, Nyarko KA, Richardson LC, Raskob GE. The economic burden of incident venous thromboembolism in the United States: a review of estimated attributable healthcare costs. Thromb Res. 2016;137:3–10.
28. Sakon M, Maehara Y, Kobayashi T, Kobayashi H, Shimazui T, Seo N, et al. Economic burden of venous thromboembolism in patients undergoing major abdominal surgery. Value Health Reg Issues. 2015;6:73–9.
29. Guyatt GH, Akl EA, Crowther M, Gutterman DD, Schuunemann HJ, American College of Chest Physicians Antithrombotic T, et al. Executive summary: antithrombotic therapy and prevention of thrombosis, 9th ed: American College of Chest Physicians Evidence-Based Clinical Practice Guidelines. Chest. 2012;141(2 Suppl):7S–47S.
30. Stevens SM, Douketis JD. Deep vein thrombosis prophylaxis in hospitalized medical patients: current recommendations, general rates of implementation, and initiatives for improvement. Clin Chest Med. 2010;31(4):675–89.
31. Agnelli G. Prevention of venous thromboembolism in surgical patients. Circulation. 2004;110(24 Suppl 1):IV4–12.
32. Geerts WH, Bergqvist D, Pineo GF, Heit JA, Samama CM, Lassen MR, et al. Prevention of venous thromboembolism: American College of Chest Physicians Evidence-Based Clinical Practice Guidelines (8th Edition). Chest. 2008;133(6 Suppl):381S–453S.
33. O'Donnell M, Weitz JI. Thromboprophylaxis in surgical patients. Can J Surg. 2003;46(2):129–35.
34. Shekelle PG, Pronovost PJ, Wachter RM, McDonald KM, Schoelles K, Dy SM, et al. The top patient safety strategies that can be encouraged for adoption now. Ann Intern Med. 2013;158(5 Pt 2):365–8.
35. Chung JW, Ju MH, Kinnier CV, Sohn MW, Bilimoria KY. Postoperative venous thromboembolism outcomes measure: analytic exploration of potential misclassification of hospital quality due to surveillance bias. Ann Surg. 2015;261(3):443–4.
36. Bilimoria KY, Chung J, Ju MH, Haut ER, Bentrem DJ, Ko CY, et al. Evaluation of surveillance bias and the validity of the venous thromboembolism quality measure. JAMA. 2013;310(14):1482–9.
37. Glynn LG, Buckley B, Reddan D, Newell J, Hinde J, Dinneen SF, et al. Multimorbidity and risk among patients with established cardiovascular disease: a cohort study. Br J Gen Pract. 2008;58(552):488–94.
38. New JP, Middleton RJ, Klebe B, Farmer CK, de Lusignan S, Stevens PE, et al. Assessing the prevalence, monitoring and management of chronic kidney disease in patients with diabetes compared with those without diabetes in general practice. Diabet Med. 2007;24(4):364–9.
39. Coresh J, Astor BC, Greene T, Eknoyan G, Levey AS. Prevalence of chronic kidney disease and decreased kidney function in the adult US population: Third National Health and Nutrition Examination Survey. Am J Kidney Dis. 2003;41(1):1–12.
40. Malhotra R, Nguyen HA, Benavente O, Mete M, Howard BV, Mant J, et al. Association between more intensive vs less intensive blood pressure lowering and risk of mortality in chronic kidney disease stages 3 to 5: a systematic review and meta-analysis. JAMA Intern Med. 2017;177(10):1498–505.

41. Kidney Disease Outcomes Quality I. K/DOQI clinical practice guidelines on hypertension and antihypertensive agents in chronic kidney disease. Am J Kidney Dis. 2004;43(5 Suppl 1):S1–290.
42. Stevens PE, Levin A, Kidney Disease: Improving Global Outcomes Chronic Kidney Disease Guideline Development Work Group M. Evaluation and management of chronic kidney disease: synopsis of the kidney disease: improving global outcomes 2012 clinical practice guideline. Ann Intern Med. 2013;158(11):825–30.
43. Kovesdy CP, Bleyer AJ, Molnar MZ, Ma JZ, Sim JJ, Cushman WC, et al. Blood pressure and mortality in U.S. veterans with chronic kidney disease: a cohort study. Ann Intern Med. 2013;159(4):233–42.
44. Mangano DT, Layug EL, Wallace A, Tateo I. Effect of atenolol on mortality and cardiovascular morbidity after noncardiac surgery. N Engl J Med. 1996;335(23):1713–21.
45. Wallace A, Layug B, Tateo I, Li J, Hollenberg M, Browner W, et al. Prophylactic atenolol reduces postoperative myocardial ischemia. McSPI Research Group. Anesthesiology. 1998;88(1):7–17.
46. Eagle KA, Berger PB, Calkins H, Chaitman BR, Ewy GA, Fleischmann KE, et al. ACC/AHA guideline update for perioperative cardiovascular evaluation for noncardiac surgery–executive summary a report of the American College of Cardiology/American Heart Association Task Force on Practice Guidelines (Committee to update the 1996 guidelines on perioperative cardiovascular evaluation for noncardiac surgery). Circulation. 2002;105(10):1257–67.
47. Lindenauer PK, Pekow P, Wang K, Mamidi DK, Gutierrez B, Benjamin EM. Perioperative beta-blocker therapy and mortality after major noncardiac surgery. N Engl J Med. 2005;353(4):349–61.
48. Task Force for Preoperative Cardiac Risk A, Perioperative Cardiac Management in Noncardiac S, European Society of C, Poldermans D, Bax JJ, Boersma E, et al. Guidelines for pre-operative cardiac risk assessment and perioperative cardiac management in non-cardiac surgery. Eur Heart J. 2009;30(22):2769–812.
49. American College of Cardiology Foundation/American Heart Association Task Force on Practice G, American Society of E, American Society of Nuclear C, Heart Rhythm S, Society of Cardiovascular A, Society for Cardiovascular A, et al. 2009 ACCF/AHA focused update on perioperative beta blockade. J Am Coll Cardiol. 2009;54(22):2102–28.
50. Group PS, Devereaux PJ, Yang H, Yusuf S, Guyatt G, Leslie K, et al. Effects of extended-release metoprolol succinate in patients undergoing non-cardiac surgery (POISE trial): a randomised controlled trial. Lancet. 2008;371(9627):1839–47.
51. Bouri S, Shun-Shin MJ, Cole GD, Mayet J, Francis DP. Meta-analysis of secure randomised controlled trials of beta-blockade to prevent perioperative death in non-cardiac surgery. Heart. 2014;100(6):456–64.
52. McDonald R, Roland M. Pay for performance in primary care in England and California: comparison of unintended consequences. Ann Fam Med. 2009;7(2):121–7.
53. Petersen LA, Woodard LD, Urech T, Daw C, Sookanan S. Does pay-for-performance improve the quality of health care? Ann Intern Med. 2006;145(4):265–72.
54. Rosenthal MB, Frank RG. What is the empirical basis for paying for quality in health care? Med Care Res Rev. 2006;63(2):135–57.
55. Rosenthal MB, Dudley RA. Pay-for-performance: will the latest payment trend improve care? JAMA. 2007;297(7):740–4.
56. Roland M, Olesen F. Can pay for performance improve the quality of primary care? BMJ. 2016;354:i4058.
57. Fiscella K, Burstin HR, Nerenz DR. Quality measures and sociodemographic risk factors: to adjust or not to adjust. JAMA. 2014;312(24):2615–6.
58. Pontarelli J. Study finds hospital ranking flawed rush university: rush; 2015. Available from: https://www.rushu.rush.edu/news/study-finds-hospital-ranking-flaws.
59. Chan DC, Huynh J, Studdert DM. Accuracy of valuations of surgical procedures in the Medicare Fee Schedule. N Engl J Med. 2019;380:1546–54.

60. Browne K, Roseman D, Shaller D, Edgman-Levitan S. Analysis & commentary. Measuring patient experience as a strategy for improving primary care. Health Aff (Millwood). 2010;29(5):921–5.
61. Schneider EC, Zaslavsky AM, Landon BE, Lied TR, Sheingold S, Cleary PD. National quality monitoring of Medicare health plans: the relationship between enrollees' reports and the quality of clinical care. Med Care. 2001;39(12):1313–25.
62. Beck KL, Larrabee JH. Measuring patients' perceptions of nursing care. Nurs Manage. 1996;27(9):32B-D.
63. Hickey ML, Kleefield SF, Pearson SD, Hassan SM, Harding M, Haughie P, et al. Payer-hospital collaboration to improve patient satisfaction with hospital discharge. Jt Comm J Qual Improv. 1996;22(5):336–44.
64. Blackington SM, McLauchlan T. Continuous quality improvement in the neonatal intensive care unit: evaluating parent satisfaction. J Nurs Care Qual. 1995;9(4):78–85.
65. Bonheur BB. Measuring satisfaction with patient education. A hospital-wide program evaluation. J Nurs Staff Dev. 1995;11(1):35–40.
66. Coulter A, Cleary PD. Patients' experiences with hospital care in five countries. Health Aff (Millwood). 2001;20(3):244–52.
67. Collins K. Developing patient satisfaction questionnaires. Nurs Stand. 1999;14(11):37–8.
68. Fottler MD, Ford RC, Bach SA. Measuring patient satisfaction in healthcare organizations: qualitative and quantitative approaches. Best Pract Benchmarking Healthc. 1997;2(6):227–39.
69. Lund CM. Benchmarking patient satisfaction. Best Pract Benchmarking Healthc. 1996;1(4):203–6.
70. O'Connell B, Young J, Twigg D. Patient satisfaction with nursing care: a measurement conundrum. Int J Nurs Pract. 1999;5(2):72–7.
71. Kravitz RL, Bell RA, Azari R, Krupat E, Kelly-Reif S, Thom D. Request fulfillment in office practice: antecedents and relationship to outcomes. Med Care. 2002;40(1):38–51.
72. Macfarlane J, Holmes W, Macfarlane R, Britten N. Influence of patients' expectations on antibiotic management of acute lower respiratory tract illness in general practice: questionnaire study. BMJ. 1997;315(7117):1211–4.
73. Marple RL, Kroenke K, Lucey CR, Wilder J, Lucas CA. Concerns and expectations in patients presenting with physical complaints. Frequency, physician perceptions and actions, and 2-week outcome. Arch Intern Med. 1997;157(13):1482–8.
74. Fenton JJ, Jerant AF, Bertakis KD, Franks P. The cost of satisfaction: a national study of patient satisfaction, health care utilization, expenditures, and mortality. Arch Intern Med. 2012;172(5):405–11.
75. Department of Health and Human Services AHRaQ. Guide to Patient Safety Indicators Rockville, MD: Agency for Healthcare Research and Quality; 2003, 2.1. Available from: https://www.qualityindicators.ahrq.gov/downloads/modules/psi/v21/psi_guide_rev2.pdf.
76. Romano PS, Geppert JJ, Davies S, Miller MR, Elixhauser A, McDonald KM. A national profile of patient safety in U.S. hospitals. Health Aff (Millwood). 2003;22(2):154–66.
77. Isaac T, Jha AK. Are patient safety indicators related to widely used measures of hospital quality? J Gen Intern Med. 2008;23(9):1373–8.
78. Thornlow DK, Stukenborg GJ. The association between hospital characteristics and rates of preventable complications and adverse events. Med Care. 2006;44(3):265–9.
79. Winters BD, Bharmal A, Wilson RF, Zhang A, Engineer L, Defoe D, et al. Validity of the agency for health care research and quality patient safety indicators and the centers for Medicare and Medicaid hospital-acquired conditions: a systematic review and meta-analysis. Med Care. 2016;54(12):1105–11.
80. Miller MR, Pronovost P, Donithan M, Zeger S, Zhan C, Morlock L, et al. Relationship between performance measurement and accreditation: implications for quality of care and patient safety. Am J Med Qual. 2005;20(5):239–52.

81. Press MJ, Scanlon DP, Ryan AM, Zhu J, Navathe AS, Mittler JN, et al. Limits of readmission rates in measuring hospital quality suggest the need for added metrics. Health Aff (Millwood). 2013;32(6):1083–91.
82. Bhalla R, Kalkut G. Could Medicare readmission policy exacerbate health care system inequity? Ann Intern Med. 2010;152(2):114–7.
83. Gorodeski EZ, Starling RC, Blackstone EH. Are all readmissions bad readmissions? N Engl J Med. 2010;363(3):297–8.
84. Joynt KE, Jha AK. Characteristics of hospitals receiving penalties under the Hospital Readmissions Reduction Program. JAMA. 2013;309(4):342–3.
85. Naylor MD, Kurtzman ET, Grabowski DC, Harrington C, McClellan M, Reinhard SC. Unintended consequences of steps to cut readmissions and reform payment may threaten care of vulnerable older adults. Health Aff (Millwood). 2012;31(7):1623–32.
86. Barnett ML, Hsu J, McWilliams JM. Patient characteristics and differences in hospital readmission rates. JAMA Intern Med. 2015;175(11):1803–12.
87. Gilman M, Hockenberry JM, Adams EK, Milstein AS, Wilson IB, Becker ER. The financial effect of value-based purchasing and the hospital readmissions reduction program on safety-net hospitals in 2014: a cohort study. Ann Intern Med. 2015;163(6):427–36.
88. Joynt KE, Orav EJ, Jha AK. Thirty-day readmission rates for Medicare beneficiaries by race and site of care. JAMA. 2011;305(7):675–81.
89. Dharmarajan K, Wang Y, Lin Z, Normand ST, Ross JS, Horwitz LI, et al. Association of changing hospital readmission rates with mortality rates after hospital discharge. JAMA. 2017;318(3):270–8.
90. Konstam MA, Upshaw J. Sisyphus and 30-day heart failure readmissions: futility in predicting a flawed outcome metric. JACC Heart Fail. 2016;4(1):21–3.
91. Khera R, Dharmarajan K, Wang Y, Lin Z, Bernheim SM, Wang Y, et al. Association of the Hospital Readmissions Reduction Program with mortality during and after hospitalization for acute myocardial infarction, heart failure, and pneumonia. JAMA Netw Open. 2018;1(5):e182777.
92. Rinne ST, Castaneda J, Lindenauer PK, Cleary PD, Paz HL, Gomez JL. Chronic obstructive pulmonary disease readmissions and other measures of hospital quality. Am J Respir Crit Care Med. 2017;196(1):47–55.
93. Centers for M, Medicaid Services HHS. Medicare program; hospital inpatient prospective payment systems for acute care hospitals and the long-term care hospital prospective payment system and fiscal year 2015 rates; quality reporting requirements for specific providers; reasonable compensation equivalents for physician services in excluded hospitals and certain teaching hospitals; provider administrative appeals and judicial review; enforcement provisions for organ transplant centers; and electronic health record (EHR) incentive program. Final rule. Fed Regist. 2014;79(163):49853–50536.
94. Fonarow GC, Alberts MJ, Broderick JP, Jauch EC, Kleindorfer DO, Saver JL, et al. Stroke outcomes measures must be appropriately risk adjusted to ensure quality care of patients: a presidential advisory from the American Heart Association/American Stroke Association. Stroke. 2014;45(5):1589–601.
95. Chernew ME, Landrum MB. Targeted supplemental data collection — addressing the quality-measurement conundrum. N Engl J Med. 2018;378(11):979–81.
96. Meyer GS, Nelson EC, Pryor DB, James B, Swensen SJ, Kaplan GS, et al. More quality measures versus measuring what matters: a call for balance and parsimony. BMJ Qual Saf. 2012;21(11):964–8.
97. Nordal KC. Letter to Andy Slavitt, Acting Administrator Centers for Medicare and Medicaid Services, Re: Proposed Rule on the Merit-Based Incentive Payment System (MIPS) and Alternative Payment Model (APM) Incentive under the Physician Fee Schedule and Criteria for Physician-Focused Payment Models. PsycEXTRA Dataset: American Psychological Association (APA); 2016.

98. Casalino LP, Gans D, Weber R, Cea M, Tuchovsky A, Bishop TF, et al. US physician practices spend more than $15.4 billion annually to report quality measures. Health Aff. 2016;35(3):401–6.
99. Saver BG, Martin SA, Adler RN, Candib LM, Deligiannidis KE, Golding J, et al. Care that matters: quality measurement and health care. PLoS Med. 2015;12(11):e1001902.
100. Glasziou PP, Buchan H, Del Mar C, Doust J, Harris M, Knight R, et al. When financial incentives do more good than harm: a checklist. BMJ. 2012;345(aug13 2):e5047-e.
101. Grady D, Redberg RF, O'Malley PG. Quality improvement for quality improvement studies. JAMA Intern Med. 2018;178(2):187.
102. Bishop TF. Pushing the outpatient quality envelope. JAMA. 2013;309(13):1353–4.
103. Pauly MV. Is it time to reexamine the patent system's role in spending growth? Health Aff (Millwood). 2009;28(5):1466–74.
104. Ovretveit J, Leviton L, Parry G. Increasing the generalisability of improvement research with an improvement replication programme. BMJ Qual Saf. 2011;20(Suppl 1):i87–91.
105. Hahlweg P, Didi S, Kriston L, Harter M, Nestoriuc Y, Scholl I. Process quality of decision-making in multidisciplinary cancer team meetings: a structured observational study. BMC Cancer. 2017;17(1):772.
106. Rhee C, Dantes R, Epstein L, Murphy DJ, Seymour CW, Iwashyna TJ, et al. Incidence and trends of Sepsis in US hospitals using clinical vs claims data, 2009–2014. JAMA. 2017;318(13):1241–9.
107. Howard DH, Karcz A, Roback JD. The accuracy of claims data for measuring transfusion rates. Transfus Med. 2016;26(6):457–9.
108. Coalition Care that Matters. Report card: blue cross blue shield AQC metrics Massachussetts: care that matters; 2018, v1.0. Available from: http://www.carethatmatters.org/.
109. Kansagara D, Fu R, Freeman M, Wolf F, Helfand M. Intensive insulin therapy in hospitalized patients: a systematic review. Ann Intern Med. 2011;154(4):268–82.
110. Yu KT, Wyer PC. Evidence-based emergency medicine/critically appraised topic. Evidence behind the 4-hour rule for initiation of antibiotic therapy in community-acquired pneumonia. Ann Emerg Med. 2008;51(5):651–62, 62.e1–2.
111. Lyu H, Wick EC, Housman M, Freischlag JA, Makary MA. Patient satisfaction as a possible indicator of quality surgical care. JAMA Surg. 2013;148(4):362–7.
112. Chang JT, Hays RD, Shekelle PG, MacLean CH, Solomon DH, Reuben DB, et al. Patients' global ratings of their health care are not associated with the technical quality of their care. Ann Intern Med. 2006;144(9):665–72.
113. Hawn MT, Itani KM, Gray SH, Vick CC, Henderson W, Houston TK. Association of timely administration of prophylactic antibiotics for major surgical procedures and surgical site infection. J Am Coll Surg. 2008;206(5):814–9; discussion 9–21.
114. Fonarow GC, Abraham WT, Albert NM, Stough WG, Gheorghiade M, Greenberg BH, et al. Association between performance measures and clinical outcomes for patients hospitalized with heart failure. JAMA. 2007;297(1):61–70.
115. Sud M, Yu B, Wijeysundera HC, Austin PC, Ko DT, Braga J, et al. Associations between short or long length of stay and 30-day readmission and mortality in hospitalized patients with heart failure. JACC Heart Fail. 2017;5(8):578–88.
116. Joynt KE, Jha AK. Thirty-day readmissions–truth and consequences. N Engl J Med. 2012;366(15):1366–9.
117. van Walraven C, Jennings A, Taljaard M, Dhalla I, English S, Mulpuru S, et al. Incidence of potentially avoidable urgent readmissions and their relation to all-cause urgent readmissions. CMAJ. 2011;183(14):E1067–72.
118. Meddings JA, Reichert H, Hofer T, McMahon LF Jr. Hospital report cards for hospital-acquired pressure ulcers: how good are the grades? Ann Intern Med. 2013;159(8):505–13.
119. Kaafarani HM, Borzecki AM, Itani KM, Loveland S, Mull HJ, Hickson K, et al. Validity of selected patient safety indicators: opportunities and concerns. J Am Coll Surg. 2011;212(6):924–34.

120. Rosen AK, Itani KM, Cevasco M, Kaafarani HM, Hanchate A, Shin M, et al. Validating the patient safety indicators in the Veterans Health Administration: do they accurately identify true safety events? Med Care. 2012;50(1):74–85.
121. Cevasco M, Borzecki AM, O'Brien WJ, Chen Q, Shin MH, Itani KM, et al. Validity of the AHRQ patient safety Indicator "central venous catheter-related bloodstream infections". J Am Coll Surg. 2011;212(6):984–90.
122. Borzecki AM, Kaafarani HM, Utter GH, Romano PS, Shin MH, Chen Q, et al. How valid is the AHRQ patient safety Indicator "postoperative respiratory failure"? J Am Coll Surg. 2011;212(6):935–45.

Index

A
Accreditation Council for Graduate Medical
        Education (ACGME), 153
Achilles' Heel of Quality Assessment, 80
ACS NSQIP Pediatric, 11
Advanced Alternative Payment Model
        (AAPM), 154
Affordable Care Act (ACA), 77, 203, 215
Agency for Healthcare Research and Quality
        (AHRQ), 5, 27, 68, 132, 139,
        189, 218
AHRQ Quality Indicators™, 6
Ambulatory physician quality
        dashboard, 206
American Academy of Hospice and Palliative
        Care Medicine (AAHPM), 109
American Association for Cancer Research,
        the American Cancer Society
        (ASCO), 92
American College of Surgeons Committee on
        Emerging Technologies and
        Education (ACS-CESTE), 34
American College of Surgeons National
        Surgical Quality Improvement
        Program (ACS NSQIP®), 11
American Diabetes Association, 219
American Heart Association's Center of
        Excellence, 154
American Heart Association's Get With The
        Guidelines Program for heart failure
        (GWTG-HF), 74
American Society of Clinical Oncology
        (ASCO), 89, 94
Annual Quality and Safety plan, 189, 191
Assessing Care of Vulnerable Elders
        (ACOVE) project, 93

Association of American Medical Colleges
        (AAMC), 152
Aurora Health, 130

B
Bell Commission, 168
Bisoprolol, 222
Blue cross blue shield AQC metrics, 216–217
Board and the quality of care and safety
        committee, 187
Board leadership, 181, 189
Board of Registration in Medicine, 186
Boards on Board program, 181
Bridging the gap, 173

C
Cancer care
        chemotherapy errors, 93
        Ensuring Quality Cancer Care, 86
        evidence-based guidelines, 86
        five-point rating scale, 92
        health equity, 91
        medical errors, 93
        national death rate, 85
        NICCQ, 88
        1999 IOM recommendations, 91
        Oncology Demonstration Projects, 89, 90
        Outcomes Quality, 87
        patient-centered approaches, 92
        patient errors, 94
        process-oriented quality measurements, 91
        Process Quality, 87, 92, 93
        QOPI, 90, 91
        quality of care, 87

Cancer care (*cont.*)
  racial gap, 91
  socioeconomic inequalities, 91
  Structural Quality, 87
  treatment decision-making, 92
  voluntary accreditation programs, 93
Cancer screening, 201, 206
Cardiac care, 63, 64
Cardiac Surgery Reporting System
    (CSRS), 70, 71
Cardiovascular quality metrics
  Achilles' Heel of Quality Assessment, 80
  balancing population-wide measurement
      strategies, 67
  balancing population-wide prevention, 64
  CABG outcomes, 70, 71
  CCP, 72
  childhood roots of cardiovascular
      diseases, 64
  CRUSADE trial, 73
  Donabedian models, 68
  GWTG-HF, 74
  HRRP, 77, 78
  HVBP, 77
  measurement and interpretation, 71
  Merit-Based Incentive Program, 78
  MHS Registry, 72
  National Quality Forum, 74, 75
  NHF project, 73
  NMIR, 72
  outcome measures, 68
  patient-centered outcomes, 74, 75
  P4P, 76
  population/risk paradox, 67
  Premier HQID, 76
  primordial prevention, 64, 66
  process measures, 68
  RCPSAP, 73
  six aims of healthcare, 68
  stakeholders, 71
  state-of-the-art risk adjustment
      techniques, 72
  statin therapy, 66
  structural measures, 68
Catheter associated urinary tract infections
    (CAUTI), 50, 58, 118
Center for Advance Palliative Care
    (CAPC), 110
Centers for Disease Control and Prevention
    (CDC), 48, 49
Centers for Disease Control and Prevention's
    National Breast and Cervical
    Cancer Early Detection Program, 92

Centers for Medicare and Medicaid Services
    (CMS), 6, 49, 88, 129, 165, 189,
    203, 215
Central line-associated bloodstream infections
    (CLABSIs), 49, 50, 118
Change Team, 206
Child Core Set, 7, 8
Children's Asthma Care (CAC), 7
Children's Health Insurance Program
    (CHIP), 7
Children's Health Insurance Program
    Reauthorization Act of 2009
    (CHIPRA), 6
Children's Hospitals' Solutions for Patient
    Safety Network, 18, 19, 185
Chronic Care Model, 203
Chronic opioid therapy, 210–212
Clavien-Dindo classification, 24, 25
Clinical Learning Environment Review
    (CLER), 169–171, 175
Congenital Heart Surgery Database
    (CHSD), 11
Cooperative Cardiovascular Project (CCP), 72
Core General Surgery Privileges, 34
Core Quality Measures Collaborative
    (CQMC), 13
Coronary artery bypass grafting (CABG)
    outcomes, 70, 71
"Crossing the Quality Chasm", 67, 165
CRUSADE trial, 73
Cystic Fibrosis (CF) Foundation, 11

D
Days away restricted/transferred
    (DART), 185
DECREASE I trial, 222
Department of Health and the Board of
    Registration in Medicine, 186
Diabetes, 201, 203, 206, 208
Diagnostic stewardship, 51
Donabedian framework of measures, 16
Donabedian models, 68
Duty of care, 182
Duty of loyalty, 182
Duty of obedience, 182

E
Educationally sensitive patient outcomes
    (ESPOs), 174
Effective patient- and systems-level
    outcomes, 170

Electronic health record (EHR) system, 94,
    201–203, 205, 207, 209–212
Emergency Department (ED CAHPS), 138
Empanelment, 205
End result system, 167
Ensuring Quality Cancer Care, 86
Environmental scan, 123
Evaluating the Quality of Medical Care, 1
Expanded measurement approach, 228

F
Financial oversight, 182
"A Framework for Effective Governance", 182

G
Global Palliative Care Quality Alliance
    (GPCQA), 109
Governance Institute, 181–183
Government's Hospital Compare website, 129
Graduate medical education (GME), 153
    ACGME response, 169, 170
    CLER, 170, 171
    competency-based assessments, 173
    ESPOs, 174
    faculty development, 172
    health care delivery, 168
    Morbidity and Mortality conference, 173
    NQMC, 175
    objective metric assessments, 174
    physical culture, 167, 168
    physician- and resident-lead quality
        improvement, 172
    physicians training, 168
    quality improvement, 172
    resident quality metrics, 174
    resident work hours, 168
    sponsoring institutions, 170

H
Harm Bubble, 121, 122
HCAHPS Quality Assurance Guidelines
    manual, 131
Healthcare-associated infection
    metrics, 53, 54
Healthcare Effectiveness Data and Information
    Set (HEDIS), 9
Healthcare Infection Control Practices
    Advisory Committee, 49
Health Care Quality Improvement (HCQI), 72
Health Grades, 129

Health Information Technology for Clinical
    and Economic Health (HITECH)
    Act, 202
Health Service Executive Quality
    Improvement Division, 187
Hidden curriculum, 168
Home Health (HH CAHPS), 138
Hospital-acquired conditions (HACs),
    185, 215–218
Hospital board of trustees
    board's fiduciary duties, 181, 182
    boards and board quality capability, 188
    decision making, 183
    duty of care, 182
    duty of loyalty, 182
    duty of obedience, 182
    goals
        costs and expenses of healthcare, 186
        data accumulation, 186
        hospital-acquired conditions, 185
        patient safety and quality, 186
        perfection, 186
        quality and safety measures, 187
        serious safety events, 185
        SREs, 187
    hospital-acquired infection, 184
    lethal medical errors, 184
    management role, 183
    policy statements, 183
    quality and safety
        Netherlands, 188
        Quality of Care Committee, 188, 189
        Scotland measurement, 188
        Taiwan, 188
        Tufts Medical Center, 188
        USA, 188
    Tufts Medical Center, 189–191
Hospital Compare website, 189
Hospital quality metrics system
    driving improvement, 123
    getting started, 117
    inconsistent scoring, 116
    measurement burden, 116
    measurement imperative, 116, 117
    measurement overload, 115
    monitoring progress, 123
    setting, 117
    validity, 116
Hospital Readmissions Reduction Program
    (HRRP), 69, 77, 78, 215, 226, 227
Hospital Value-Based Purchasing (HVBP)
    program, 77, 215
Hyperglycemia, 218–220

Hypertension, 201, 203, 205, 206, 208, 209
Hypoglycemia, 220

I
Improve Care Now (ICN), 12
Infection prevention quality metrics
  CAUTIs, 58
  diagnostic stewardship, 51, 52
  healthcare-associated infection
    metrics, 53, 54
    reporting, 50, 51
  hierarchy of intervention effectiveness, 57
  history, 48, 49
  National Action Plan, 50
  performance improvement, 54, 57, 58
Institute of Medicine (IOM), 49, 86, 87
Integrating Quality (IQ), 152
Intensive insulin therapy, 218–220
International Classification of Diseases (ICD)
    codes, 225
International Consortium for Health Outcomes
    Measurement (ICHOM), 231
Intra-institutional data sources, 24–27

J
Joint Commission on Accreditation of
    Healthcare Organizations (JCAHO),
    69, 224, 226
Joint Commission on Accreditation of
    Hospitals (JCAH), 70
Joint Commission's Certification for Primary
    Stroke Centers, 154
Journal of the American Medical Association
    (JAMA), 230

L
Lean, 156
Leapfrog Hospital Survey, 189
Leonard and Frankel's system, 33

M
Massachusetts Department of Public Health
    (DPH), 187
Massachusetts General Law, 187
MassHealth, 203
Medical errors, 215
Medical School Quality Improvement and
    Healthcare Systems
    Curriculum, 157

Medicare Access and CHIP
    Reauthorization Act of 2015
    (MACRA), 154, 228
Medicare Accountable Care Organization
    (ACO) model, 203–205, 210, 212
Medicare and Medicaid Services 2015
    Value-based Purchasing
    program, 220
Medicare's merit-based incentive payment
    system (MIPS), 228
Merit-based Incentive Payment System
    (MIPS), 78, 154
Methicillin-resistant *Staphylococcus aureus*
    (MRSA), 50
Morbidity and Mortality conference
    (M&M), 168, 173

N
National Action Plan, 50
National Cancer Database, 85
National Committee for Quality
    Assurance (NCQA), 9, 189,
    202, 203, 224–225
National Consensus Project's Clinical Practice
    (NCP), 102
National Healthcare Safety Network
    (NHSN), 48, 49
National Heart Failure (NHF) project, 73
National Initiative for Cancer Care Quality
    (NICCQ), 87, 88
National Kidney Foundation Kidney
    Disease Outcome Quality
    Initiative (NKF K/DOQI), 221
National Myocardial Infarction Registry
    (NMIR), 72
National Palliative Care Research Center
    (NPCRC), 109
National Quality Forum (NQF),
    8, 74, 75, 110, 181, 187, 220, 222
National Quality Measures Clearinghouse
    (NQMC), 175
National Quality Strategy (NQS), 16, 17
National Surgical Quality Improvement
    Program (NSQIP), 23, 28–30,
    174, 224
Newsday Freedom of Information Act, 70
NICE-SUGAR trial, 220
Nightingale's impact on healthcare quality
    measures, 64
Novel targeted supplemental data collection
    approach, 229
Nursing Homes (LTC CAHPS), 138

O
Oncology Care Model (OCM), 89
Oncology Demonstration Projects, 89, 90
Oncology Nursing Society (ONS), 94
Operating Room (S CAHPS), 138
Organized Program to Initiate Lifesaving
          Treatment in Hospitalized Patients
          With Heart Failure
          (OPTIMIZE-HF), 73

P
Palliative care
    CAPC registry, 107, 109
    challenges, 100, 101
    clinical research, 100
    continuous performance improvement, 100
    evaluating, 99
    health care system, 100
    high-value quality measures, 102, 106
    improving, 99
    opportunities, 101
    optimal clinical care, 100
    policy standpoint, 100
Palliative Care Outcomes Collaboration
          (PCOC), 109, 110
Patient and Family Reported Outcome
          Measures (PROM), 110
Patient Care Assessment (PCA)
          Program, 186
Patient-centered medical home (PCMH),
          154, 202, 203
Patient-centered outcomes research
          (PCOR), 158
Patient family advisory council, 189
Patient Protection and Affordable Care
          Act, 226
Patient registry, 203, 210
Patient safety indicators (PSIs), 220, 221,
          225, 226
Patient satisfaction metrics
    business case
        CMS, 129
        healthcare providers, 130
        hospital compare patient
          experience, 129
        malpractice risk, 130
        referral patterns to hospitals, 129
        vouchers, 130
        web-based physician grading
          platforms, 129
    compliance with treatment
          recommendations, 128, 129
    disadvantages, 146–148
    improvements
        AIDET, 145
        colleagues and staff management, 145
        effective communication, 145
        eliminating wasteful steps, 144
        high-impact improvements, 144
        measuring patient experience, 143
        patient centric culture, 143
        staff satisfaction, 146
        team involvement, 143
        top drivers, 144
        value stream mapping, 144
    improving human condition, 128
    inpatient experience metrics
        CAHPS patient satisfaction
          metrics, 138
        case transition, 138
        discharge information, 138
        doctor communication, 136
        hospital rating, 138
        medication communication, 137, 138
        nurse communication, 136
        pain management, 137
        Press Ganey survey, 138
        quietness, 137
        recommendation, 138
        room cleanliness, 137
        staff responsiveness, 136
    medical care quality, 127
    outpatient metrics
        CG CAHPS, 139–142
        patient complaints, 143
        phone metrics, 142
        Press Ganey survey, 142
    relieving suffering, 128
    validity of the metrics, 131, 132, 136
Patient satisfaction surveys, 131
Pay-for-performance (P4P) program, 76, 203,
          215, 218, 223, 224
Pediatric Quality Indicators (PDI), 6
Pediatric Quality Measurement Program
          (PQMP), 7
Pediatric quality measures
    ACS NSQIP Pediatric, 11
    AHRQ Quality Indicators™, 6
    benchmarking databases and disease
          registries, 9
    CAC, 7
    CF Foundation, 11
    Child Core Set, 7, 8
    CHIP, 7
    CHIPRA, 6, 7

Pediatric quality measures (*cont.*)
   classification, 13, 16–18
   condition-focused QI network, 12
   CQMC, 13
   development of, 5
   governmental metrics, 7
   HEDIS, 9
   home management plan of care
      (CAC3), 7, 9
   ICN, 12
   NCQA, 9
   obesity rates, 9, 10
   ORYX®, 7
   outcome measures, 15
   pediatric specialty- /condition-focused
      networks, 11, 12
   PQMP, 7
   process measures, 13–15
   purpose of, 18–20
   structure measures, 16
   Virtual Pediatric Systems, 10
   VON, 9
Peer review protections, 23
Penicillin-resistant *Staphylococcus aureus*
      infections, 48
Philanthropy, 182
Phone metrics, 142
Physician Compare website, 129
Physician Quality Reporting System
      (PQRS), 154
Plan-Do-Study-Act (PDSA) cycle, 156, 159
Point-of-care (POC) hemoglobin A1c (HbA1c)
      testing, 206–208
POISE randomized trial, 222
Policy statements, 183
Population management in adult primary care
   ambulatory quality measures
      challenges, 201
      electronic health record, 201, 202
      HITECH act, 202
      PCMH, 202
   Change Team, 206
   data transparency and reporting, 205
   empanelment, 205
   guiding principles, 204, 205
   hypertension control, 208, 209
   opioids
      EHR, 211
      patient registry, 210
      risk-assessment algorithm, 210
      standardization of chronic opioid, 210
      team-based case management, 210
   POC HbA1c testing, 206–208

quality improvement, 204
Practice-Based Learning and Improvement
      (PBLI), 169
Premier Hospital Quality Incentive
      Demonstration (HQID), 76
Press Ganey survey, 138, 142
Primary care provider, 201, 203, 205
Public reporting strategy,
      218, 220, 224, 226

Q
Quadruple Aim, 203, 204, 212
Quality and Patient Safety Division
      (QPSD), 186
Quality dashboard
   public agencies, 118
   STEEP, 118–120
Quality Improvement Knowledge Application
      Tool (QIKAT), 162
Quality In-Training Initiative (QITI), 174
Quality metrics, 1, 2
Quality of Care and Safety Committee, 181,
      186, 188, 189
Quality of quality measures
   beta-blockers in non-cardiac
      surgery, 221–223
   blood pressure, chronic kidney
      disease, 221
   Blue cross blue shield AQC
      metrics, 216–217
   clinical research for efficacy and
      safety, 230
   complications, 218, 219
   expanded measurement approach, 228
   flawed methodology and statistical
      designs, 223, 224
   generalizability of measures across
      specialties, 231, 232
   intensive insulin therapy in critically-ill
      patients, 218–220
   medical errors, 215
   novel targeted supplemental data
      collection approach, 229
   outcomes, 218, 231
   P4P, 215, 218, 223, 224
   patient safety indicators, 225, 226
   patient satisfaction, 224, 225
   post-operative venous thromboembolism,
      220, 221
   public reporting, 218, 220
   readmission rates, 226, 227
   reduced reliance on claims data, 232

relative costs, 231
responsiveness to patient preference, 231
scaling back approach, 228, 229
Quality Oncology Practice Initiative
(QOPI), 90, 91
Quality Payment Programs (QPP), 110

R
Raw data, 186
Relative Value Scale Update Committee
(RUC), 224
Risk adjustment, 2
Role of governance, 183
Root cause analysis (RCA), 156, 159, 161
Royal College of Physicians Stroke Audit
Package (RCPSAP), 73

S
Safety incident analysis, 159
Scaling back approach, 228, 229
Secretary of Health and Human Services, 7
Serious reportable events (SREs), 187
Serious safety events (SSEs), 185
Six Sigma methodology, 156
Society of Thoracic Surgeons (STS) National
Database, 10–11
Specific surgical site infections (SSIs), 50
Sponsoring Institutions, 167, 170, 175
Stakeholders, 157–159
Standardized infection ratios (SIRs), 118
Strategy development and
implementation, 182
Study on the Effectiveness of Nosocomial
Infection Control (SENIC), 48
Surgery quality and safety improvement
programs
accurate granular risk-adjusted data, 24
AHRQ data, 27, 28
attributes, 26
benchmarking, 24
briefing, 39, 40
checklist, 35, 36, 39
Clavien-Dindo classification, 24, 25
credentialing and privileging, 34, 35
Departmental and Institutional
Structure, 31
departmental leadership, 24
incident reporting systems, 26, 27
individual accountability, 33
intra-institutional data sources, 24–27
Leonard and Frankel's system errors, 33

NSQIP, 28–30
performance dashboard, 40
perioperative pneumonias, 40, 42, 43
psychological safety, 24
root cause analysis, 26
SQSC, 31, 32
trend analysis, 24
Surgical Quality and Safety Committee
(SQSC), 31, 32
Surgical Quality Officer (SQO), 31
Sustainable grown rate (SGR) formula, 78
Systems-based practice (SBP), 169

T
"Teaching for Quality: Report of an
Expert Panel", 155
TEAMS model, 152
Toyota Production System, 156
Transparent data, 186
Triple Aim, 201–204
Tufts Medical Center, 181, 188–191

U
Undergraduate medical
education (UME)
aim of, 151
ancillary skill sets to prepare learners
for, 157
core competency, 153
lean, 156
longitudinal assessment of learners,
161, 162
MIPS/AAPM, 154
PDSA cycle, 155, 156
PQRS, 154
purpose, 152
role, 152
root cause analysis, 156, 159, 160
safety incident analysis, 161
Six Sigma methodology, 156
stakeholder engagement, 159
stakeholders to share and use data
for, 157–159
US Agency for Healthcare Research and
Quality (AHRQ), 118
U.S. Department of Health & Human
Services, 189
US National Institutes of Health PROMIS
program, 231
US Preventative Services Task Force
(USPSTF), 232

V
Value stream mapping, 144
Venous thromboembolism (VTE), 220
Vermont Oxford Network (VON), 9
Virtual Pediatric Systems (VPS), 10
Vital Signs, 129
Vizient Quality and Accountability Study, 189

W
World Report Best Hospital Rankings, 224

Y
Yelp! and Angie's List, 129

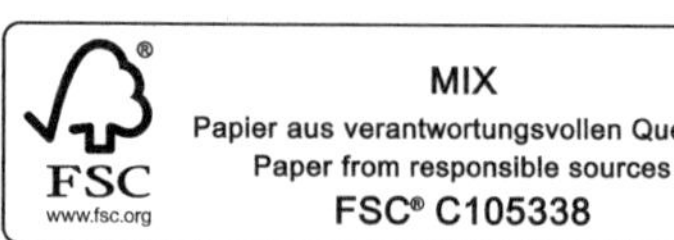

®
MIX
Papier aus verantwortungsvollen Quellen
Paper from responsible sources
FSC
www.fsc.org
FSC® C105338